Chronic Pain Management

Chronic Pain Management

Editor

Mark I. Johnson

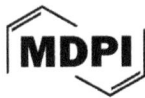

Basel • Beijing • Wuhan • Barcelona • Belgrade • Novi Sad • Cluj • Manchester

Editor
Mark I. Johnson
Leeds Beckett University
Leeds
United Kindom

Editorial Office
MDPI
St. Alban-Anlage 66
4052 Basel, Switzerland

This is a reprint of articles from the Special Issue published online in the open access journal *Medicina* (ISSN 1648-9144) (available at: https://www.mdpi.com/journal/medicina/special_issues/chronic_pain_management).

For citation purposes, cite each article independently as indicated on the article page online and as indicated below:

Lastname, A.A.; Lastname, B.B. Article Title. *Journal Name* **Year**, *Volume Number*, Page Range.

ISBN 978-3-7258-1119-9 (Hbk)
ISBN 978-3-7258-1120-5 (PDF)
doi.org/10.3390/books978-3-7258-1120-5

© 2024 by the authors. Articles in this book are Open Access and distributed under the Creative Commons Attribution (CC BY) license. The book as a whole is distributed by MDPI under the terms and conditions of the Creative Commons Attribution-NonCommercial-NoDerivs (CC BY-NC-ND) license.

Contents

About the Editor vii

Preface ix

Mark I. Johnson
The Landscape of Chronic Pain: Broader Perspectives
Reprinted from: *Medicina* **2019**, *55*, 182, doi:10.3390/medicina55050182 1

Carole A. Paley and Mark I. Johnson
Acupuncture for the Relief of Chronic Pain: A Synthesis of Systematic Reviews
Reprinted from: *Medicina* **2020**, *56*, 6, doi:10.3390/medicina56010006 20

Ayappa V. Subramaniam, Ashwaq Hamid Salem Yehya and Chern Ein Oon
Molecular Basis of Cancer Pain Management: An Updated Review
Reprinted from: *Medicina* **2019**, *55*, 584, doi:10.3390/medicina55090584 68

Valeriu Ardeleanu, Alexandra Toma, Kalliopi Pafili, Nikolaos Papanas, Ion Motofei, Camelia Cristina Diaconu, et al.
Current Pharmacological Treatment of Painful Diabetic Neuropathy: A Narrative Review
Reprinted from: *Medicina* **2020**, *56*, 25, doi:10.3390/medicina56010025 87

Helen Radford, Karen H. Simpson, Suzanne Rogerson and Mark I. Johnson
A Single Site Population Study to Investigate CYP2D6 Phenotype of Patients with Persistent Non-Malignant Pain
Reprinted from: *Medicina* **2019**, *55*, 220, doi:10.3390/medicina55060220 97

Lorenzo Panella, Laura Volontè, Nicola Poloni, Antonello Caserta, Marta Ielmini, Ivano Caselli, et al.
Pharmacogenetic Testing in Acute and Chronic Pain: A Preliminary Study
Reprinted from: *Medicina* **2019**, *55*, 147, doi:10.3390/medicina55050147 120

Hee Yong Kang, Chung Hun Lee, Sang Sik Choi, Mi Kyoung Lee, Yeon Joo Lee and Jong Sun Park
Comparison of the Analgesic Effect of Ropivacaine with Fentanyl and Ropivacaine Alone in Continuous Epidural Infusion for Acute Herpes Zoster Management: A Retrospective Study
Reprinted from: *Medicina* **2020**, *56*, 22, doi:10.3390/medicina56010022 129

Dong Yoon Park, Seok Kang and Joo Hyun Park
Factors Predicting Favorable Short-Term Response to Transforaminal Epidural Steroid Injections for Lumbosacral Radiculopathy
Reprinted from: *Medicina* **2019**, *55*, 162, doi:10.3390/medicina55050162 140

Yutaka Owari and Nobuyuki Miyatake
Prediction of Chronic Lower Back Pain Using the Hierarchical Neural Network: Comparison with Logistic Regression—A Pilot Study
Reprinted from: *Medicina* **2019**, *55*, 259, doi:10.3390/medicina55060259 151

Soleika Salvioli, Andrea Pozzi and Marco Testa
Movement Control Impairment and Low Back Pain: State of the Art of Diagnostic Framing
Reprinted from: *Medicina* **2019**, *55*, 548, doi:10.3390/medicina55090548 159

Juan Nieto-García, Luis Suso-Martí, Roy La Touche and Mónica Grande-Alonso
Somatosensory and Motor Differences between Physically Active Patients with Chronic Low Back Pain and Asymptomatic Individuals
Reprinted from: *Medicina* **2019**, *55*, 524, doi:10.3390/medicina55090524 180

Jung-Min Park, Sihwa Park and Yong-Seok Jee
Rehabilitation Program Combined with Local Vibroacoustics Improves Psychophysiological Conditions in Patients with ACL Reconstruction
Reprinted from: *Medicina* **2019**, *55*, 659, doi:10.3390/medicina55100659 193

Peter Francis, Isobel Thornley, Ashley Jones and Mark I. Johnson
Pain and Function in the Runner a Ten (din) uous Link
Reprinted from: *Medicina* **2020**, *56*, 21, doi:10.3390/medicina56010021 205

Alexios Pitsillides and Dimitrios Stasinopoulos
The Beliefs and Attitudes of Cypriot Physical Therapists Regarding the Use of Deep Friction Massage
Reprinted from: *Medicina* **2019**, *55*, 472, doi:10.3390/medicina55080472 215

Alexios Pitsillides and Dimitrios Stasinopoulos
Cyriax Friction Massage—Suggestions for Improvements
Reprinted from: *Medicina* **2019**, *55*, 185, doi:10.3390/medicina55050185 227

Yuta Sakamoto, Takeru Oka, Takashi Amari and Satoshi Simo
Factors Affecting Psychological Stress in Healthcare Workers with and without Chronic Pain: A Cross-Sectional Study Using Multiple Regression Analysis
Reprinted from: *Medicina* **2019**, *55*, 652, doi:10.3390/medicina55100652 232

Yuta Sakamoto, Takeru Oka, Takashi Amari and Satoshi Shimo
Factors Affecting Psychological Stress in Healthcare Workers with and without Chronic Pain: A Cross-Sectional Study Using Multiple Regression Analysis
Reprinted from: *Medicina* **2020**, *56*, 7, doi:10.3390/medicina56010007 247

Jieun Lee, Jaewon Beom, Seoyun Choi, Seulgi Lee Amy Wachholtz and Jang-Han Lee
Chronic Pain Patients' Gaze Patterns toward Pain-Related Information: Comparison between Pictorial and Linguistic Stimuli
Reprinted from: *Medicina* **2019**, *55*, 530, doi:10.3390/medicina55090530 248

Carlos Suso-Ribera, Verónica Martínez-Borba, Alejandro Viciano, Francisco Javier Cano-García and Azucena García-Palacios
Empathic Accuracy in Chronic Pain: Exploring Patient and Informal Caregiver Differences and Their Personality Correlates
Reprinted from: *Medicina* **2019**, *55*, 539, doi:10.3390/medicina55090539 262

About the Editor

Mark I. Johnson

Professor Mark I. Johnson, PhD, is a Professor of Pain and Analgesia and Director of the Centre for Pain Research at Leeds Beckett University, U.K. Professor Johnson has been investigating the science of pain and its management for over 35 years and has published over 300 research articles and book chapters. Professor Johnson conducts research in laboratory, clinical, and non-clinical settings, using quantitative, qualitative, and literature-based methodologies.

Professor Johnson is recognised for his research on factors influencing pain, response to treatments such as electrophysical agents (e.g., transcutaneous electrical nerve stimulation (TENS), acupuncture, low-level laser therapy, and kinesiology taping), perceptual embodiment, pain education, and the epidemiology of pain. Professor Johnson's current interests include art and pain, community-based pain services, and socio-ecological factors that make pain 'sticky', including the concept of the painogenic environment and salutogenic approaches to assist recovery. Professor Johnson is a longstanding member of the International Association for the Study of Pain and offers expert consultancy services for both the public and private sectors. Professor Johnson teaches a variety of university courses, including the supervision of over 25 PhD candidates, and is passionate about engaging the public about pain and its prevention, treatment, and management.

Preface

This reprint contains a collection of articles on contemporary research and scholarship in the field of chronic pain management. Chronic pain is defined as pain that persists or recurs for more than three months, with a global point prevalence estimated to be greater than 20% of the adult population. Chronic pain has a significant financial impact on society in terms of healthcare costs, sickness benefits, and lost productivity; however, healthcare policies have overlooked chronic pain because, unlike other diseases and functional impairments, pain is not visible.

The International Classification of Diseases (ICD-11) categorises chronic pain as either primary or secondary. Chronic secondary pain is sub-divided as follows: cancer-related, postsurgical and post-traumatic, secondary musculoskeletal, secondary visceral, neuropathic, and secondary headache and orofacial. Chronic primary pain is associated with significant emotional distress or functional disability that cannot be explained by other conditions, and includes widespread chronic pain, fibromyalgia, non-specific musculoskeletal pain, complex regional pain syndrome, and irritable bowel syndrome. Hence, chronic pain is multifaceted, with a variety of modifiable and non-modifiable risk factors. A biopsychosocial framework and stepped model of care are optimal. This involves multidisciplinary teams that work with patients to co-create explanations for pain and utilise pharmacological and non-pharmacological treatments. Drug medication dominates clinical practice, partly due to the constraints of health service delivery, which has led to open-ended prescribing and widespread opioid abuse and overdose deaths in some countries. The use of non-pharmacological treatments, such as manual therapies (e.g., massage, manipulation, and mobilisation) and complementary therapies (e.g., acupuncture), is hindered by uncertain evidence regarding their efficacy and effectiveness.

The first article in this reprint is a review of the landscape of chronic pain from the perspective of evolutionary mismatch, contextualising chronic pain and its management in modern world settings. This is followed by an overview of systematic reviews evaluating the effectiveness of acupuncture and reviews on the molecular basis of cancer pain, as well as the treatment of painful diabetic neuropathy. The articles then navigate through CYP2D6 polymorphism and codeine, pharmacogenetic testing, and factors influencing diagnosis and treatment responses. The contributions focus on non-specific low back pain, lumbosacral radiculopathy, tendinopathy, anterior cruciate ligament reconstruction, acute herpes zoster, epidural ropivacaine with fentanyl, steroid injection, local body vibration with built-in vibroacoustic sound, Cyriax friction massage, biomechanics, psychological stress, empathy, and eye-gaze patterns. Thus, this reprint provides the reader with a rich tapestry of contemporary research and scholarship about chronic pain and its management.

Mark I. Johnson
Editor

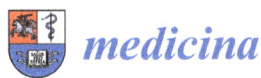

Review

The Landscape of Chronic Pain: Broader Perspectives

Mark I. Johnson

Centre for Pain Research, School of Clinical and Applied Sciences, City Campus, Leeds Beckett University, Leeds LS1 3HE, UK; M.Johnson@leedsbeckett.ac.uk

Received: 15 March 2019; Accepted: 16 May 2019; Published: 21 May 2019

Abstract: Chronic pain is a global health concern. This special issue on matters related to chronic pain aims to draw on research and scholarly discourse from an eclectic mix of areas and perspectives. The purpose of this non-systematic topical review is to précis an assortment of contemporary topics related to chronic pain and its management to nurture debate about research, practice and health care policy. The review discusses the phenomenon of pain, the struggle that patients have trying to legitimize their pain to others, the utility of the acute–chronic dichotomy, and the burden of chronic pain on society. The review describes the introduction of chronic primary pain in the World Health Organization's International Classification of Disease, 11th Revision and discusses the importance of biopsychosocial approaches to manage pain, the consequences of overprescribing and shifts in service delivery in primary care settings. The second half of the review explores pain perception as a multisensory perceptual inference discussing how contexts, predictions and expectations contribute to the malleability of somatosensations including pain, and how this knowledge can inform the development of therapies and strategies to alleviate pain. Finally, the review explores chronic pain through an evolutionary lens by comparing modern urban lifestyles with genetic heritage that encodes physiology adapted to live in the Paleolithic era. I speculate that modern urban lifestyles may be painogenic in nature, worsening chronic pain in individuals and burdening society at the population level.

Keywords: chronic pain; analgesia; pain perception; sensory illusions; embodied pain; painogenic environment; evolutionary mismatch hypothesis

1. Introduction

Chronic pain is a global health concern with evidence that patients are receiving inadequate care, due in part to deficits in knowledge and skills of health care professionals [1,2]. Chronic pain is a biopsychosocial phenomenon, yet pain education for health professionals continues to focus on biomedical aspects of pain [3]. The purpose of this topical review is to précis an assortment of contemporary issues related to chronic pain and its management to reveal the landscape of current knowledge and thinking in the field. My intention is to bring certain issues to light through commentary rather than comprehensive in-depth objective appraisal of research literature. The review is narrative in style and I have based the direction and content of the review on what I find interesting and controversial. I have attempted to integrate knowledge from a variety of disciplines including philosophy, phenomenology, epidemiology, biomedicine, psychology, evolutionary biology and health promotion. My approach is ambitious. Arguments are anthropomorphic in nature and cannot be generalized to non-human species. I appreciate that the non-systematic approach to review is vulnerable to selection and evaluation biases and opinion-oriented arguments, so I direct readers to key references for comprehensive coverage of topics of further interest. I hope that some of the issues discussed in the review prompts scholarly debate about future directions for research, practice and health care policy.

2. The Paradox of Pain

"To live in pain is not only to suffer aversive sensations but to be caught in a web of paradoxes"
Leder [4], p. 2.

2.1. Defining Pain

Historically, clinicians viewed pain as a secondary symptom of injury and disease and focused treatment on removing the precipitating (primary) cause. Relief of pain was of secondary concern. Nowadays the importance of alleviating pain is widely accepted. The International Association for the Study of Pain (IASP) defines pain as: '*An unpleasant sensory and emotional experience associated with actual or potential tissue damage, or described in terms of such damage.*' [5]. The association between tissue damage and pain is at the core of the definition, although the clause ' ... *or described in terms of such damage*' avoids *always* binding pain to the stimulus (i.e., potential or actual tissue damage). This is because pain is a psychological state produced by the brain in response to a multitude of biopsychosocial inputs of which activity in nociceptive (noxious detecting) pathways is but one. Often, scientists and clinicians view pain as a technical problem solvable by biomedical interventions (e.g., drugs and surgery) that target physiology, pharmacology, biochemistry, and molecular biology of the nociceptive system. This approach has proven successful at advancing our understanding of the pathophysiology of pain and identifying novel biomedical targets to alleviate pain. The focus on a biomedical approach has been at the expense of the contribution of psychosocial and environmental factors in the lived experience of pain. This may be one reason why management of chronic pain remains a challenge and the burden of chronic pain on society continues to rise. Pain is complex.

2.2. The Lived Experience of Pain

The lived experience of pain is a perplexing mix of sensory, emotional and cognitive phenomenon that fluctuate in and out of conscious awareness. The unpleasant nature of pain demands attention, explanation and action to resolve actual or potential damage of the body. An assortment of biopsychosocial and environmental factors influence the appearance, severity, character, and time course of pain, although often pain is unpredictable. Pain may occur in response to noxious stimuli, innocuous stimuli or in the absence of any apparent stimuli. From a phenomenological perspective people report their experience of pain to fluctuate in the present and the past and the future; to be localized and radiating everywhere; to be productive and destructive of value and meaning; and to be never changing and ever-changing [4]. Often pain is amorphous.

2.3. Why Do We Communicate Pain?

Expression of pain is at the core of human group dynamics, serving to inform other individuals that you are injured or ill. In modern society expressing pain has the potential to generate empathy in others to motivate them to offer aid. Individuals evaluate a person's expression of pain to determine the extent of their disability and whether the person can fulfill their responsibilities. It seems plausible that expression of pain was beneficial for our human ancestors living as hunter-gatherers in the Paleolithic era [6]. Hunter-gatherer groups need to keep moving to search for food and avoid predation. Providing assistance or care to group members who were injured or ill could be detrimental to a group's ability to acquire sufficient food or remain safe. Thus, the ability to legitimize pain to others would have been important when trying to persuade others to provide care and assistance. Interestingly, individuals could use this to their advantage by claiming to be in pain when in fact they were not, to avoid dangerous tasks such as hunting trips. Legitimizing pain to others is particularly challenging in the absence of visible cues of injury or illness because other group members may believe that the person is expressing pain to seek an unfair advantage. It seems plausible that evolution has hardwired the nervous system to exaggerate expression of pain (to be believed) and paradoxically hardwired the nervous system to be skeptical about the existence of pain in others (to prevent being duped). This paradox plays out in the adversary struggle that chronic pain patients experience when trying to legitimise their pain in the health care system [7–10].

3. The Struggle to Legitimize Pain

"To have pain is to have certainty; to hear about pain is to have doubt"
Scarry [11], p. 13.

3.1. Disproving Pain

Communicating the complex, dynamic, and multidimensional nature of pain experience is a challenge. The amorphous character of pain does not sit comfortably with the objective nature of medical practice and evidence suggests that chronic pain patients have difficulties convincing health care professionals of the existence of pain [7,9,10]. Pain is a perceptual experience that is personal to the individual and by definition unobservable by another person. The subjective nature of pain makes it is impossible to prove or disprove a person's pain and therefore it is not possible to distinguish a person's report of pain experience from that of tissue damage. A person's report of pain should be accepted if their sensory and emotional experience of pain is expressed in the same ways as that caused by tissue damage. This was recognised in 1968 by McCaffery who defined pain as '... *whatever the experiencing person says it is, existing whenever the experiencing person says it does*' [12]. Hence, conveying pain experience depends on an ability to use language and/or behavioral action to communicate the internal state of one's body. It also depends on an ability to persuade others of the existence of pain in oneself. Likewise, the observer needs to be receptive to what is being communicated, including being able to interpret the meaning and importance of both verbal and behavioral information. This can be challenging for individuals with limited verbal expression such as infants or with compromised cognitive ability such as individuals with dementia. A recent systematic review of pain management for community-dwelling people with dementia found that informal caregivers were more likely to report pain on behalf of the person with dementia and pain-focused behavioral observation assessment was infrequently used by practitioners [13]. Multimodal assessment of pain that includes self-reported and non-self-reported measures have been developed to capture the complexity of pain experience [14], although it is important to note that behavioral signs, effort testing, self-reported questionnaires, or symptom validity tests have been shown to be unable to identify malingering [15].

3.2. The Tenuous Link between Pain and Pathology

Skepticism about the legitimacy of another person's pain is at its height when there is an absence of evidence of injury or disease [16]. For example, pain may be driven by central sensitization and/or abnormal functioning of the nociceptive system, and/or altered higher level processing such as fear-avoidance behavior. Unlike many illnesses, pain is not visible or measurable using objective means and clinicians have to rely on patients' self-report, coupled with observation. Subjective and objective assessment, including the patient's report of symptoms, examinations of functional capacity, and diagnostic tests, contribute to pain diagnoses. When legitimizing pain and constructing logical explanations for pain, patients and non-pain specialist practitioners tend to give credence to positive diagnostic tests related to tissue pathology, at the expense of alterations in physiological processing associated with pain se (e.g., central sensitisation). Diagnostic imaging techniques are critical for detecting sinister pathology in patients presenting with pain. However, tissue pathology may be present in the absence of pain [17] so paradoxically, evidence of tissue pathology may be counterproductive when searching for causes of pain in some circumstances Thus, in some instances the relationship between pain, injury and disease may be tenuous.

Pain may occur in the absence of injury. A clinical anecdote by Fisher et al. [18] described the case of a builder who presented to accident and emergency complaining of severely disabling pain due to a 15-cm nail that had penetrated his boot. The builder needed strong analgesia and sedation before physicians were able to remove the nail from the boot. On removing the boot from the foot, they discovered that the nail had lodged between the toes without causing tissue damage! Pain may occur in the presence of minor injuries. A sliver of metal embedded in the skin of a finger is a good example. Paradoxically, serious injuries may be devoid of pain. Beecher et al.'s seminal paper reported that over 50% of soldiers with fresh combat wounds reported mild or no pain [19]. Evidence suggests that high proportions of individuals without pain have pathological changes associated with aging [17]. Clinical care pathways for some chronic pain conditions do not recommend diagnostic imaging in the absence of red flags (e.g., non-specific low back pain [20]). Pathology may not always be driving pain.

3.3. Pain is Not a Unitary Phenomenon

Clearly, the dynamic, multidimensional, and amorphous nature of pain is challenging to capture with any degree of specificity and precision. Commonly, pain is reduced to a unitary phenomenon measured by numerical intensity rating scales. This approach is convenient and psychometric research evidence suggests that data gathered from scales is valid and reliable [21–23]. However, rating scales do not measure pain objectively and can give a false impression of the level of measurement precision (e.g., 1 mm on 100-mm visual analogue scale). Scales presume linearity of subjective report between scale ends and use anchors that are nebulous (e.g., 'The worst-ever pain' or 'The worst pain imaginable'). Patients have been known to extend scale ends to incorporate incidents that have provoked pain beyond the worst they had previously thought imaginable [24]. The measurement of pain in this way is not only imprecise but is also fails to capture the complex and subjective nature of pain. To overcome the restrictions associated with numeric scaling Wideman et al. [14] have offered a multimodal assessment model of pain that describes quantitative aspects of pain such as self-reported and non-self-reported measures, and importantly, qualitative aspects of pain such as the words and behaviors of the patient's narrative. This practical framework assists the integration of the subjectivity of pain within assessment. The inclusion of, and importance paid to, the narrative report captures more fully an individual's pain experience helping to legitimize pain for both patient and practitioner. This promotes a compassion-based consultation and provides much information that enriches assessment of the underlying processes contributing to pain.

4. Chronic Pain

4.1. Reassessing the Acute–Chronic Dichotomy?

Traditionally, service delivery and clinical practice views pain through an acute or chronic lens. Acute pain is pain persisting less than twelve weeks. Chronic pain is often secondary to disease or traumatic injury and initially considered a symptom. Chronic pain is pain that persists or recurs for twelve weeks or more, or beyond the expected time for healing. Recently, Loser argued that the acute–chronic dichotomy is so entrenched in pain parlance that it has escaped critical scrutiny [25]. There are no temporal correlates of physiological processes associated with pain based on time points used to distinguish acute and chronic. Loser argues that we should describe pain syndromes based on physiological mechanisms, including peripheral or centrally generated perspectives as originally discussed by John Bonica in the 1950s.

From an evolutionary perspective, hypersensitivity of the nervous system serves to assist the healing process by amplifying and prolonging pain. This discourages use of, and contact with, injured tissue. Peripheral sensitization is driven by the release and production of biochemical mediators at the site of tissue damage that lower the threshold of activation of transducer ion channel receptors expressed in nociceptor terminals. Sometimes the adaptive function of peripheral sensitization is lost as is the case for some autoimmune diseases such as rheumatoid arthritis that generates ongoing inflammation, peripheral sensitization and pain hypersensitivity even though healing does not occur.

Central sensitization is centrally mediated amplification of pain irrespective of mechanism or location. Central sensitization is triggered by noxious (excitatory) input arising from direct activation of nociceptors (nociceptive) or from damaged or dysfunctional neuronal fibers (neuropathic). Nerve injury can reduce segmental and/or extrasegmental inhibitory influences on central nociceptive transmission (i.e., disinhibition) through a loss of interneurons, loss of descending pathways, altered connectivity and microglial activation. These mechanisms lower the threshold of excitation of central nociceptive transmission neurons, amplifying their output to noxious and non-noxious stimuli [26]. The molecular mechanisms are multifactorial and complex with NMDA (N-Methyl D-Aspartate) receptors having a critical role, in a process similar to long-term potentiation associated with memory formation. The receptive fields of central nociceptive transmission neurons also expand so that they become responsive to stimuli applied to areas of tissue that do not normally activate them. Thus, central sensitization increases the area of pain hypersensitivity across body parts.

Central sensitization manifests primary and secondary hyperalgesia and allodynia and sometimes pain presents spontaneously in the absence of nociceptive stimuli. Patients may present with widespread pain in multiple body regions and pain arising after mundane activities such as walking or cooking. Yunus coined the term central sensitivity syndrome to describe pain-related conditions without obvious tissue pathology, that have similar comorbid symptoms (e.g., poor sleep hygiene, fatigue, and slowness of cognition) and include fibromyalgia and irritable bowel syndrome [27].

4.2. Nociplastic Pain: A New Mechanistic Descriptor?

Presently, mechanistic categories of pain are; *nociceptive pain*, resulting from activation of nociceptors by a noxious stimulus that is damaging or threatens damage to healthy tissues (other than neural structures); and *neuropathic pain* resulting from a lesion or disease of the somatosensory nervous system. Recently, Kosek et al. [28] have proposed consideration of a third mechanistic descriptor, *nociplastic pain* (other candidate terms offered were algopathic or nocipathic pain), to describe pain arising from altered central nociceptive processing in the absence of tissue damage. Kosek et al. argue that inclusion of nociplastic pain, or some other equivalent, in the vocabulary of pain would raise awareness that pain may present without detectable tissue damage and promote screening for signs of nociceptive dysfunction to improve diagnosis and treatment. Nociceptive and neuropathic mechanisms that contribute to pain are proven and can be detected using various techniques including biochemical investigations, radiology, nerve conduction tests and imaging of the nervous system. It is important to recognize that the terms nociplastic, nociceptive and neuropathic are not diagnoses or exclusive categorical labels but descriptors of concurrent potential mechanistic drivers of pain. Nevertheless, the term nociplastic pain could help patients create explanatory models of their pain experience to legitimize their pain to others.

4.3. The Burden of Chronic Pain

Most literature discusses pain from an acute–chronic dichotomy. Chronic pain affects between 15–30% of the general adult population [29–31], with severe, debilitating chronic pain affecting 10–15% of adults [32]. Healthcare and socioeconomic costs of chronic pain is high and estimated to be 3–10% of gross national domestic product in Europe [33]. In the United States annual costs related to health care delivery and lower worker productivity due to chronic pain is estimated to be between $560 and $635 billion dollars and greater than heart disease ($309 billion), cancer ($243 billion), and diabetes ($188 billion) [34].

People do not die directly of pain, and unlike functional impairment, pain is not visible. Pain is often secondary to other medical conditions. Health care policies often focus on curing or slowing progression of the primary disease as a means to improve functional outcome, and may neglect pain management. For example, pain is underdiagnosed and inadequately managed in neurological conditions [35,36], despite high prevalence (e.g., Parkinson's disease (40–85% (range) [37]), multiple sclerosis (55–70% (95% confidence intervals (CI)) [38]), motor neuron disease (19–85% (95% CI) [36]) and Alzheimer's disease (38–75% (95% CI) [36]). There has been a long-standing debate whether chronic pain should be considered a disease entity in its own right under certain circumstances [39].

4.4. International Classification of Diseases: Chronic Primary Pain

The 11th edition of the World Health Organization's International Classification of Diseases (ICD-11) categorises chronic pain as secondary to other conditions: chronic cancer-related pain, chronic neuropathic pain, chronic secondary visceral pain, chronic posttraumatic and postsurgical pain, chronic secondary headache and orofacial pain, and chronic secondary musculoskeletal pain [40]. The ICD-11 recognises that in some circumstances, chronic pain may not be explained by the presence of another condition and require special treatment and care in its own right. Thus, ICD-11 includes a category for chronic primary pain to reflect in part that pain should be regarded as a pathologic entity in its own right and characterized by a dysfunctional nervous system with persistent central sensitization (for review of the history of this debate see Raffaeli, and Arnaudo [39]).

Chronic primary pain defies classical pathological based classification and is described as pain as the primary complaint in one or more regions of the body and causing significant emotional distress or functional disability. Specific examples include chronic widespread pain, fibromyalgia, irritable bowel syndrome and non-specific chronic low back pain. Chronic primary pain draws attention to the much broader spectrum of possible biological, psychological and social causes and consequences than tissue damage or on going disease. The premise that pain is a biosychosocial phenomenon is widely accepted but social components of pain are often absent from pain definitions. Recently, Williams and Craig have called for the IASP to re-consider its definition of pain to highlight the contribution of social elements in pain experience, as follows: ' ... *a distressing experience associated with actual or potential tissue damage with sensory, emotional, cognitive, and social components*' [41] (p. 2420). This would draw further attention to the need to deliver holistic models of care.

5. Desirable Models of Care

It is recommended that patients with chronic pain are managed using a biopsychosocial model of care with pharmacological and non-pharmacological interventions tailored to the needs of the individual [42]. Care plans should promote physical and psychological wellbeing through lifestyle adjustments (e.g., in diet and physical activity), psychological interventions (e.g., cognitive behavioral therapy), and non-pharmacological adjuncts such as manual therapies, transcutaneous electrical nerve stimulation (TENS), thermal therapies, acupuncture, low level laser therapy, mirror therapy and virtual reality. The World Health Organization promotes the use of multidisciplinary teams working in partnership with patients to co-create explanations about pain and construct care plans that empower individuals to be active participants in their treatment because it creates self-efficacy [42–44]. Traditionally, first line treatment for pain involves the use of analgesic and adjuvant drugs that modulate nociceptive system processing, and the simplicity, convenience and partial success of this approach has meant that it dominates service delivery in many parts of the world.

5.1. The Analgesic Ladder

The World Health Organization's analgesic ladder, initially developed for cancer pain [45], advocates a stepwise approach to prescribing starting with mild analgesics and increasing dosage or switching to powerful analgesics if pain is not adequately managed. Paracetamol or nonsteroidal anti-inflammatory drugs (Non-Steroidal Anti-Inflammatory Drugs (NSAIDs), e.g., diclofenac and ibuprofen) are prescribed for mild to moderate non-neuropathic pain, stepping up to weak opioids (e.g., codeine and dihydrocodeine) for moderate pain, and strong opioids (e.g., morphine and oxycodone) for moderate to severe pain. Prescribers also use local anesthetics for mild pain (e.g., mouth ulcers), and for moderate to severe pain (e.g., during and post-surgery). Adjuvants are drugs whose primary use was not originally for relief of pain and are used to manage neuropathic pain (e.g., amitriptyline, duloxetine, gabapentin or pregabalin) or muscle spasm (e.g., baclofen).

Analgesic drugs interact with nociceptive pathways to inhibit the onward transmission of noxious information from the site of injury to the brain in order to alleviate pain. Non-steroidal anti-inflammatory drugs inhibit cyclooxygenase reducing the production of prostaglandins that normally sensitize nociceptors; opioids prevent onward transmission of nociceptive transmission in the central nervous system; and local anesthetics block sodium channels reducing transmission of nerve impulses in nociceptive fibers. Analgesic and adjuvant medications are extremely valuable for short-term management of pain and used cautiously in the long-term. The largest pan European survey of chronic pain found that 64% of participants stated that medication did not adequately control pain [2]. It may be difficult for some health care professionals to accept that long-term drug medication may not be the best option and that the multidimension nature of pain means that response to drug intervention is highly malleable. This malleability is demonstrated in research using open-hidden paradigms. A review of experimental evidence by Benedetti [46] provided evidence that the efficacy of analgesic drugs is modulated by cognitive and affective state. Administering a placebo (fake) drug coupled with the suggestion that it is an analgesic drug increases analgesia and administering an analgesic drug with the suggestion that it is a placebo (fake) drug reduces analgesic outcome. The addition of open-label placebo treatment as an adjunct to treatment for chronic lower back pain has been shown to be safe and effective at reducing pain raising interesting ethical debates about the role of placebos in treatment [47].

5.2. Overprescribing

Concerns have been expressed about detrimental consequences to individuals and society of over diagnosis and over prescribing for chronic long-term illnesses, including chronic pain [48,49]. Abuse of prescription opioids is a major problem in some Western countries [50], although paradoxically, restricted access to opioids impedes pain management in parts of Asia, Africa, and Middle East [51]. The use of prescription opioid medication in the United States has risen from 4.1% in 1999–2000 to 6.8% in 2013–2014, with long-term users rising from 45.1% of all opioid users in 1999–2000 to 79.4% in 2013–2014 [52]. Social, economic and environmental variables are as influential in the opioid epidemic as health and biomedical factors. Recently, cross-sectional analyses of individual and county-level demographic and economic factors have found that elevated mortality from opioid overdose due to increased opioid prescribing was positively associated with direct marketing of opioid medication to physicians [53], and that chronic opioid use was positively associated with presidential voting patterns in USA counties [54]. Abuse of prescription opioids demonstrates the need for greater caution and selectivity in prescribing of long-term opioid therapy. Ironically, as one drug loses favor others come into view.

5.3. Novel Centrally Acting Drugs

There is a debate whether plant-based cannabis preparations could replace opioids [55]. There is low-level evidence that cannabinoids alleviate neuropathic pain and insufficient evidence to recommend their clinical use for other types of pain [56,57]. Presently, professional bodies recommend that cannabinoids be considered in exceptional circumstances for neuropathic pain, chronic non-malignant pain and cancer pain when patients are not responding to other treatment [58]. Centrally acting psychedelic drugs such as lysergic acid diethylamide and psilocybin have also attracted interest for the management of chronic pain [59]. Psychedelics act as agonists at $5-HT_{2A}$ receptors and may modulate pain through action in the rostral ventromedial medulla enhancing descending pain inhibitory pathway activity [60]. Psychedelics influence metacognitive interpretation of pain including the resting state of awareness mediated by the default mode network in the brain [61]. Pain interferes with activity in the default mode network causing intrusive cognition and the breakdown of normal self [62]. Only a few small studies without controls exist that suggest potential benefit of psychedelics for cluster headache and malignant and neuropathic pain [59].

6. Service Delivery in Primary Care

The value of analgesic medication is undisputed providing it is within a biopsychosocial model of care. Adams and Turk [63] suggest that a biopsychosocial perspective, rather than a singular biomedical, or psychological, or social perspective, is necessary to fully understand the lived experiences of people with chronic central sensitivity pain syndrome. A comprehensive approach to assessment is optimal to address physical, emotional, and social functioning and a palliative approach is optimal to manage pain and distressing symptoms because there are no curative treatments. However, resource pressures often hinder the delivery of a truly biopsychosocial model of care by multidisciplinary teams in primary care settings.

6.1. Shared Appointments and First Points of Contact

Employing multidisciplinary teams of physicians, nurses, physiotherapists, psychologists, dietitians and occupational therapists can be financially costly. Traditionally, the first point of contact is the primary care (general) physician (GP) who conducts a short one-on-one ten-minute consultation with the patient to assess, diagnose, agree appropriate treatment and discuss difficult concepts. This consultation often feels rushed with GPs having similar consultations with different patients over the course of a day. Shared appointments may be a more cost-effective model of service delivery than one-to-one consultations and have been successful for the management of diabetes, and obesity [64]. Shared appointments involve each patient consulting with the clinical team, with elements of group education and discussion between patients, and peer support by learning from the experiences of other patients. Patients impart information more readily in shared appointments and engagement with patients with similar conditions provides motivation for health behavior change. There is increasing use of shared medical appointments for persistent pain [64]. Moreover, physiotherapists and nurses may be better suited than GPs as a first point of contact to diagnose and advise patients with non-complex chronic pain [65].

6.2. Social Prescribing

Some countries have adopted programmes of social prescribing to provide patients in primary care with sources of support within their community. Social prescribing enables healthcare professionals to refer patients to non-medical personnel who work with the patient to co-design a nonclinical social prescription to improve health and well-being [66]. Social prescriptions include access to practical information and advice, community activity, and physical activities provided by voluntary and community sectors. A systematic review of 15 evaluations of social prescribing schemes in UK settings could not reliably judge effectiveness or value for money because evaluations had a paucity of data and methodological limitations, although conclusions of individual evaluations were generally positive [67]. Social prescribing schemes seem to be an ideal fit for the management of many chronic pain conditions because social prescribing addresses psychological, social and environmental factors affecting health and well-being associated with pain.

7. Pain Perception: Active Top-Down Processing?

Classically, a 'bottom-up' stimulus-organism-response model describes the physiological processes involved in producing pain sensation. The model inadvertently implies that pain is an inevitable consequence of activity in the nociceptive system driven by tissue damage. This stimulus-organism-response model has been refined to incorporate changes in the sensitivity of the nociceptive system and top-down processes that facilitate and inhibit nociceptive transmission [68,69]. Melzack suggested that the multidimensional experience of pain resulted from characteristic patterns of nerve impulses (i.e., a neurosignature) produced within multiple widely distributed neural networks in the brain that are genetically determined and modified by sensory experience (i.e., body-self neuromatrix theory of pain) [70]. Melzack suggested that multiple factors influenced the output patterns of the body-self neuromatrix, of which noxious input was only one. This would explain why pain sometimes arises and/or persists despite limited noxious input.

7.1. Maleability of Perceived Properties of the Body

Predictions and expectations are a core feature of the central nervous system processing enabling the brain to generate perceptual experiences based on snippets of multisensory input. This 'perceptual inference' is involved in the generation of the sense of ownership of body parts, and in the location of sensory events, including pain, within the body. The perceptual qualities associated with the sense of body ownership are malleable as demonstrated by somatosensory illusions.

The rubber hand illusion demonstrates how rapidly the brain can update assumptions about the location of stimuli and 'ownership' of body parts. An individual watches a rubber hand stroked with a brush whilst their real hand is stroked in synchrony but hidden out of view [71]. Within minutes, the sensation of stroking feels as if it is arising from the rubber hand and the individual experiences a sense that the rubber hand has become part of their body (i.e., the rubber hand has been embodied and the real hand disembodied) [72]. Approaching a perceptually embodied rubber hand with a threatening stimuli may elicit somatosensations in some individuals including pain, subjective anxiety and skin conductance responses that are similar in magnitude to that experienced when a real hand is threatened [73,74].

The marble hand illusion demonstrates how the brain can update assumptions of the material qualities of the body. The illusion involves gently hitting the hand with a hammer and progressively replacing the sound of hammer blow on skin with a hammer blow on marble. Within five minutes the hand feels stiffer, heavier, harder, less sensitive and unnatural [75]. Protecting a virtual limb with a virtual iron armor cover can reduce electrically evoked pain [76] and hearing a creaky door when moving a stiff joint or back increases the need to protect the spine whereas hearing a gentle whoosh reduces the need to protect [77]. In fact, perceptual stiffness in the back was found not to be a representation of biomechanical properties of tissue but rather a perceptual inference error of stiffness, in other words, "... *feeling stiff does not equate to being stiff in chronic low back pain*" [77] [p2]. Thus, the brain operates to reduce threat and preserve coherent behavior according to situational context and these perceptual inferences can operate in both directions, i.e., pain or analgesia [78,79].

7.2. Multisensory Perceptual Inference as a Protector

Pain is never motivationally neutral. Pain is a potent driver of action in much the same way as thirst drives drinking and hunger drives eating, because the cost of ignoring pain may result in tissue damage, disrupted homeostasis and threat to life. Outcomes of behaviors that do not meet predictions (i.e., are unexpected with a large prediction error) have a major influence on future behavior. Unexpected pain, such as a severe lancinating shooting pain during an innocuous movement, is likely to have a disproportionately large effect on the expected intensity of future encounters with the same stimuli. Unexpected pain is likely to amplify multisensory perceptual inference serving to protect the integrity of tissue by creating, for example, fear-avoidance of movement (i.e., the motivational-decision model of pain [80]). Individuals experiencing pain over-estimate the distance and the effort needed to walk to a target [81] and perceive targets to be further away [82] (i.e., economy of action hypothesis), although potential scaling of spatial perceptions during pain have not been consistently demonstrated [83]. Actions that fail to restore coherence of behavior may also contribute to perceptual dysfunctions accompanying pain. Examples include phantom limbs stuck in one position [84], and painful limbs feeling excessively large in complex regional pain syndrome [85,86], or excessively small in osteoarthritis [87]. Contemporary models of pain perception are attempting to integrate sensory, affective, cognitive, social, and bodily cues interpreted within social, environmental and evolutionary contexts, including previous experiences, from the perspective of embodied cognition.

7.3. The Theory of Embodied Pain

The embodied theory of pain designates pain as arising from situations that *infer* bodily threat to drive behaviors to reduce the impact of the threat on the integrity of tissues (i.e., defensive) whilst maintaining the integrity of rational behavior [88]. The embodied theory describes pain as a dynamic, motor experience rather than a passive, sensory experience and blurs the distinction between perception and action: "*Pain is always about action.*" ([88], p. 3). The embodied theory of pain places the body and its ability to investigate the environment through a dynamic exchange of information between nervous system and environment at the core of pain experience. Thus, the brain uses information about previous encounters with pain and previous behaviors on pain to 'flavour' pain experience. For example, individuals report thermal stimuli to be hotter and more painful when delivered in synchrony with a red light (often associated with heat) compared with a blue light [89]. Appreciating that the brain uses multisensory perceptual inference to predict likely consequences of undertaking defensive behaviors offers opportunities for therapeutic interventions [88,90–93].

7.4. Multisensory Perceptual Inference to Alleviate Pain

Therapeutic opportunities can arise from manipulating the environment and context to reinstate coherence of behavior and normalize perception. Mirrors, lenses, and virtual reality have been used to alleviate pain and improve function through visual distraction, 'normalizing' the appearance of dysmorphic painful body parts, reducing threat associated with moving painful body parts, and aligning ownership and agency of body parts through visual, proprioceptive, and tactile congruency. Therapeutic success is varied and research findings from systematic reviews of controlled clinical studies are inconsistent due to a paucity of robust primary studies [94–97].

Advanced technologies that couple visual, auditory, and haptic (tactile) stimuli, such as vibration in hand held game controllers and force feedback systems for medical and military training are being adapted to manipulate the multisensory environment impinging on the body influencing embodied and embedded perceptual experience. Immersive virtual reality technology using head-sets and non-immersive virtual reality technology using computer screens can be used in combination with motion tracking systems so that movements of an individual's real limb can be used to control the movement of a virtual limb. Pain may be modulated when individuals are immersed in different virtual reality environments [98,99]. Virtual and augmented reality technologies providing enriched practice environments tailored to individual needs are being used in recovery and rehabilitation after brain damage or injury to facilitate motor learning and neural plasticity. Virtual reality offers several opportunities for pain management including distraction from painful body parts, providing contexts that reduce perceived threat, resizing of painful dysmorphic body parts, re-embodiment of alienated and/or disowned painful body parts, and modulation of agency to facilitate movement of painful body parts accompanied by fear-avoidance of movement.

Task-oriented virtual reality provides opportunities to reduce the sense of threat associated with moving painful body parts accompanied by fear-avoidance of movement [100–103]. For example, Ortiz-Catalan et al. [104] designed a virtual environment as a rehabilitation training aid for individuals with amputated upper limbs. Surface electrodes were used to record muscle activation over the stump of the residual limb whilst individuals tried to voluntarily control a virtual phantom limb that was displayed in real-time on a computer screen. Motor volition was decoded using myoelectric pattern recognition software whilst the patient matched random target postures or attempted to drive a virtual car using the virtual limb. Improvements in phantom limb pain occurred after 12 training sessions that was sustained for six months post-training.

8. Social and Environmental Contexts

At the core of multisensory perceptual inference of pain is the social context in which an individual lives, including previous experiences associated with pain. Thus, an individual's pain experience is embedded in environmental settings.

8.1. Lifestyle and Chronic Pain

Increasingly, modern human lifestyles are embedded in urban environments. Modern urban lifestyles are associated with mortality and morbidity of noncommunicable 'lifestyle' diseases, such as cardiovascular diseases (heart attacks and stroke), chronic respiratory diseases (chronic obstructed pulmonary disease and asthma), diabetes and cancer [105]. Chronic pain is a secondary consequence of many of these non-communicable diseases causing suffering, disability and a significant impact on quality of life. The Global Burden of Disease Study 2013, found that chronic low back pain had the highest number of years lived with disability [106]. Some lifestyle behaviours are risk factors for non-communicable diseases including sedentary activity, unhealthy diet, anxiety and depression, smoking, lack of sunshine, disrupted sleep, unemployment, living in adverse socioeconomic circumstances, and previous history of abuse or violence [107–109]. The relationship between these lifestyle factors and chronic pain is complex and unclear with causal processes likely to be acting in both directions.

Built and food environments are known to promote obesity in populations and has been described as obesogencity of urban environments [110]. The concept of an obesogenic environment has helped to focus attention upstream on whole systems public health solutions including the design of urban environments [111]. There are similarities between obesity and chronic pain [112]. Both conditions disproportionately affect poorer people society; are associated with high economic and social costs; are influenced by biopsychosocial factors including physical activity and diet; and are managed using pharmacological, educational and behavioural interventions. This raises the possibility that modern urban environments may be painogenic in nature [113].

8.2. Painogenicity of Modern Urban Living

Painogenicity is the sum of influences that the surroundings, opportunities or conditions of life have on promoting persistent pain in individuals or populations [113]. Modern urban environments generally consist of air polluted with toxic emissions and particulates, high population densities, limited green open space and readily available processed foodstuffs. Consequently, there has been a shift toward sedentary lifestyles and high calorie diets of over processed food with excess sucrose, salt, fat and additives, both known to contribute to noncommunicable 'lifestyle diseases' (c.f. Sick City Syndrome, Modern Urban Living Syndrome) [114]. The shift to modern urban living is more rapid than physiological adaptation resulting in a potential evolutionary mismatch [114,115]. An evolutionary lens has been used to explore the biological role of sensitization and hyperalgesia in chronic pain [78,116–118] but little is written about the contribution of evolutionary mismatch to chronic pain [113].

8.3. Chronic Pain and Evolutionary Mismatch

Evolutionary mismatch may provide insights to potential painogencity of modern urban environments. Our genetic heritage encodes physiology adapted for hominin ancestors that existed in the Paleolithic era, circa 4–7 million years ago with clean air, exposure to microorganisms and lifestyles consisting of walking, climbing, lifting, carrying and bending and diets of fresh vegetables, fruit and raw meat (i.e., hunter-gatherer lifestyles). Paleolithic ancestors existed in calorie-limited environments and were adapted to minimize energy expenditure wherever possible and maximise consumption of fat, sugar and salt driven by cravings. Paleolithic ancestors existed in outdoor environments with direct exposure to microorganisms and parasites through contact with soil, plants, and animals resulting in a diversity of microorganisms thriving on the skin and within the gastrointestinal tract (i.e., the human microbiota) [119]. The symbiotic relationship between the human microbiota, acquired after birth, and the immune system drives protective responses to pathogens and tolerance to innocuous antigens.

In contrast, modern urban dwellers exist in towns and cities and have lifestyles that are indoors and involve consumption of over-processed foods, and prescription and recreational drugs. Modern urban lifestyles are becoming increasingly sedentary with excessive amounts of time being physically inactive leading to 'disuse syndromes' (e.g., 'walking deficiency syndrome', 'hyper-sitting syndrome') and an increased risk of non-specific chronic musculoskeletal pain [120–122]. The shift to urban living is associated with a decline nutritional diversity due to consumption of fewer vegetables, fruits, antioxidants and omega-3 fatty acids and a rise in consumption of high calorie over-processed foods creating diet-induced proinflammatory states [123]. The gastrointestinal microbiota–brain axis of modern humans has been disrupted by the shift to indoor living with environmentally controlled air, sanitation, processed foodstuffs, and the use of pharmaceuticals to eradicate infections and parasites. Reduced exposure to microorganisms in childhood results in immune systems unable to differentiate pathogens that confer benefit or harm and this may contribute to inappropriate immune (allergic) responses to harmless allergens associated with a disrupted microbiota resulting in inflammatory responses and peripheral and central sensitization of the nociceptive system [124]. Evidence suggests that abnormal immune responses may directly influence processes associated with sensitization of the peripheral and central nociceptive system through atypical regulation and output of the hypothalamic–pituitary–adrenal axis including downstream signaling that sensitizes nociceptive afferents [125]. These processes may be contributory factors in visceral pain resulting from inflammatory bowel disease, celiac disease, and metabolic syndrome [119] and idiopathic pain disorders manifesting with persistent central sensitization such as fibromyalgia, chronic pelvic pain, and migraine [125].

Current models of care for chronic pain, especially related to the musculoskeletal system, promote lifestyle adjustment. In essence, they are attempting to rebalance this evolutionary mismatch. Physical activity and diet is at the core of lifestyle adjustment (e.g., for non-specific chronic low back pain [20]). Diet therapies that increase consumption of antioxidants and omega-3 fatty acids, and reduce consumption of exocitoxic substances (e.g., monosodium glutamate, hydrolyzed protein, protein isolates/concentrates, yeast extract, aspartame) and foodstuffs (e.g., bran, nuts, soybean, and aged cheeses) may alleviate chronic pain [126–128]. Dietary interventions such as probiotics and prebiotics may prove beneficial to alleviate visceral hypersensitivity associated with a disrupted microbiota [119,129]. However, adherence to long-term lifestyle adjustment is poor and this may be due to the social and environmental conditions in which patients live.

9. Upstream for Solutions

Clinical guidelines recommend that practitioners counsel people living with persistent pain to undertake healthy lifestyles. Pain education about the nature of lifestyle adjustments is prominent in pain discourse but incongruous social and environmental conditions may hinder long-term behaviour change. Consideration of upstream solutions may help to reduce chronic pain at both individual and population level.

9.1. Social Models of Health Promotion

People with chronic pain prioritize justice-related issues within the context of their personal concerns and needs [130]. Low socioeconomic status, poor working conditions or unemployment, unstable home life, low levels of education, and living in deprived environments are associated with increased pain [108]. People with chronic pain believe that treatment of chronic pain is unfair [131]. Interpretative phenomenological analyses demonstrate that chronic pain patients from lower socioeconomic groups express concerns associated with unfair advantages of others, whereas those from middle socioeconomic groups are concerned with a battle for quality of life, and those from upper socioeconomic groups with the quality of care [130].

Social models of health promotion have been used successfully to tackle social injustices detrimental to health and wellbeing, such as poverty, provision of inexpensive foodstuffs that encourage healthy diets, poor housing and lack of employment [132]. There is however, limited discourse about the use of social models of health promotion within pain literature [133].

9.2. Evolutionary-Concordant Environments

There are also constraints of healthy living imposed by the nature of built environments. Often, urban environments are not conducive to undertaking physical activity outdoors due to limited greenspace, fear for personal safety, and air and noise pollution. Indoor activities may introduce additional issues such as transportation to and from a gym, financial expense to use a gym, and chronic overuse injuries such as strains and tendonitis from, for example, jogging on treadmills in restrictive shoes [134]. The Evolutionary Determinants of Health program launched in 2014 provides a framework for debate of evolutionary-concordant healthy cities and social regimes for urban societies, with green, open spaces and clean air to encourage individuals to be physically active [135]. However, there needs to be commitment on the part of policy makers to address social injustices and construct healthy urban environments to enable patients and individuals to live healthy lifestyles.

10. Conclusions

Chronic pain remains a major health care problem posing numerous challenges for researchers, practitioners, policy makers and patients alike. In this review, I have used a broad lens to explore a variety of contemporary matters associated with chronic pain. I have argued that pain is perplexing, subjective and amorphous and some patients feel that health care providers do not believe that they have significant pain. I have argued that it is not possible to disprove a person's pain and that the association between pain and pathology may be tenuous in some circumstances. I described the consequences of long-term prescribing of analgesic medication and offered examples of service delivery that may promote a biopsychosocial model of care at the first point of contact in primary care.

Ultimately, pain is a psychological construct arising from physiological processes occurring in the brain. I have described pain as a top-down perceptual inference that integrates sensory, motor, affective, cognitive, social and environmental contexts to update the final experience of pain. I argue that pain does not faithfully reflect tissue status but serves instead to *infer* bodily threat and drive behaviors to reduce the impact of threat on the integrity of the body. I have provided examples of the malleability of pain perception and offered examples of interventions that manipulate context to alleviate pain. Finally, I have speculated that modern urban environments are painogenic in nature and incompatible with Paleolithic physiology encoded by our genetic heritage. I believe that exploration of pain through the lens of evolutionary mismatch may provide novel insights to why patients have difficulties adhering to healthy lifestyles and provide upstream strategies to reduce the burden of chronic pain on society.

Funding: This research received no external funding.

Acknowledgments: I wish to express gratitude to Gareth Jones and Priscilla Wittkopf for commenting on drafts of the manuscript

Conflicts of Interest: Mark I. Johnson's institution has received research and consultancy funding for work that he has undertaken for GlaxoSmithKline.

References

1. International Association for the Study of Pain. Declaration of Montreal. Declaration That Access to Pain Management Is a Fundamental Human Right. Available online: https://www.iasp-pain.org/DeclarationofMontreal (accessed on 8 March 2019).
2. Breivik, H.; Collett, B.; Ventafridda, V.; Cohen, R.; Gallacher, D. Survey of chronic pain in Europe: Prevalence, impact on daily life, and treatment. *Eur. J. Pain* **2006**, *10*, 287–333. [CrossRef] [PubMed]

3. Thompson, K.; Johnson, M.I.; Milligan, J.; Briggs, M. Twenty-five years of pain education research-what have we learned? Findings from a comprehensive scoping review of research into pre-registration pain education for health professionals. *Pain* **2018**, *159*, 2146–2158. [CrossRef] [PubMed]
4. Leder, D. The Experiential Paradoxes of Pain. *J. Med. Philos.* **2016**, *41*, 444–460. [CrossRef] [PubMed]
5. International Association for the Study of Pain. IASP Terminology: Pain. Available online: https://www.iasp-pain.org/terminology?navItemNumber=576#Pain (accessed on 8 March 2019).
6. Sullivan, M.D. Clarifying our cultural contest about chronic pain. *Pain* **2019**, *160*, 279–280. [CrossRef] [PubMed]
7. Toye, F.; Seers, K.; Allcock, N.; Briggs, M.; Carr, E.; Andrews, J.; Barker, K. Patients' experiences of chronic non-malignant musculoskeletal pain: A qualitative systematic review. *Br. J. Gen. Pract.* **2013**, *63*, e829–e841. [CrossRef] [PubMed]
8. Toye, F.; Seers, K.; Allcock, N.; Briggs, M.; Carr, E.; Andrews, J.; Barker, K. *A Meta-Ethnography of Patients' Experience of Chronic non-Malignant Musculoskeletal Pain*; NIHR Journals Library: Southampton, UK, 2013.
9. Toye, F.; Seers, K.; Barker, K. A meta-ethnography of patients' experiences of chronic pelvic pain: Struggling to construct chronic pelvic pain as 'real'. *J. Adv. Nurs.* **2014**, *70*, 2713–2727. [CrossRef]
10. Toye, F.; Seers, K.; Barker, K.L. Meta-ethnography to understand healthcare professionals' experience of treating adults with chronic non-malignant pain. *BMJ Open* **2017**, *7*, e018411. [CrossRef]
11. Scarry, E. *The Body in Pain: The Making and Unmaking of the World*; Oxford University Press: New York, NY, USA, 1985.
12. McCaffery, M. *Nursing Practice Theories Related to Cognition, Bodily Pain, and Man-Environment Interactions*; University of California (UCLA Students' Store): Los Angeles, CA, USA, 1968; p. 207.
13. Bullock, L.; Bedson, J.; Jordan, J.L.; Bartlam, B.; Chew-Graham, C.A.; Campbell, P. Pain assessment and pain treatment for community-dwelling people with dementia: A systematic review and narrative synthesis. *Int. J. Geriatr. Psychiatry* **2019**, *34*, 807–821. [CrossRef]
14. Wideman, T.H.; Edwards, R.R.; Walton, D.M.; Martel, M.O.; Hudon, A.; Seminowicz, D.A. The Multimodal Assessment Model of Pain: A Novel Framework for Further Integrating the Subjective Pain Experience Within Research and Practice. *Clin. J. Pain* **2019**, *35*, 212–221. [CrossRef]
15. Tuck, N.L.; Johnson, M.H.; Bean, D.J. You'd Better Believe It: The Conceptual and Practical Challenges of Assessing Malingering in Patients With Chronic Pain. *J. Pain* **2019**, *20*, 133–145. [CrossRef]
16. Ojala, T.; Hakkinen, A.; Karppinen, J.; Sipila, K.; Suutama, T.; Piirainen, A. Although unseen, chronic pain is real-A phenomenological study. *Scand. J. Pain* **2015**, *6*, 33–40. [CrossRef] [PubMed]
17. Brinjikji, W.; Luetmer, P.H.; Comstock, B.; Bresnahan, B.W.; Chen, L.E.; Deyo, R.A.; Halabi, S.; Turner, J.A.; Avins, A.L.; James, K.; et al. Systematic literature review of imaging features of spinal degeneration in asymptomatic populations. *AJNR Am. J. Neuroradiol.* **2015**, *36*, 811–816. [CrossRef]
18. Fisher, J.P.; Hassan, D.T.; O'Connor, N. Minerva. *BMJ* **1995**, *310*, 70. [CrossRef]
19. Beecher, H.K. Anesthesia for Men Wounded in Battle. *Ann. Surg.* **1945**, *122*, 807–819. [CrossRef] [PubMed]
20. National Institute for Health and Care Excellence (NICE). *Low Back Pain and Sciatica in over 16s: Assessment and Management. Clinical Guideline [NG59]*; National Institute for Health and Care Excellence (NICE): London, UK, 2016; pp. 1–18.
21. Ferreira-Valente, M.A.; Pais-Ribeiro, J.L.; Jensen, M.P. Validity of four pain intensity rating scales. *Pain* **2011**, *152*, 2399–2404. [CrossRef]
22. Dworkin, R.H.; Turk, D.C.; Farrar, J.T.; Haythornthwaite, J.A.; Jensen, M.P.; Katz, N.P.; Kerns, R.D.; Stucki, G.; Allen, R.R.; Bellamy, N.; et al. Core outcome measures for chronic pain clinical trials: IMMPACT recommendations. *Pain* **2005**, *113*, 9–19. [CrossRef]
23. Dworkin, R.H.; Turk, D.C.; McDermott, M.P.; Peirce-Sandner, S.; Burke, L.B.; Cowan, P.; Farrar, J.T.; Hertz, S.; Raja, S.N.; Rappaport, B.A.; et al. Interpreting the clinical importance of group differences in chronic pain clinical trials: IMMPACT recommendations. *Pain* **2009**, *146*, 238–244. [CrossRef]
24. Royal, K.D.; Brosh, A. A More Accurate Pain Scale? *Rasch Meas. Trans.* **2013**, *26*, 1398.
25. Loeser, J.D. A new way of thinking about pain. *Pain Manag* **2018**. [CrossRef]
26. Woolf, C.J. Pain amplification—A perspective on the how, why, when, and where of central sensitization. *J. Appl. Behav. Res.* **2018**, *23*. [CrossRef]

27. Yunus, M.B. Central sensitivity syndromes: A new paradigm and group nosology for fibromyalgia and overlapping conditions, and the related issue of disease versus illness. *Semin. Arthritis Rheum.* **2008**, *37*, 339–352. [CrossRef]
28. Kosek, E.; Cohen, M.; Baron, R.; Gebhart, G.F.; Mico, J.A.; Rice, A.S.; Rief, W.; Sluka, A.K. Do we need a third mechanistic descriptor for chronic pain states? *Pain* **2016**, *157*, 1382–1386. [CrossRef] [PubMed]
29. Elzahaf, R.A.; Tashani, O.A.; Unsworth, B.A.; Johnson, M.I. The prevalence of chronic pain with an analysis of countries with a Human Development Index less than 0.9: A systematic review without meta-analysis. *Curr. Med. Res. Opin.* **2012**, *28*, 1221–1229. [CrossRef]
30. Jackson, T.; Thomas, S.; Stabile, V.; Shotwell, M.; Han, X.; McQueen, K. A Systematic Review and Meta-Analysis of the Global Burden of Chronic Pain Without Clear Etiology in Low- and Middle-Income Countries: Trends in Heterogeneous Data and a Proposal for New Assessment Methods. *Anesth. Analg.* **2016**, *123*, 739–748. [CrossRef]
31. Macfarlane, G.J. The epidemiology of chronic pain. *Pain* **2016**, *157*, 2158–2159. [CrossRef] [PubMed]
32. Fayaz, A.; Croft, P.; Langford, R.M.; Donaldson, L.J.; Jones, G.T. Prevalence of chronic pain in the UK: A systematic review and meta-analysis of population studies. *BMJ Open* **2016**, *6*, e010364. [CrossRef]
33. Breivik, H.; Eisenberg, E.; O'Brien, T. The individual and societal burden of chronic pain in Europe: The case for strategic prioritisation and action to improve knowledge and availability of appropriate care. *BMC Public Health* **2013**, *13*, 1229. [CrossRef]
34. Gaskin, D.J.; Richard, P. The economic costs of pain in the United States. *J. Pain* **2012**, *13*, 715–724. [CrossRef]
35. Borsook, D. Neurological diseases and pain. *Brain* **2012**, *135*, 320–344. [CrossRef]
36. De Tommaso, M.; Arendt-Nielsen, L.; Defrin, R.; Kunz, M.; Pickering, G.; Valeriani, M. Pain in Neurodegenerative Disease: Current Knowledge and Future Perspectives. *Behav. Neurol.* **2016**, *2016*, 7576292. [CrossRef]
37. Broen, M.P.; Braaksma, M.M.; Patijn, J.; Weber, W.E. Prevalence of pain in Parkinson's disease: A systematic review using the modified QUADAS tool. *Mov. Disord.* **2012**, *27*, 480–484. [CrossRef]
38. Foley, P.L.; Vesterinen, H.M.; Laird, B.J.; Sena, E.S.; Colvin, L.A.; Chandran, S.; MacLeod, M.R.; Fallon, M.T. Prevalence and natural history of pain in adults with multiple sclerosis: Systematic review and meta-analysis. *Pain* **2013**, *154*, 632–642. [CrossRef] [PubMed]
39. Raffaeli, W.; Arnaudo, E. Pain as a disease: An overview. *J. Pain Res.* **2017**, *10*, 2003–2008. [CrossRef]
40. Treede, R.D.; Rief, W.; Barke, A.; Aziz, Q.; Bennett, M.I.; Benoliel, R.; Cohen, M.; Evers, S.; Finnerup, N.B.; First, M.B.; et al. Chronic pain as a symptom or a disease: The IASP Classification of Chronic Pain for the International Classification of Diseases (ICD-11). *Pain* **2019**, *160*, 19–27. [CrossRef]
41. Williams, A.C.; Craig, K.D. Updating the definition of pain. *Pain* **2016**, *157*, 2420–2423. [CrossRef]
42. International Association for the Study of Pain. Desirable Characteristics of National Pain Strategies. Available online: https://www.iasp-pain.org/DCNPS?navItemNumber=655 (accessed on 8 March 2019).
43. Lorig, K.R.; Holman, H. Self-management education: History, definition, outcomes, and mechanisms. *Ann. Behav. Med. Publ. Soc. Behav. Med.* **2003**, *26*, 1–7. [CrossRef]
44. Boyers, D.; McNamee, P.; Clarke, A.; Jones, D.; Martin, D.; Schofield, P.; Smith, B.H. Cost-effectiveness of self-management methods for the treatment of chronic pain in an aging adult population: A systematic review of the literature. *Clin. J. Pain* **2013**, *29*, 366–375. [CrossRef]
45. Leung, L. From ladder to platform: A new concept for pain management. *J. Prim. Health Care* **2012**, *4*, 254–258. [CrossRef] [PubMed]
46. Benedetti, F.; Carlino, E.; Pollo, A. Hidden administration of drugs. *Clin. Pharmacol. Ther.* **2011**, *90*, 651–661. [CrossRef]
47. Carvalho, C.; Caetano, J.M.; Cunha, L.; Rebouta, P.; Kaptchuk, T.J.; Kirsch, I. Open-label placebo treatment in chronic low back pain: A randomized controlled trial. *Pain* **2016**, *157*, 2766–2772. [CrossRef] [PubMed]
48. Brodersen, J.; Kramer, B.S.; Macdonald, H.; Schwartz, L.M.; Woloshin, S. Focusing on overdiagnosis as a driver of too much medicine. *BMJ* **2018**, *362*, k3494. [CrossRef]
49. Le Fanu, J. Mass medicalisation is an iatrogenic catastrophe. *BMJ* **2018**, *361*, k2794. [CrossRef]
50. Shipton, E.A.; Shipton, E.E.; Shipton, A.J. A Review of the Opioid Epidemic: What Do We Do About It? *Pain Ther.* **2018**, *7*, 23–36. [CrossRef]

51. Duthey, B.; Scholten, W. Adequacy of opioid analgesic consumption at country, global, and regional levels in 2010, its relationship with development level, and changes compared with 2006. *J. Pain Symptom Manag.* **2014**, *47*, 283–297. [CrossRef] [PubMed]
52. Mojtabai, R. National trends in long-term use of prescription opioids. *Pharmacoepidemiol. Drug Saf.* **2017**. [CrossRef]
53. Hadland, S.E.; Rivera-Aguirre, A.; Marshall, B.D.L.; Cerda, M. Association of Pharmaceutical Industry Marketing of Opioid Products with Mortality from Opioid-Related Overdoses. *JAMA Netw. Open* **2019**, *2*, e186007. [CrossRef]
54. Goodwin, J.S.; Kuo, Y.F.; Brown, D.; Juurlink, D.; Raji, M. Association of Chronic Opioid Use with Presidential Voting Patterns in US Counties in 2016. *JAMA Netw. Open* **2018**, *1*, e180450. [CrossRef]
55. Humphreys, K.; Saitz, R. Should Physicians Recommend Replacing Opioids with Cannabis? *JAMA* **2019**. [CrossRef]
56. Mucke, M.; Phillips, T.; Radbruch, L.; Petzke, F.; Hauser, W. Cannabis-based medicines for chronic neuropathic pain in adults. *Cochrane Database Syst. Rev.* **2018**, *3*, CD012182. [CrossRef] [PubMed]
57. Urits, I.; Borchart, M.; Hasegawa, M.; Kochanski, J.; Orhurhu, V.; Viswanath, O. An Update of Current Cannabis-Based Pharmaceuticals in Pain Medicine. *Pain Ther.* **2019**. [CrossRef] [PubMed]
58. British Pain Society. BPS Position Statement on the Medicinal Use of Cannabinoids in Pain Management. Available online: https://www.britishpainsociety.org/static/uploads/resources/files/BPS_Position_Statement_on_the_medicinal_use_of_cannabinoids_in_pain_management.pdf (accessed on 27 February 2019).
59. Whelan, A.; Johnson, M.I. Lysergic acid diethylamide and psilocybin for the management of patients with persistent pain: A potential role? *Pain Manag.* **2018**, *8*, 217–229. [CrossRef]
60. De Gregorio, D.; Comai, S.; Posa, L.; Gobbi, G. d-Lysergic Acid Diethylamide (LSD) as a Model of Psychosis: Mechanism of Action and Pharmacology. *Int. J. Mol. Sci.* **2016**, *17*, 1953. [CrossRef] [PubMed]
61. Carhart-Harris, R.L.; Roseman, L.; Bolstridge, M.; Demetriou, L.; Pannekoek, J.N.; Wall, M.B.; Tanner, M.; Kaelen, M.; McGonigle, J.; Murphy, K.; et al. Psilocybin for treatment-resistant depression: fMRI-measured brain mechanisms. *Sci. Rep.* **2017**, *7*, 13187. [CrossRef]
62. Baliki, M.N.; Geha, P.Y.; Apkarian, A.V.; Chialvo, D.R. Beyond feeling: Chronic pain hurts the brain, disrupting the default-mode network dynamics. *J. Neurosci. Off. J. Soc. Neurosci.* **2008**, *28*, 1398–1403. [CrossRef]
63. Adams, L.D.; Turk, D.C. Central sensitization and the biopsychosocial approach to understanding pai. *J. Appl. Behav. Res.* **2018**, *23*, e12125. [CrossRef]
64. Coates, J.; Gething, F.; Johnson, M.I. Shared medical appointments for managing pain in primary care settings? *Pain Manag.* **2017**, *7*, 223–227. [CrossRef]
65. Goodwin, R.W.; Hendrick, P.A. Physiotherapy as a first point of contact in general practice: A solution to a growing problem? *Prim. Health Care Res. Dev.* **2016**, *17*, 489–502. [CrossRef]
66. Morton, L.; Ferguson, M.; Baty, F. Improving wellbeing and self-efficacy by social prescription. *Public Health* **2015**, *129*, 286–289. [CrossRef]
67. Bickerdike, L.; Booth, A.; Wilson, P.M.; Farley, K.; Wright, K. Social prescribing: Less rhetoric and more reality. A systematic review of the evidence. *BMJ Open* **2017**, *7*, e013384. [CrossRef]
68. Melzack, R.; Wall, P.D. Pain mechanisms: A new theory. *Science* **1965**, *150*, 971–979. [CrossRef]
69. Woolf, C.J. The dorsal horn: State-dependent sensory processing and the generation of pain. In *Textbook of Pain*; Wall, P.D., Melzack, R., Eds.; Churchill-Livingstone: Edinburgh, UK, 1994; pp. 101–112.
70. Melzack, R. Phantom limbs and the concept of a neuromatrix. *Trends Neurosci.* **1990**, *13*, 88–92. [CrossRef]
71. Botvinick, M.; Cohen, J. Rubber hands 'feel' touch that eyes see. *Nature* **1998**, *391*, 756. [CrossRef] [PubMed]
72. Lewis, E.; Lloyd, D.M. Embodied experience: A first-person investigation of the rubber hand illusion. *Phenomenol. Cogn. Sci.* **2010**, *9*, 317–339. [CrossRef]
73. Ehrsson, H.H.; Wiech, K.; Weiskopf, N.; Dolan, R.J.; Passingham, R.E. Threatening a rubber hand that you feel is yours elicits a cortical anxiety response. *Proc. Natl. Acad. Sci. USA* **2007**, *104*, 9828–9833. [CrossRef] [PubMed]
74. Johnson, M.I.; Smith, E.; Yellow, S.; Mulvey, M.R. A preliminary investigation into psychophysiological effects of threatening a perceptually embodied rubber hand in healthy human participants. *Scand. J. Pain* **2016**, *11*, 1–8. [CrossRef] [PubMed]

75. Senna, I.; Maravita, A.; Bolognini, N.; Parise, C.V. The Marble-Hand Illusion. *PLoS ONE* **2014**, *9*, e91688. [CrossRef]
76. Weeth, A.; Muhlberger, A.; Shiban, Y. Was it less painful for knights? Influence of appearance on pain perception. *Eur. J. Pain* **2017**, *21*, 1756–1762. [CrossRef] [PubMed]
77. Stanton, T.R.; Moseley, G.L.; Wong, A.Y.L.; Kawchuk, G.N. Feeling stiffness in the back: A protective perceptual inference in chronic back pain. *Sci. Rep.* **2017**, *7*, 9681. [CrossRef]
78. Williams, A.C. What can evolutionary theory tell us about chronic pain? *Pain* **2016**, *157*, 788–790. [CrossRef]
79. Melzack, R. From the gate to the neuromatrix. *Pain* **1999**, *82* (Suppl. 6), S121–S126. [CrossRef]
80. Fields, H.L. How expectations influence pain. *Pain* **2018**, *159* (Suppl. 1), S3–S10. [CrossRef]
81. Witt, J.K.; Proffitt, D.R.; Epstein, W. Perceiving distance: A role of effort and intent. *Perception* **2004**, *33*, 577–590. [CrossRef] [PubMed]
82. Witt, J.K.; Linkenauger, S.A.; Bakdash, J.Z.; Augustyn, J.S.; Cook, A.; Proffitt, D.R. The long road of pain: Chronic pain increases perceived distance. *Exp. Brain Res.* **2009**, *192*, 145–148. [CrossRef]
83. Tabor, A.; O'Daly, O.; Gregory, R.W.; Jacobs, C.; Travers, W.; Thacker, M.A.; Moseley, G.L. Perceptual inference in chronic pain: An investigation into the economy of action hypothesis. *Clin. J. Pain* **2016**, *32*, 588–593. [CrossRef] [PubMed]
84. Giummarra, M.J.; Georgiou-Karistianis, N.; Nicholls, M.E.; Gibson, S.J.; Bradshaw, J.L. The phantom in the mirror: A modified rubber-hand illusion in amputees and normals. *Perception* **2010**, *39*, 103–118. [CrossRef]
85. Lewis, J.S.; Kersten, P.; McCabe, C.S.; McPherson, K.M.; Blake, D.R. Body perception disturbance: A contribution to pain in complex regional pain syndrome (CRPS). *Pain* **2007**, *133*, 111–119. [CrossRef] [PubMed]
86. Moseley, G.L. Distorted body image in complex regional pain syndrome. *Neurology* **2005**, *65*, 773. [CrossRef] [PubMed]
87. Gilpin, H.R.; Moseley, G.L.; Stanton, T.R.; Newport, R. Evidence for distorted mental representation of the hand in osteoarthritis. *Rheumatology (Oxf.)* **2015**, *54*, 678–682. [CrossRef]
88. Tabor, A.; Keogh, E.; Eccleston, C. Embodied pain-negotiating the boundaries of possible action. *Pain* **2017**, *158*, 1007–1011. [CrossRef]
89. Moseley, G.L.; Arntz, A. The context of a noxious stimulus affects the pain it evokes. *Pain* **2007**, *133*, 64–71. [CrossRef]
90. Tabor, A.; Thacker, M.A.; Moseley, G.L.; Körding, K.P. Pain: A Statistical Account. *PLoS Comput. Biol.* **2017**, *13*. [CrossRef]
91. Anchisi, D.; Zanon, M. A Bayesian Perspective on Sensory and Cognitive Integration in Pain Perception and Placebo Analgesia. *PLoS ONE* **2015**, *10*. [CrossRef] [PubMed]
92. Nicholas, M.K.; Ashton-James, C. Embodied pain: Grasping a thorny problem? *Pain* **2017**, *158*, 993–994. [CrossRef] [PubMed]
93. Di Lernia, D.; Serino, S.; Riva, G. Pain in the body. Altered interoception in chronic pain conditions: A systematic review. *Neurosci. Biobehav. Rev.* **2016**, *71*, 328–341. [CrossRef] [PubMed]
94. Kenney, M.P.; Milling, L.S. The Effectiveness of Virtual Reality Distraction for Reducing Pain: A Meta-Analysis. *Psychol. Conscious. Theory Res. Pract.* **2016**, *3*, 199–210. [CrossRef]
95. Boesch, E.; Bellan, V.; Moseley, G.L.; Stanton, T.R. The effect of bodily illusions on clinical pain: A systematic review and meta-analysis. *Pain* **2016**, *157*, 516–529. [CrossRef]
96. Wittkopf, P.G.; Lloyd, D.M.; Johnson, M.I. Managing pain using virtual representations of body parts: A systematic review of clinical and experimental studies. *Disabil. Rehabil.* **2018**, *5*, 1–15. [CrossRef] [PubMed]
97. Wittkopf, P.G.; Lloyd, D.M.; Johnson, M.I. The effect of visual feedback of body parts on pain perception: A systematic review of clinical and experimental studies. *Eur. J. Pain* **2018**, *22*, 647–662. [CrossRef]
98. Shahrbanian, S.; Simmonds, M.J. Effects of Different Virtual Reality Environments on Experimental Pain Rating in Post-stroke Individuals With and Without Pain in Comparison to Pain-free Healthy Individuals. *Cyberpsychol. Behav.* **2009**, *12*, 106–106.
99. Simmonds, M.; Shahrbanian, S. Effects of different virtual reality environments on experimental pain threshold in individuals with pain following stroke. In Proceedings of the 7th ICDVRAT with ArtAbilitation, Maia, Portugal, 8–11 September 2008; pp. 87–94.

100. Roosink, M.; Robitaille, N.; McFadyen, B.J.; Hebert, L.J.; Jackson, P.L.; Bouyer, L.J.; Mercier, C. Real-time modulation of visual feedback on human full-body movements in a virtual mirror: Development and proof-of-concept. *J. Neuroeng. Rehabil.* **2015**, *12*, 2. [CrossRef]
101. Osumi, M.; Ichinose, A.; Sumitani, M.; Wake, N.; Sano, Y.; Yozu, A.; Kumagaya, S.; Kuniyoshi, Y.; Morioka, S. Restoring movement representation and alleviating phantom limb pain through short-term neurorehabilitation with a virtual reality system. *Eur. J. Pain* **2017**, *21*, 140–147. [CrossRef] [PubMed]
102. Villiger, M.; Bohli, D.; Kiper, D.; Pyk, P.; Spillmann, J.; Meilick, B.; Curt, A.; Hepp-Reymond, M.C.; Hotz-Boendermaker, S.; Eng, K. Virtual reality-augmented neurorehabilitation improves motor function and reduces neuropathic pain in patients with incomplete spinal cord injury. *Neurorehabil. Neural Repair.* **2013**, *27*, 675–683. [CrossRef]
103. Harvie, D.S.; Broecker, M.; Smith, R.T.; Meulders, A.; Madden, V.J.; Moseley, G.L. Bogus visual feedback alters onset of movement-evoked pain in people with neck pain. *Psychol. Sci.* **2015**, *26*, 385–392. [CrossRef]
104. Ortiz-Catalan, M.; Guethmundsdottir, R.A.; Kristoffersen, M.B.; Zepeda-Echavarria, A.; Caine-Winterberger, K.; Kulbacka-Ortiz, K.; Widehammar, C.; Eriksson, K.; Stockselius, A.; Ragno, C.; et al. Phantom motor execution facilitated by machine learning and augmented reality as treatment for phantom limb pain: A single group, clinical trial in patients with chronic intractable phantom limb pain. *Lancet* **2016**, *388*, 2885–2894. [CrossRef]
105. World Health Organization. The Top 10 Causes of Death. Available online: www.who.int/en/news-room/fact-sheets/detail/the-top-10-causes-of-death (accessed on 25 February 2019).
106. Rice, A.S.; Smith, B.H.; Blyth, F.M. Pain and the global burden of disease. *Pain* **2016**, *157*, 791–796. [CrossRef] [PubMed]
107. Smuck, M.; Kao, M.C.; Brar, N.; Martinez-Ith, A.; Choi, J.; Tomkins-Lane, C.C. Does physical activity influence the relationship between low back pain and obesity? *Spine J.* **2014**, *14*, 209–216. [CrossRef] [PubMed]
108. Van Hecke, O.; Torrance, N.; Smith, B.H. Chronic pain epidemiology—Where do lifestyle factors fit in? *Br. J. Pain* **2013**, *7*, 209–217. [CrossRef]
109. Dean, E.; Soderlund, A. What is the role of lifestyle behaviour change associated with non-communicable disease risk in managing musculoskeletal health conditions with special reference to chronic pain? *BMC Musculoskelet. Disord.* **2015**, *16*, 87. [CrossRef]
110. Swinburn, B.; Egger, G.; Raza, F. Dissecting obesogenic environments: The development and application of a framework for identifying and prioritizing environmental interventions for obesity. *Prev. Med.* **1999**, *29*, 563–570. [CrossRef]
111. Townshend, T.; Lake, A. Obesogenic environments: Current evidence of the built and food environments. *Perspect. Public Health* **2017**, *137*, 38–44. [CrossRef]
112. Riskowski, J.L. Associations of socioeconomic position and pain prevalence in the United States: Findings from the National Health and Nutrition Examination Survey. *Pain Med.* **2014**, *15*, 1508–1521. [CrossRef] [PubMed]
113. Johnson, M. Opinions on Paleolithic physiology living in painogenic environments: Changing the perspective through which we view chronic pain. *Pain Manag.* **2019**, in press.
114. Riggs, J.E. Stone-age genes and modern lifestyle: Evolutionary mismatch or differential survival bias. *J. Clin. Epidemiol.* **1993**, *46*, 1289–1291. [CrossRef]
115. Lieberman, D.E. *The Story of the Human Body: Evolution, Health and Disease*; Penguin Books: London, UK, 2014.
116. Walters, E.T. Injury-related behavior and neuronal plasticity: An evolutionary perspective on sensitization, hyperalgesia, and analgesia. *Int. Rev. Neurobiol.* **1994**, *36*, 325–427. [PubMed]
117. Price, T.J.; Dussor, G. Evolution: The advantage of 'maladaptive' pain plasticity. *Curr. Biol.* **2014**, *24*, R384–R386. [CrossRef]
118. Mogil, J.S. Social modulation of and by pain in humans and rodents. *Pain* **2015**, *156* (Suppl. 1), S35–S41. [CrossRef]
119. Young, V.B. The role of the microbiome in human health and disease: An introduction for clinicians. *BMJ* **2017**, *356*, j831. [CrossRef] [PubMed]
120. Bortz, W.M., 2nd. The disuse syndrome. *Western J. Med.* **1984**, *141*, 691–694.
121. Van Wilgen, C.P.; Dijkstra, P.U.; Versteegen, G.J.; Fleuren, M.J.; Stewart, R.; van Wijhe, M. Chronic pain and severe disuse syndrome: Long-term outcome of an inpatient multidisciplinary cognitive behavioural programme. *J. Rehabil. Med.* **2009**, *41*, 122–128. [CrossRef]

122. Chen, S.M.; Liu, M.F.; Cook, J.; Bass, S.; Lo, S.K. Sedentary lifestyle as a risk factor for low back pain: A systematic review. *Int. Arch. Occup. Environ. Health* **2009**, *82*, 797–806. [CrossRef]
123. Seaman, D.R. The diet-induced proinflammatory state: A cause of chronic pain and other degenerative diseases? *J. Manip. Physiol. Ther.* **2002**, *25*, 168–179. [CrossRef]
124. Rook, G.A. Regulation of the immune system by biodiversity from the natural environment: An ecosystem service essential to health. *Proc. Natl. Acad. Sci. USA* **2013**, *110*, 18360–18367. [CrossRef]
125. Eller-Smith, O.C.; Nicol, A.L.; Christianson, J.A. Potential Mechanisms Underlying Centralized Pain and Emerging Therapeutic Interventions. *Front. Cell. Neurosci.* **2018**, *12*, 35. [CrossRef]
126. De Gregori, M.; Muscoli, C.; Schatman, M.E.; Stallone, T.; Intelligente, F.; Rondanelli, M.; Franceschi, F.; Arranz, L.I.; Lorente-Cebrian, S.; Salamone, M.; et al. Combining pain therapy with lifestyle: The role of personalized nutrition and nutritional supplements according to the SIMPAR Feed Your Destiny approach. *J. Pain Res.* **2016**, *9*, 1179–1189. [CrossRef] [PubMed]
127. Rondanelli, M.; Faliva, M.A.; Miccono, A.; Naso, M.; Nichetti, M.; Riva, A.; Guerriero, F.; De Gregori, M.; Peroni, G.; Perna, S. Food pyramid for subjects with chronic pain: Foods and dietary constituents as anti-inflammatory and antioxidant agents. *Nutr. Res. Rev.* **2018**, *31*, 131–151. [CrossRef] [PubMed]
128. Brain, K.; Burrows, T.L.; Rollo, M.E.; Chai, L.K.; Clarke, E.D.; Hayes, C.; Hodson, F.J.; Collins, C.E. A systematic review and meta-analysis of nutrition interventions for chronic noncancer pain. *J. Hum. Nutr. Diet.* **2018**. [CrossRef]
129. Rea, K.; O'Mahony, S.M.; Dinan, T.G.; Cryan, J.F. The Role of the Gastrointestinal Microbiota in Visceral Pain. *Handb. Exp. Pharmacol.* **2017**, *239*, 269–287. [CrossRef]
130. McParland, J.L.; Eccleston, C.; Osborn, M.; Hezseltine, L. It's not fair: An Interpretative Phenomenological Analysis of discourses of justice and fairness in chronic pain. *Health (Lond.)* **2011**, *15*, 459–474. [CrossRef]
131. McParland, J.; Hezseltine, L.; Serpell, M.; Eccleston, C.; Stenner, P. An investigation of constructions of justice and injustice in chronic pain: A Q-methodology approach. *J. Health Psychol.* **2011**, *16*, 873–883. [CrossRef] [PubMed]
132. Johnson, M.I.; Dixey, R. Should pain be on the health promotion agenda? *Glob. Health Promot.* **2012**, *19*, 41–44. [CrossRef]
133. Johnson, M.I.; Briggs, M.; Dixey, R. Should health promotion be on the pain agenda? *Pain Manag.* **2014**, *4*, 385–388. [CrossRef] [PubMed]
134. Lieberman, D.E.; Venkadesan, M.; Werbel, W.A.; Daoud, A.I.; D'Andrea, S.; Davis, I.S.; Mang'eni, R.O.; Pitsiladis, Y. Foot strike patterns and collision forces in habitually barefoot versus shod runners. *Nature* **2010**, *463*, 531–535. [CrossRef] [PubMed]
135. Milne, G. The Evolutionary Determinants of Health Programme: Urban Living in the 21st Century from a Human Evolutionary Perspective. *Archaeol. Int.* **2015**, *18*, 84–96. [CrossRef]

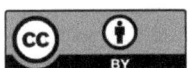

© 2019 by the author. Licensee MDPI, Basel, Switzerland. This article is an open access article distributed under the terms and conditions of the Creative Commons Attribution (CC BY) license (http://creativecommons.org/licenses/by/4.0/).

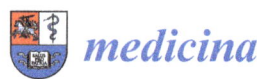

Review

Acupuncture for the Relief of Chronic Pain: A Synthesis of Systematic Reviews

Carole A. Paley [1,2,*] **and Mark I. Johnson** [2]

[1] Research and Development Dept, Airedale National Health Service (NHS) Foundation Trust, Skipton Road, Steeton, Keighley BD20 6TD, UK
[2] Centre for Pain Research, School of Clinical and Applied Sciences, Leeds Beckett University, City Campus, Leeds LS1 3HE, UK; M.Johnson@leedsbeckett.ac.uk
* Correspondence: carole.paley@nhs.net

Received: 24 October 2019; Accepted: 6 December 2019; Published: 24 December 2019

Abstract: *Background and Objectives*: It is estimated that 28 million people in the UK live with chronic pain. A biopsychosocial approach to chronic pain is recommended which combines pharmacological interventions with behavioural and non-pharmacological treatments. Acupuncture represents one of a number of non-pharmacological interventions for pain. In the current climate of difficult commissioning decisions and constantly changing national guidance, the quest for strong supporting evidence has never been more important. Although hundreds of systematic reviews (SRs) and meta-analyses have been conducted, most have been inconclusive, and this has created uncertainty in clinical policy and practice. There is a need to bring all the evidence together for different pain conditions. The aim of this review is to synthesise SRs of RCTs evaluating the clinical efficacy of acupuncture to alleviate chronic pain and to consider the quality and adequacy of the evidence, including RCT design. *Materials and Methods*: Electronic databases were searched for English language SRs and meta-analyses on acupuncture for chronic pain. The SRs were scrutinised for methodology, risk of bias and judgement of efficacy. *Results*: A total of 177 reviews of acupuncture from 1989 to 2019 met our eligibility criteria. The majority of SRs found that RCTs of acupuncture had methodological shortcomings, including inadequate statistical power with a high risk of bias. Heterogeneity between RCTs was such that meta-analysis was often inappropriate. *Conclusions*: The large quantity of RCTs on acupuncture for chronic pain contained within systematic reviews provide evidence that is conflicting and inconclusive, due in part to recurring methodological shortcomings of RCTs. We suggest that an enriched enrolment with randomised withdrawal design may overcome some of these methodological shortcomings. It is essential that the quality of evidence is improved so that healthcare providers and commissioners can make informed choices on the interventions which can legitimately be provided to patients living with chronic pain.

Keywords: acupuncture; pain; systematic review; evidence synthesis

1. Introduction

The World Health Organisation (WHO) recognises chronic pain as a long-term condition in its own right and as a secondary consequence of other long-term conditions [1]. It has been estimated that 28 million adults in the UK (43%) are affected by chronic pain and that the pain of 7.9 million of these adults is moderately or severely limiting [2]. The prevalence of chronic pain is higher in older age groups, with an estimated 62% of people over 75 being affected [2]. Individuals living with pain often experience a very poor quality of life, it affects their ability to work, socialise, sleep and maintain good relationships and can lead to depressive illness, decreased motivation and a reduction in physical activity [3]. As such, chronic pain represents a major challenge for health service provision and government policy.

Current guidance from the International Association for the Study of Pain (IASP) recommends a biopsychosocial approach to pain utilising a multidisciplinary, multimodal, stepwise approach which combines pharmacological interventions with behavioural and non-pharmacological treatments [4]. Non-pharmacological interventions are recommended as part of a comprehensive pain management programme, including lifestyle adjustments, pain education, and physical, psychological and complementary therapies.

In the UK, acupuncture has been available in some parts of the National Health Service (NHS) for decades as a non-pharmacological intervention to manage acute or chronic pain. In the NHS, acupuncture is administered by Allied Health Professionals, Nurses or Doctors. Outside the NHS, acupuncture is available from a variety of sources, including 'traditional' acupuncturists, sports therapists, osteopaths and chiropractors.

Acupuncture is an age-old technique which became part of modern medicine in the 1970s. In modern medicine, traditional forms of acupuncture, based on the ancient Chinese concept of qi and meridians, have been superseded by acupuncture based on a neurophysiological model [5,6]. The unique identity of acupuncture lies in the process of inserting needles ('acu') in the skin ('puncture'), although a modern definition should include the need to do this at specific points in accordance with known physiological or anatomical rationale [7].

Over the past two decades, the quantity of clinical studies on the use of acupuncture for various types of pain has significantly increased. In 2013, it was estimated that over 3000 clinical trials had been published [8] with over one hundred systematic reviews (SRs) (some with meta-analyses) attempting to synthesise available evidence. Many SRs of randomised controlled trials (RCTs) of acupuncture have been inconclusive and this has created uncertainty in clinical policy and practice. This uncertainty was highlighted in 2016 when the National Institute for Health and Care Excellence (NICE) reversed its 2009 recommendation to offer acupuncture as a first line treatment for non-specific, chronic low back pain because evidence indicated that it was no more effective than sham acupuncture [9–11]. Interestingly, there had been no significant change in evidence provided by RCTs between 2009 and 2016. Presently, NICE only recommends acupuncture as a prophylactic treatment for chronic tension-type headache and migraine [12,13].

In the face of conflicting evidence and continually changing guidance, it is unsurprising that acupuncture practitioners are finding that an intervention that, anecdotally at least, is often well received by patients in the clinic and appears to have good results, is rejected by commissioners and policy makers and regarded in some quarters as a 'theatrical placebo' [8,14]. One reason for this uncertainty may be related to the clinical research methodologies used to determine clinical efficacy.

Policy makers give credence to the findings of RCTs because they are the 'gold standard' methodology for evaluating clinical efficacy. RCTs enable isolation of the effects (benefit and harm) associated with the active ingredient of a treatment from effects associated with the act of receiving a treatment, i.e., believing that an active ingredient of a treatment has been received. This is operationalised by using needles to puncture the skin at defined points compared with pretending to puncture the skin at defined points (i.e., a 'placebo' or 'sham' intervention).

Systematic reviews and meta-analyses of multiple RCTs provide an indicator of consistency of findings between RCTs and allow for generalisability of findings [15]. Practitioners and policy makers may feel overwhelmed by the volume of SRs on acupuncture, suggesting a need to bring all this evidence together. In doing so, there is an opportunity to appraise RCT design and whether it is fit for purpose.

The aim of this review is to synthesise evidence from previously published SRs of RCTs evaluating the clinical efficacy of acupuncture to alleviate chronic pain from any source. We have made judgements from a Western medical perspective. Our approach is to outline research findings through commentary rather than a comprehensive objective appraisal of SRs. We appreciate that the non-systematic approach is vulnerable to selection and evaluation biases and opinion-orientated arguments. Nevertheless, our approach enables consideration of issues surrounding the quality and adequacy of the evidence, including RCT design, and provides practitioners and policy makers with a comprehensive source of SRs published to date.

2. Materials and Methods

A search of electronic databases (MEDLINE, the Database of Abstracts of Reviews of Effects (DARE) and the Cochrane Library) was conducted in April 2019 and updated in July 2019 using free text search terms 'acupuncture', 'chronic pain', 'analgesia', 'pain management', 'systematic review' and/or 'meta-analysis'. The search was restricted to English language databases. Systematic reviews and meta-analyses were screened for eligibility.

2.1. Inclusion Criteria

Search results were screened by the authors, CAP and MIJ. All SRs with or without meta-analyses of studies using manual acupuncture, electro-acupuncture, dry needling or auriculotherapy (ear acupuncture) for any chronic pain condition were included. Reviews were included where acupuncture was compared with sham or placebo acupuncture, no treatment, or another intervention (pharmacological and non-pharmacological). We included Cochrane and non-Cochrane reviews and overviews of SRs. Systematic reviews containing non-RCT studies were included in order that information from RCTs could be extracted.

2.2. Exclusion Criteria

Reviews were excluded if they did not evaluate invasive acupuncture (e.g., reviews on acupressure or laser acupuncture). Systematic reviews were excluded if they evaluated acute pain but not chronic pain (e.g., specifically focusing on postoperative pain or pain in the emergency setting). Reviews focusing on additional elements such as bee venom were also excluded. Non-English reviews were included if they contained an English abstract. However, non-English reviews were not translated.

2.3. Evidence Synthesis

One review author (CAP) extracted information from reviews including type of pain, number of RCTs, treatments, conclusion and quality of evidence stated by the authors of each included review taken as a direct quote from the Conclusion, Abstract or Discussion sections of their manuscript. In addition, we ascribed a judgement of efficacy of each review according to whether the sample size met criteria based on the work of Moore et al. [16,17] and adopted by the Pain, Palliative and Supportive Care group from Cochrane Collaboration in their risk of bias assessment. They suggest that trial arms with fewer than 200 participants in RCTs or fewer than 500 participants in meta-analyses are at a high risk of bias, which seriously undermines confidence in findings. Thus, reviews were categorized as meeting our criteria for adequacy if they contained a pooled analysis of 500 events or at least one RCT with >200 participants in each arm of the trial. We categorised efficacy as: Sufficient evidence and in favour of acupuncture (+), sufficient evidence in favour of control/placebo (−), sufficient evidence but conflicting/inconclusive (=) and insufficient evidence to make a judgement (?). We also noted statements within manuscripts about RCT methodology across the following themes:

- The nature of placebo/sham interventions.
- Quality and risk of bias (including blinding).
- Sample size in relation to treatment effect. We used criteria developed by Dechartres [18] when commenting on adequacy of sample size as: adequately powered (≥200 patients per treatment arm), moderately powered (100–199 patients per treatment arm) and underpowered <100 patients per treatment arm).

3. Results

A total of 177 reviews of acupuncture for pain relief published between 1989 to September 2019 were included (Table 1). There were two overviews of Cochrane reviews, ten overviews of non-Cochrane SRs and 145 non-Cochrane SRs. The earliest systematic reviews were published in 1989 by ter Riet [19–21]. There were 20 Cochrane SRs (including updates), with the earliest published in 2000 by Tulder et al. [22] and the most recent published in 2018 by Choi et al. [23]. Findings are presented according to the most frequent evaluations of acupuncture for different types of pain and described chronologically to provide a sense of the evolution of evidence over time. A statement of current clinical guidance from NICE is provided where available.

3.1. Chronic Pain Irrespective of Aetiology or Pathophysiology

The earliest SR that evaluated the efficacy of acupuncture across chronic pain conditions irrespective of aetiology or pathophysiology was published in 2000 and was inconclusive, although it was claimed that six or more sessions of acupuncture were more likely to be associated with positive outcomes [24]. The first overview of SRs was published in 2006 and concluded that acupuncture was not shown to be efficacious for a variety of pain conditions [25].

We found four other overviews of SRs of acupuncture for chronic pain irrespective of aetiology or pathophysiology. In 2010, Ernst and Lee published an overview of 30 SRs of acupuncture (319 RCTs) for 'rheumatic conditions' and judged there to be some evidence to support efficacy in routine care of patients with pain associated with osteoarthritis, low back pain and lateral elbow pain [26]. Hopton et al. pooled data from eight meta-analyses of acupuncture for chronic pain and concluded that acupuncture was more effective than a placebo, despite an absence of statistical significance for individual conditions, except osteoarthritis of the knee and headache [27]. Two overviews published in 2011 concluded that there was tentative evidence that acupuncture might be effective for headache, peripheral joint osteoarthritis and neck pain (overview of eight Cochrane Reviews [28], overview of 57 SRs [29]), although reviewers agreed that the quality of the primary studies was poor, with a high risk of bias.

We found 20 SRs of acupuncture for chronic pain irrespective of aetiology or pathophysiology. In 2014, SRs reported that evidence supported the efficacy of wrist-ankle acupuncture and auricular acupuncture for alleviating chronic pain [30,31]. Since then, SRs were generally inconclusive because of methodological shortcomings and small sample sizes in primary studies [32–36]. In 2018, Vickers et al. concluded that evidence supported the efficacy of acupuncture for various chronic pain conditions associated with musculoskeletal disorders, headache and osteoarthritis, with beneficial effects persisting at long-term follow-up (39 RCTs, [37]). The long-term effects of acupuncture were consistent with evidence from an earlier SR by MacPherson et al. [38].

Evidence from SRs suggests that there are insufficient high-quality RCTs to judge the efficacy of acupuncture for chronic pain associated with various medical conditions. There is no specific NICE guidance about the use of acupuncture for chronic pain conditions irrespective of aetiology or pathophysiology, although some guidance exists for specific pain conditions (see respective sections below). Guidance by NICE on chronic pain assessment and management is currently being developed (GID-NG10069) with publication expected in August 2020.

Table 1. Systematic reviews of Acupuncture (acup) for Chronic Pain Conditions.

Condition	Reference	Type of Review	Treatments Evaluated	No of RCTs in Review	Systematic Reviewers' Conclusion of Efficacy *	Our Judgement of Efficacy **	Systematic Reviewers' Conclusion of Quality of Available Evidence ***	Our Comments
CHRONIC PAIN IRRESPECTIVE OF AETIOLOGY OR PATHOPHYSIOLOGY	Vickers et al., 2018 [37]	Non-Cochrane Systematic Review	Chronic Pain	39	'We conclude that acupuncture is effective for the treatment of chronic pain, with treatment effects persisting over time.'	+	'… in keeping with the original analyses, significant heterogeneity was found in 5 out of 7 comparisons.'	Large studies with arms >200 participants were included for headache, low back pain, OA and shoulder pain.
	MacPherson et al., 2017 [38]	Non-Cochrane Systematic Review	Chronic Pain (persistence of acupuncture effects over time)	29	'The effects of a course of acupuncture treatment for patients with chronic pain do not appear to decrease importantly over 12 months.'	+	'… strict inclusion criteria required evidence of unambiguous allocation concealment, leading to our inclusion of only higher quality trials.'	Dataset of almost 18,000 patients, including some high-quality studies with >200 participants per trial arm.
	Gattie et al., 2017 [36]	Non-Cochrane Systematic Review	Musculoskeletal conditions	13	'… evidence suggests that dry needling is more effective than no treatment, sham dry needling, and other treatments …'	?	'… overall quality of the evidence was considered to be very low to moderate using the GRADE approach.'	Included studies all had arms of <200 participants.
	Zhang et al., 2017 [39]	Non-Cochrane Systematic Review	Pain conditions	23	'Cupping therapy and acupuncture are potentially safe, and they have similar effectiveness in relieving pain.'	N/A	'… no study was evaluated as low risk of bias, studies unclear risk of bias, and the remaining 15 studies, high risk of bias.'	This was a comparative SR between acupuncture and cupping. None of included studies had arms of >200 participants
	Cox et al., 2016 [32]	Non-Cochrane Systematic Review	Musculoskeletal Disorders of the Extremities	15	'Evidence for the effectiveness of acupuncture for musculoskeletal disorders of the extremities was inconsistent.'	=	'Ten of 15 RCTs had a low risk of bias … . Five of 15 RCTs had a high risk of bias.'	Effect sizes were small. One large study with >200 participants per treatment arm and low risk of bias.
	Yuan et al., 2016 [33]	Non-Cochrane Systematic Review	Musculoskeletal pain	61	'Our review provided low-quality evidence that acupuncture has a moderate effect (approximately a 12-point pain reduction on the VAS 100 mm) on relieving pain associated with musculoskeletal disorders.'	=	'The main weakness of this study was the relative paucity of high-quality RCTs. About half of the trials did not perform intention to treat analyses or correct allocation concealments.'	This review included several large studies with pooled events of >500

Table 1. Cont.

Condition	Reference	Type of Review	Treatments Evaluated	No of RCTs in Review	Systematic Reviewers' Conclusion of Efficacy *	Our Judgement of Efficacy **	Systematic Reviewers' Conclusion of Quality of Available Evidence ***	Our Comments
	Wong et al., 2015 [34]	Non-Cochrane Systematic Review	Chronic MSK pain	19	'This review showed moderate evidence of local or distant points stimulation in reducing pain at the end of the treatment when compared with control groups.'	?	'The 19 studies were of moderate quality.'	Comparison between local and distal acup stimulation. No included studies had arms of >200 participants.
	Zhao et al., 2015 [35]	Non-Cochrane Systematic Review	Chronic pain	15	'Due to the significant clinical heterogeneity and methodological flaws identified in the analysed trials, the current evidence on AT for chronic pain management is still limited.'	?	'The significant methodological flaws identified ... contributed to high risk of bias of the included studies.'	Auricular therapy studies (not all acup). No included studies had arms of >200 participants.
	Yeh et al., 2014 [31]	Non-Cochrane Systematic Review	Pain management	22	'... AA (auricular acup), was found to be a significant method of pain relief when compared to the sham or control group.'	?	'In the studies included in this meta-analysis, 91% were rated as good [quality] ...'	No included studies had arms of >200 participants. Publication bias was detected.
	Zhu et al., 2014 [30]	Non-Cochrane Systematic Review	Pain symptoms (Wrist-ankle acup (WAA))	33	'... the efficacy of WAA or WAA adjuvants was much better than Western medicine, sham acupuncture, or body acupuncture.'	?	'... higher quality and more rigorously designed clinical trials with large enough sample sizes are needed ...'	All studies were Chinese. No included studies had arms of >200 participants.
	Vickers et al., 2012 [40]	Non-Cochrane Systematic Review	Chronic pain	29	'Acupuncture is effective for the treatment of chronic pain and is therefore a reasonable referral option. Significant differences between true and sham acupuncture indicate that acupuncture is more than a placebo.'	+	'Neither study quality nor sample size appear to be a problem for this meta-analysis, on the grounds that only high-quality studies were eligible, and the total sample size is large.'	Authors looked at musculoskeletal (MSK) pain, osteoarthritis (OA), headache and shoulder pain. Six studies included with arms of >200 participants.
	Ernst & Lee 2011 [29]	Systematic review of systematic reviews	Multiple pain conditions	57 SR	'In conclusion, numerous systematic reviews have generated little truly convincing evidence that acupuncture is effective in reducing pain.'	−	'For indications where only one systematic review was available, definitive conclusions were usually prevented by the paucity or poor quality of the primary studies or the poor quality of the reviews.'	Four out of 57 reviews were of excellent quality. Primary studies variable in sample sizes.

Table 1. Cont.

Condition	Reference	Type of Review	Treatments Evaluated	No of RCTs in Review	Systematic Reviewers' Conclusion of Efficacy *	Our Judgement of Efficacy **	Systematic Reviewers' Conclusion of Quality of Available Evidence ***	Our Comments
	Lee & Ernst 2011 [28]	Overview of Cochrane reviews	Pain	8 SR	'All of these reviews were of high quality. Their results suggest that acupuncture is effective for some but not all types of pain.'	?	'Many primary studies that were included ... had a high risk of bias. This often means that the current evidence is limited, insufficient, or inconclusive.'	All these Cochrane Reviews are of high quality. Acupuncture effective for only some types of pain.
	Asher et al., 2010 [41]	Non-Cochrane Systematic Review	8 perioperative, 4 acute, and 5 chronic pain	17	'Auriculotherapy may be effective for the treatment of a variety of types of pain, especially postoperative pain.'	?	'... we believe our results likely reflect the results of higher quality studies and reduced publication bias.'	Auricular therapy only. Six studies were rated as 'good' quality. Study arms all had <200 participants.
	Ernst & Lee 2010 [26]	Overview of systematic reviews	Rheumatic conditions	30 SR	'Only for OA, low back pain and lateral elbow pain is the evidence sufficiently sound to warrant positive recommendations of this therapy ... '	=	'SRs of acupuncture have been noted to be limited by the often poor-quality of the primary data ... '	Studies of variable quality and primary studies of various sample sizes.
	Hopton & MacPherson 2010 [27]	Systematic review of pooled data from meta-analyses	Chronic Pain	8 SR	'The accumulating evidence from recent reviews suggests that acupuncture is more than a placebo ... '.	=	'... the reviews we are reporting include small-scale trials, with some variability in quality ... '	Positive score for OA knee and headache only. Number of pooled participants >1000 in 3 of 5RSs.
	Madsen et al., 2009 [42]	Non-Cochrane Systematic Review	Pain conditions	13	'We found a small analgesic effect of acupuncture that seems to lack clinical relevance and cannot be clearly distinguished from bias.'	−	'The review is fairly large, includes several trials of high methodological quality ... '	One study with arms >200 participants and pooled events of >500.
	Ernst et al., 2009 [43]	Systematic review of Cochrane reviews	Multiple conditions, including pain.	32 SR	'It is concluded that Cochrane reviews of acupuncture do not suggest that this treatment is effective for a wide range of conditions.'	−	'.... acupuncture trials are ... often poorly designed and badly reported.'	Included 10 SRs on chronic pain conditions, representing 95 primary RCTs.
	Derry et al., 2006 [25]	Systematic review of systematic reviews 1996-2005	Multiple pain conditions	35 SR	'Systematic reviews ... provide no robust evidence that acupuncture works for any indication.'	−	'Many reviews included studies with designs known to be associated with bias and overestimation of treatment effects.'	Included SRs on non-pain conditions, e.g., nausea and vomiting. 24 out of 35 reviews had information on less than 1000 patients.

Table 1. Cont.

Condition	Reference	Type of Review	Treatments Evaluated	No of RCTs in Review	Systematic Reviewers' Conclusion of Efficacy *	Our Judgement of Efficacy **	Systematic Reviewers' Conclusion of Quality of Available Evidence ***	Our Comments
	Ezzo et al., 2000 [24]	Non-Cochrane Systematic Review	Chronic pain	51	'There is limited evidence that acupuncture is more effective than no treatment for chronic pain, and inconclusive evidence that acupuncture is more effective than placebo, sham acupuncture or standard care.'	?	'Two-thirds of the studies … received a low-quality score and low-quality trials were significantly associated with positive results … High-quality studies were associated with … risk of false negative (type II) errors …'	Fifty-one RCTs representing 2423 chronic pain patients. The median sample size per group was 18 and the mode was 15.
HEADACHE								
(a) Tension-type								
	Linde et al., 2016 [44]	Cochrane Review	Episodic or chronic tension-type headache	12	'… acupuncture is effective for treating frequent episodic or chronic tension-type headaches …'	+	'Overall, the quality of the evidence assessed using GRADE was moderate or low ….'	Includes 2 studies with >200 participants in each study arm
	Linde et al., 2009 [45]	Cochrane review	Episodic or chronic tension-type headache	11	'… acupuncture could be a valuable non-pharmacological tool in patients with frequent episodic or chronic tension-type headaches.'	+	'… sequence generation, allocation concealment, handling of dropouts and withdrawals and reporting of findings were adequate.'	Includes 2 studies with >200 participants in each study arm
	Davis et al., 2008 [46]	Non-Cochrane Systematic Review	Non-migrainous headache	8	'… limited efficacy for the reduction of headache frequency'	−	'… all included studies to be of high quality, with scores of 3 or 4 ….'	One study with >200 participants per arm. Pooled analysis not significant
	Vernon et al, 1999 [47]	Non-Cochrane Systematic Review	Tension-type and cervicogenic headache	8	'Acupuncture does not appear to be more effective than a course of physiotherapy.'	?	'Two of four higher quality studies reported negative results ….'	None of included studies has >200 participants in each arm
	Sun et al., 2008 [48]	Non-Cochrane Systematic Review	Chronic headache	31	'… acupuncture is superior to sham acupuncture and medication therapy in improving headache intensity, frequency, and response rate.'	+	'The quality of the more recent trials is higher than the older trials, with more emphasis on proper randomization, allocation concealment, and description of patient dropout.'	Three studies with >200 participants in each arm. Pooled events >500
	Ter Riet et al., 1989 [20]	Non-Cochrane Systematic Review	Tension-type headache and migraine	10	'It is not … possible to draw a conclusion that acupuncture works for migraine and/or tension headache'.	?	'… number of patients and the methodological level of the experiments are … low.'	None of included studies has >200 participants in each arm

Table 1. Cont.

Condition	Reference	Type of Review	Treatments Evaluated	No of RCTs in Review	Systematic Reviewers' Conclusion of Efficacy *	Our Judgement of Efficacy **	Systematic Reviewers' Conclusion of Quality of Available Evidence ***	Our Comments
(b) Migraine								
	Linde et al., 2016 [49]	Cochrane review	Episodic migraine	22	'... a course of acupuncture consisting of at least six treatment sessions can be a valuable option ... .'	+	'Overall the quality of the evidence was moderate.'	Number of pooled events >500 and 3 studies with >200 participants in each arm
	Yang et al., 2016 [50]	Non-Cochrane Systematic Review	Migraine	10	'... verum acupuncture is superior to sham acupuncture in migraine'	?	'The majority of the included studies were considered to be of generally high methodological quality ... .'	All study arms <200 participants and pooled events <500
	Linde et al., 2009 [51]	Cochrane review	Migraine	22	'... acupuncture is at least as effective as, or possibly more effective than, prophylactic drug treatment, and has fewer adverse effects.'	+	'Methods for sequence generation, allocation concealment, handling of dropouts and withdrawals and reporting of findings were adequate in most of the recent trials.'	Number of pooled events >500 and 3 studies with >200 participants in each arm
(c) Other headache								
	Melchart et al., 2001 [52]	Cochrane review	Idiopathic headache	26	'... the existing evidence supports the value of acupuncture for the treatment of idiopathic headaches.'	?	'... the quality and amount of evidence are not fully convincing.'	None of included studies has >200 participants in each arm. Pooled events <500
	Manias et al., 2000 [53]	Non-Cochrane Systematic Review	Primary headaches	27	'In the majority of the trials (23 of the 27 trials), it was concluded that acupuncture offers benefits in the treatment of headaches.'	?	The authors did not make a statement of study validity.	Insufficient information available regarding sample sizes.
	Melchart et al., 1999 [54]	Non-Cochrane Systematic Review	Recurrent headache	22	'... no straightforward recommendation for clinical practice can be made.'	?	'... most trials were small and were either inadequately reported or had identifiable methodological flaws.'	None of included studies has >200 participants in each arm. Pooled events < 500
OSTEOARTHRITIS (OA)								
(a) Knee								
	Li et al., 2019 [55]	Overview of Systematic Reviews	OA Knee	12 SRs	'According to the high-quality evidence, we concluded that acupuncture may have some advantages in treating KOA.'	+	'... there are some risk of bias and reporting deficiencies still needed to be improved.'	Two of the largest SRs were deemed to have the highest reporting quality.

Table 1. Cont.

Condition	Reference	Type of Review	Treatments Evaluated	No of RCTs in Review	Systematic Reviewers' Conclusion of Efficacy *	Our Judgement of Efficacy **	Systematic Reviewers' Conclusion of Quality of Available Evidence ***	Our Comments
	Sun et al., 2019 [56]	Non-Cochrane Systematic Review	Symptom management in OA knee	8	'The effect of acupuncture may be associated with dose of acupuncture, with a higher dosage related to better treatment outcomes … .'	+	'The results of this study rely largely on high-quality primary RCTs. However, they are inevitably limited by the small number of included trials … .'	One included study with >200 participants and one with 189–191 per trial arm.
	Li et al., 2018 [57]	Non-Cochrane Systematic Review	Symptom management in OA knee	16	'… acupuncture with heat pain or electrical stimulation might be suggested as the better choices … … .'	+	'The methodological quality evaluation was low … .'	Network meta-analysis. One study with >200 participants and two with 189–191 per sample arm.
	Chen et al., 2017 [58]	Non-Cochrane Systematic Review	Knee OA (KOA)—Electro acupuncture (EA) studies only	11	'… EA is a great opportunity to remarkably alleviate the pain … .'	?	'… more high quality RCTs with rigorous methods of design, measurement and evaluation are needed.'	Meta-analysis with <500 pooled events.
	Lin et al., 2016 [59]	Non-Cochrane Systematic Review	OA knee	10	'… only short-term pain relief in patients with chronic knee pain due to osteoarthritis.'	?	'Significant publication bias was not detected (p > 0.05), but the heterogeneity of the studies was substantial.'	Insufficient information available on sample sizes of primary studies.
	Corbett et al., 2013 [60]	Non-Cochrane Systematic Review	OA knee	11	'… acupuncture can be considered as one of the more effective physical treatments for alleviating osteoarthritis knee pain in the short-term.'	+	'Around three-quarters of the studies were classed as being of poor quality.'	Network meta-analysis (2794 acup patients). Eleven "better-quality" acupuncture studies included.
	Cao et al., 2012 [61]	Non-Cochrane Systematic Review	OA knee	14	'Acupuncture provided significantly better relief from knee osteoarthritis pain and a larger improvement in function than sham acupuncture, standard care treatment, or waiting for further treatment.'	+	'According to the Cochrane Back Review Group scale, 11 RCTs had high internal validity and 3 RCTs had low internal validity.'	One study with >200 participants and four with >100 per trial arm. Pooled events > 500.
	Selfe et al., 2008 [62]	Non-Cochrane Systematic Review	OA knee	10	'… acupuncture is an effective treatment for pain and physical dysfunction associated with osteoarthritis of the knee.'	+	Authors did not make any assessment of quality.	Included 1 study with >200 participants per trial arm and 2 with >100.
	Bjordal et al., 2007 [63]	Non-Cochrane Systematic Review	OA knee	7	'… an intensive regimen of 2–4 weeks with TENS, EA or low-level laser therapy (LLLT) seems to safely induce statistically significant and clinically relevant short-term pain relief.'	?	'Trials were generally of medium to high quality ($\geq$3) … .' (Jadad)	Insufficient pooled events in EA studies (<500) which reduced validity of conclusions.

Table 1. *Cont.*

Condition	Reference	Type of Review	Treatments Evaluated	No of RCTs in Review	Systematic Reviewers' Conclusion of Efficacy *	Our Judgement of Efficacy **	Systematic Reviewers' Conclusion of Quality of Available Evidence ***	Our Comments
	Manheimer et al., 2007 [64]	Non-Cochrane Systematic Review	OA knee	11	'Waiting list-controlled trials suggest clinically relevant benefits, some of which may be due to placebo or expectation effects.'	?	'Because of heterogeneity and small effects, current estimates should be regarded as preliminary.'	One study with >200 participants and three with >100 per trial arm. No information on number of pooled events.
	Ferrándaz Infante et al., 2002 [65]	Non-Cochrane Systematic Review	OA knee	4	'... not enough evidence to recommend acupuncture as a treatment for knee pain.'	−	'Only one study presented a high-quality level ... .'	None of the included studies had sample sizes of >100
	Ezzo et al., 2001 [66]	Non-Cochrane Systematic Review	OA knee	7	'The existing evidence suggests that acupuncture may play a role in the treatment of knee OA.'	?	'More than half of the trials (n = 4) received a low-quality rating.'	None of included studies had trial arms of >200 participants
(b) Hip								
	Manheimer et al., 2018 [67]	Cochrane review	Hip OA	16	'Acupuncture probably has little or no effect in reducing pain or improving function relative to sham acupuncture in people with hip osteoarthritis.'	−	'Overall the evidence was limited, with only six RCTs of five different comparisons, with small sample sizes, and at high risk of bias, especially for the criteria of blinding.'	None of included studies had trial arms of <200 participants. Pooled events were <500.
(c) Other								
	Manyanga et al., 2014 [68]	Non-Cochrane Systematic Review	OA—Various	12	'The use of acupuncture is associated with significant reductions in pain intensity, improvement in functional mobility and quality of life.'	+	'... limited by methodological challenges... From the included trials, 75% were adjudicated to be of unclear or high risk of bias.'	One study >200 participants. Pooled events > 500. However, effect estimates might be inflated due to risk of bias in some studies.
	Manheimer et al., 2010 [69]	Cochrane review	Peripheral joint OA	16	'Waiting list-controlled trials ... suggest statistically significant and clinically relevant benefits ... which may be due to expectation or placebo effects.'	+	'... we considered the five [studies] with the highest quality ratings on the Cochrane Back Review Group scale. Only two of the five had any obvious methodological flaws ... .'	Pooled events were >500
	Kwon et al., 2006 [70]	Non-Cochrane Systematic Review	Peripheral joint OA	18	'.... acupuncture seems an option worthy of consideration particularly for knee OA.'	=	'Even though the total number of 18 RCTs is encouraging, it is too small considering the heterogeneity of the overall dataset.'	14 studies on OA knee. One large study including >200 participants in trial arms. Pooled events < 500.

Table 1. Cont.

Condition	Reference	Type of Review	Treatments Evaluated	No of RCTs in Review	Systematic Reviewers' Conclusion of Efficacy *	Our Judgement of Efficacy **	Systematic Reviewers' Conclusion of Quality of Available Evidence ***	Our Comments
CHRONIC KNEE PAIN (NON-SPECIFIC)	Ernst 1997 [71]	Non-Cochrane Systematic Review	OA	9 (13 studies)	'... the notion that acupuncture is superior to sham-needling in pain associated with OA is not supported by published data from controlled clinical trials.'	−	'Most trials suffer from methodological flaws.'	Sample sizes for all studies < 100 participants, therefore insufficient.
	Zhang et al., 2017 [72]	Non-Cochrane Systematic Review	Chronic knee pain	17	'... we are currently unable to draw any strong conclusions regarding the effectiveness and safety of acupuncture for chronic knee pain.'	−	'... the overall methodological quality of the included trials was not satisfactory.'	One study with trial arms of >200 participants and one with arms of 190/189.
	White et al., 2007 [73]	Non-Cochrane Systematic Review	Chronic knee pain	13	'Acupuncture that meets criteria for adequate treatment is significantly superior to sham acupuncture and to no additional intervention ...'	+	'The evidence appears to be robust enough to encourage wider use of acupuncture for chronic knee pain ...'	Included 3 large studies of high quality. Two with trial arms >200 participants and one with >189 participants.
LOW BACK PAIN (a) Chronic	Xiang et al., 2019 [74]	Non-Cochrane Systematic Review	Non-specific low back pain	14	'... there is moderate evidence of efficacy for acupuncture in terms of pain reduction immediately after treatment ... when compared to sham or placebo acupuncture'.	=	'... trials included were heterogeneous regarding the needling sites, the needling manipulation and the duration of acupuncture sessions, and the type of sham ...'	One study with trial arms of >200 participants.
	Hu et al., 2018 [75]	Non-Cochrane Systematic Review	Chronic LBP	16	'... current evidence is not robust to draw a firm conclusion regarding the efficacy and safety of DN for LBP.'	−	'... methodological shortcomings ... greatly reduced the quality of evidence.'	No studies with trial arms of >200. Pooled events < 500.
	Tang et al., 2018 [76]	Non-Cochrane Systematic Review	Lumbar disc herniation	30	There is tentative evidence that acupuncture is more beneficial at alleviating pain than lumbar traction, drug therapy or Chinese herbal medicine.	=	There was insufficient robust evidence to draw firm conclusions because of methodological shortcomings.	Pooled events > 500 participants. GRADE evidence assessed by authors was LOW or VERY LOW for all studies.

Table 1. Cont.

Condition	Reference	Type of Review	Treatments Evaluated	No of RCTs in Review	Systematic Reviewers' Conclusion of Efficacy *	Our Judgement of Efficacy **	Systematic Reviewers' Conclusion of Quality of Available Evidence ***	Our Comments
	Yeganeh et al., 2017 [77]	Non-Cochrane Systematic Review	Low back pain (in Iran)	3 (7 in total)	'In conclusion, overall, the lack of studies with a low risk of bias precludes any strong recommendations.'	?	'The methodological quality of the studies was generally poor.'	None of the 3 acup studies had arms of >200 participants and pooled events insufficient (<500)
	Liu et al., 2015 [78]	Overview of systematic reviews	Chronic low back pain	16 SR	'… consistent evidence shows that acupuncture is more effective for pain relief and functional improvement at short-term follow-ups.'	+	'… three systematic reviews were considered as high quality, eight as moderate quality, and five as low quality …'	Number of pooled participants in moderate to high quality SRs were >500
	Close et al., 2014 [79]	Non-Cochrane Systematic Review	Low back and pelvic pain in pregnancy	6 (8 in total)	'At present, we simply do not have enough high-quality trials on CAM for managing Low back and pelvic pain in pregnancy.'	–	'The restricted availability of high-quality studies, combined with the very low evidence strength, makes it impossible to make evidence-based recommendations …'	Overall strength of evidence graded VERY LOW. Study arms had sample sizes of <200.
	Kim et al., 2013 [80]	Non-Cochrane Systematic Review	Lumbar spinal stenosis	12 (6 RCT)	'We found no conclusive evidence of the effectiveness and safety of acupuncture …'	?	'The current evidence found in this review is seriously limited by high or uncertain risk of bias.'	All studies had arms with <200 participants
	Lam et al., 2013 [81]	Non-Cochrane Systematic Review	Chronic, non-specific low back pain	32	'… acupuncture is effective in providing long-term relief of chronic low back pain, but this effect is produced by non-specific effects that arise from skin manipulation.'	=	'Given the clinical heterogeneity of other treatments for chronic low back pain, it is not surprising that a consistent conclusion could not be made …'	Two studies had trial arms with >200 participants, however, the results were not conclusive.
	Xu et al., 2013 [82]	Non-Cochrane Systematic Review	Chronic low back pain	13	'Compared with no treatment, acupuncture achieved better outcomes in terms of pain relief, disability recovery and better quality of life, but these effects were not observed when compared to sham acupuncture…'	=	No specific statement on quality included. The authors state 'The main biases that affected the results were performance bias and detection bias.'	Two studies had trial arms with >200 participants, however, the results were not conclusive.
	Hutchinson et al., 2012 [83]	Non-Cochrane Systematic Review	Chronic, non-specific low back pain	7	'This review provides some evidence to support acupuncture as more effective than no treatment …'	–	No specific statement on quality of studies.	3 studies with trial arms of >200 participants but these studies did not demonstrate a significant difference between acupuncture and sham.

Table 1. *Cont.*

Condition	Reference	Type of Review	Treatments Evaluated	No of RCTs in Review	Systematic Reviewers' Conclusion of Efficacy *	Our Judgement of Efficacy **	Systematic Reviewers' Conclusion of Quality of Available Evidence ***	Our Comments
	Standaert, et al., 2011 [84]	Non-Cochrane Systematic Review	Chronic low back pain	2	'... insufficient evidence to comment on the relative benefit of acupuncture compared with either structured exercise or SMT ...'	?	'The overall strength of the evidence ... was "insufficient."'	Results of only one acup RCT included therefore there was insufficient evidence.
	Trigkilidas 2010 [85]	Non-Cochrane Systematic Review	Chronic low back pain	4	'acupuncture can be superior to usual care in treating chronic low back pain, especially, when patients have positive expectations about acupuncture.'	=	No specific statement on quality was made but study designs introduced bias.	3 out of 4 studies had trial arms of >200 participants but results not conclusive.
	Yuan et al., 2008 [86,87]	Non-Cochrane Systematic Review	Chronic low back pain	23	'There is moderate evidence that acupuncture is more effective than no treatment, and strong evidence of no significant difference between acupuncture and sham acupuncture, for short-term pain relief.'	=	'... although 16/23 of the studies (70%) scored highly on the Van Tulder scale, only 8/23 had more than 40 patients per group of which 2 studies had high dropouts leaving only 6/23 high quality studies.'	2 studies had trial arms of >200 participants. Both scored 8 or above on the Van Tulder scale. Results are conflicting.
	Furlan et al., 2005 [88]	Cochrane review	Low back pain	35	'The data do not allow firm conclusions about the effectiveness of acupuncture for acute low-back pain.'	=	'The methodologic quality of the included RCTs ... was poor. There were two studies with fatal flaws ... '	One study had trial arms of >200 participants.
	Manheimer et al., 2005 [89]	Non-Cochrane Systematic Review	Chronic low back pain	33	'Acupuncture effectively relieves chronic low back pain. No evidence suggests that acupuncture is more effective than other active therapies.'	?	No statement on methodological quality was included.	All of the studies included had trial arms of <100 participants.
	Yuan et al., 2004 [90]	Non-Cochrane Systematic Review	Non-specific low back pain	10	'This review has provided strong evidence that there is no significant difference between acupuncture and sham acupuncture ... '	–	'Ten high-quality studies, with a mean Van Tulder score of 6.6/11, met the inclusion criteria ... '	Includes two studies of high quality with trial arms of >200
	Henderson 2002 [91]	Non-Cochrane Systematic Review	Chronic low back pain	5 (11 studies in total)	'Systematic examination of these articles did not provide definitive evidence to support or refute the use of acupuncture ... '	?	No quality assessment conducted.	One study with n = 262 was inconclusive. Only one other RCT with positive results had n = 28.
	van Tulder et al., 1999 [92]	Cochrane review	Non-specific low back pain	11	'The evidence ... does not indicate that acupuncture is effective for the treatment of back pain.'	?	'The methodological quality was low. Only two trials were of high quality.'	All studies had small sample sizes of 100 or less.

Table 1. Cont.

Condition	Reference	Type of Review	Treatments Evaluated	No of RCTs in Review	Systematic Reviewers' Conclusion of Efficacy *	Our Judgement of Efficacy **	Systematic Reviewers' Conclusion of Quality of Available Evidence ***	Our Comments
	Strauss et al., 1999 [93]	Non-Cochrane Systematic Review	Chronic low back pain	4	'One cannot necessarily conclude from this review whether acupuncture is an effective treatment.'	?	'… all the trials were of poor quality.'	Minimal information on primary studies included in review including study design and number of patients.
	Ernst & White 1998 [94]	Non-Cochrane Systematic Review	Low back pain	12	'… insufficient evidence to state whether it is superior to placebo.'	?	'… Only 2 trials … were of low quality. Thus, the present meta-analysis is based largely on rigorous research.'	All samples sizes were less than 100.
(b) Mixed								
	Cherkin et al., 2003 [95]	Non-Cochrane Systematic Review	Acute and chronic back pain	6	'Because the quality of the research evaluating the effectiveness of the most popular CAM therapies used for low back pain is generally poor, clear conclusions are difficult to reach … .'	?	'The trials had serious limitations, including small sample sizes, inadequate acupuncture treatment, and high dropout rates.'	The largest included study had n = 262. All others were <100.
	van Tulder et al., 1999 [96]	Non-Cochrane Systematic Review	Low back pain (acute and chronic)	11	'… this systematic review did not clearly indicate that acupuncture is effective in the management of back pain … .'	?	'Overall, the methodologic quality was low. Only two studies met the pre-set "high-quality" level for this review.'	All included studies had sample sizes of <100
(c) Back and neck Pain								
	Griswold et al., 2019 [97]	Non-Cochrane Systematic Review	Spine-related painful conditions	12	'Both superficial and deep needling resulted in clinically meaningful changes in pain scores over time.'	?	'The included studies demonstrated an unclear to high risk of bias recommending a cautious interpretation of the results.'	This article has a delayed release (embargo) and will be available in 2020
	Yuan et al., 2015 [98]	Non-Cochrane Systematic Review	Chronic neck and low back pain (CNP and CLBP)	30 (48 studies in total)	'Acupuncture, acupressure, and cupping could be efficacious in treating the pain and disability associated with CNP or CLBP in the immediate term.'	?	'In summary, many more studies with higher quality and longer-term follow-ups are warranted.'	All trial arms had <200 participants and pooled events <500
	Smith et al., 2000 [99]	Non-Cochrane Systematic Review	Chronic neck and back pain	13	'There is no convincing evidence for the analgesic efficacy of acupuncture for back or neck pain.'	?	'With acupuncture for chronic back and neck pain, we found that the most valid trials tended to be negative.'	Trial arms all had <200 participants.

Table 1. Cont.

Condition	Reference	Type of Review	Treatments Evaluated	No of RCTs in Review	Systematic Reviewers' Conclusion of Efficacy *	Our Judgement of Efficacy **	Systematic Reviewers' Conclusion of Quality of Available Evidence ***	Our Comments
NECK PAIN	Ter Riet et al., 1989 [19]	Non-Cochrane Systematic Review	Neck and back pain	16 (22 studies)	'… it is impossible to draw definite conclusions.' The authors noted the presence of publication bias.	?	'The quality was generally low and low therefore no definitive conclusions can be drawn.'	Sample sizes insufficient. One study with trial arm ≥50 participants
	Seo et al., 2017 [100]	Non-Cochrane Systematic Review		16	'Acupuncture and conventional medicine for chronic neck pain have similar effectiveness on pain and disability…'	?	'… a lot of the results were evaluated to have low level of evidence, making it difficult to draw clear conclusions …'	Trial arms <200 participants, pooled events < 500.
	Moon et al., 2014 [101]	Non-Cochrane Systematic Review	Whiplash-associated disorder	6	'In conclusion, the evidence for the effectiveness of acupuncture therapy for whiplash associated disorder is limited.'	?	'Most of the included RCTs have serious methodological flaws.'	No trials arms with >200 participants
	Wang et al., 2011 [102]	Non-Cochrane Systematic Review	Cervical spondylosis	8	'At the present, there has been no sufficient evidence to ensure that … abdominal acupuncture therapy is superior …'	?	'Attention should be paid to the randomized controlled study of larger samples and qualified design.'	Paper in Chinese therefore information taken from abstract. Small sample sizes.
	Fu et al., 2009 [103]	Non-Cochrane Systematic Review		14	'The quantitative meta-analysis … confirmed the short-term effectiveness and efficacy of acupuncture in the treatment of neck pain.'	+	'… evidence supporting the main hypothesis that acupuncture was effective in the treatment of neck pain was stronger than the evidence denying this …'	Only one study with sufficient power including >200 participants per trial arm.
	Trinh et al., 2006 [104]	Cochrane review	Neck disorders	10	'Individuals with chronic neck pain who received acupuncture reported, on average, better pain relief immediately after treatment and in the short-term than those who received sham…'	?	'… the overall quality of these studies was not considered high, with only 40% of the studies (4/10) considered as high quality …'	None of included studies had arms >200
	White & Ernst 1999 [105]	Non-Cochrane Systematic Review	Neck pain	14	'… the hypothesis that acupuncture is efficacious … is not based on the available evidence from sound clinical trials.'	?	'… the methodological quality of the studies, as assessed by the three criteria of the modified Jadad score for clinical trials, was disappointing.'	Included studies all had arms with <100 participants.

Table 1. Cont.

Condition	Reference	Type of Review	Treatments Evaluated	No of RCTs in Review	Systematic Reviewers' Conclusion of Efficacy *	Our Judgement of Efficacy **	Systematic Reviewers' Conclusion of Quality of Available Evidence ***	Our Comments
MYOFASCIAL PAIN/TRIGGER POINTS (MTPs)	Espejo-Antúnez et al., 2017 [106]	Non-Cochrane Systematic Review	MTPs	15	'Our review suggests a short-term positive impact of dry needling on pain intensity and insufficient evidence on the long-term effectiveness, in line with the findings of previous systematic reviews.'	?	'The 15 randomized controlled trials had a mean method quality score of 7.53 ± 1.30 out of 10, ranging from 5 to 9 in the PEDro scale.'	Dry needling studies. Included studies all had arms with <100 participants.
	Li et al., 2017 [107]	Non-Cochrane Systematic Review	Myofascial Pain syndrome	33	'… most acupuncture therapies, including acupuncture combined with other therapies, showed superiority over the other single physical therapies … '.	?	'The quality of this analysis is restricted by the quality of the underlying data.'	Included studies all had arms with <100 participants.
	Wang et al., 2017 [108]	Non-Cochrane Systematic Review	Myofascial pain syndrome (MPS)	10	'… we have demonstrated favourable efficacy of MA in terms of pain relief as well as the reduction of muscle irritability due to MPS when myofascial trigger points (but not acupuncture points) are stimulated …'	?	'High RoB, variable duration of symptoms and differences in the severity of initial conditions may partly influence the validity of the conclusions.'	Included studies all had arms with <100 participants.
	Rodriguez-Mansilla et al., 2016 [109]	Non-Cochrane Systematic Review	Myofascial pain syndrome	10	'… Dry needling was more effective in decreasing pain comparing to no treatment, it was not significantly different from placebo in decreasing pain.'	?	Authors report that methodological quality was variable from good to poor.	Dry needling studies. Included studies all had arms with <100 participants.
	Cagnie et al., 2015 [110]	Non-Cochrane Systematic Review	Trigger Points the upper trapezius in patients with neck pain	15	'There is moderate evidence for ischemic compression and strong evidence for dry needling to have a positive effect on pain intensity.'	?	'Six articles were of low quality and were not further included in the analysis; 9, of moderate quality; and 6, of good quality.'	Dry needling and ischaemic compression. Included studies all had arms with <100 participants.
	Ong et al., 2014 [111]	Non-Cochrane Systematic Review	MTPs in neck and shoulders	5	'… there is no significant difference between dry needling and lidocaine …'.	?	'Four out of five RCTs were rated as high-quality (≥6/10); only one RCT rated as low-quality evidence (≤5/10).'	Included studies all had arms with <100 participants. Pooled events < 500

Table 1. *Cont.*

Condition	Reference	Type of Review	Treatments Evaluated	No of RCTs in Review	Systematic Reviewers' Conclusion of Efficacy *	Our Judgement of Efficacy **	Systematic Reviewers' Conclusion of Quality of Available Evidence ***	Our Comments
	Kietrys et al., 2013 [112]	Non-Cochrane Systematic Review	Upper quarter myofascial pain	12	'… we recommend dry needling, compared to sham or placebo, for decreasing pain immediately after treatment and at 4 weeks … '	?	'… variance in comparison groups, control conditions, dosage of intervention, outcomes, outcome measurement tools, times to outcomes, and internal validity … '	Included studies all had arms with <200 participants.
	Tough & White 2011 [113]	Non-Cochrane Systematic Review	MTP pain	3	'There is limited evidence that direct MTrP (myofascial trigger points) dry needling has an overall treatment effect when compared with standard care.'	?	'… there is still a need for large scale, adequately powered, high-quality placebo-controlled trials to provide a more conclusive result.'	Included studies all had arms with <100 participants.
	Cotchett et al., 2010 [114]	Non-Cochrane Systematic Review	MTrPs associated with plantar heel pain	3 (non-RCT)	'There is limited evidence for the effectiveness of dry needling and/or injections of MTrPs associated with plantar heel pain.'	?	'… the poor quality and heterogeneous nature of the included studies precludes definitive conclusions being made.'	Included studies all had arms with <50 participants.
	Tough et al., 2009 [115]	Non-Cochrane Systematic Review	MTP pain	7	'… limited evidence deriving from one study that deep needling directly into myofascial trigger points has an overall treatment effect … '	?	'… the limited sample size and poor quality of these studies highlights and supports the need for large scale, good-quality placebo-controlled trials …'	One study with n = 296. All other studies with small sample sizes.
	Cummings et al., 2001 [116]	Non-Cochrane Systematic Review	MTP pain	23	'… the hypothesis that needling therapies have efficacy beyond placebo is neither supported nor refuted by the evidence from clinical trials.'	?	'No trials were of sufficient quality or design to test the efficacy of any needling technique beyond placebo in the treatment of myofascial pain.'	One study with n = 296. All other studies with small sample sizes.
CANCER PAIN								
	Chiu et al., 2017 [117]	Non-Cochrane Systematic Review	Malignancy-related, surgery-related or other treatment-related pain.	29	'Acupuncture is effective in relieving cancer-related pain, particularly malignancy-related and surgery-induced pain.'	?	'… methodological limitations … affected the strength of evidence and limited the internal validity of this review.'	Included studies all had arms with <100 participants.
	Hu et al., 2016 [118]	Non-Cochrane Systematic Review	Cancer-related pain	20	'Acupuncture plus drug therapy is more effective than conventional drug therapy alone for cancer-related pain.'	?	'… GRADE analysis revealed that the quality of all outcomes about acupuncture plus drug therapy was very low.'	Included studies all had arms with <100 participants.

Table 1. *Cont.*

Condition	Reference	Type of Review	Treatments Evaluated	No of RCTs in Review	Systematic Reviewers' Conclusion of Efficacy *	Our Judgement of Efficacy **	Systematic Reviewers' Conclusion of Quality of Available Evidence ***	Our Comments
	Paley et al., 2015 [119]	Cochrane review	Cancer pain	5	'We conclude that there is insufficient evidence to judge whether acupuncture is effective in relieving cancer pain in adults.'	?	'… the available evidence is of low quality. Therefore, a judgement on whether acupuncture is effective cannot be made.'	Included studies all had arms with <100 participants.
	Lian et al., 2014 [120]	Non-Cochrane Systematic Review	Palliative care symptoms including pain	6 (33 in total)	'The result … suggested that the effectiveness of acupuncture in palliative care for cancer patients is promising, especially in reducing … cancer pain.'	?	'Although the RCTs included in this study have relatively high quality, nearly half of them still rated as Jadad score 2 or below.'	Included studies all had arms with <50 participants.
	Garcia et al., 2013 [121]	Non-Cochrane Systematic Review	Cancer care (8 symptoms including pain)	11	'… appropriate adjunctive treatment for chemotherapy-induced nausea/vomiting. … For other symptoms' management, efficacy remains undetermined.'	?	'Of the 11 trials examining acupuncture for pain, nine were positive, but eight had high ROB (risk of bias).'	Included studies all had arms with <100 participants.
	Choi et al., 2012 [122]	Non-Cochrane Systematic Review	Cancer pain	15	'The total number of RCTs included in the analysis and their methodological quality were too low to draw firm conclusions.'	?	'As suggested by previous systematic reviews … methodological flaws suggest that caution should be taken when interpreting the results of these studies …'	Included studies all had arms with <100 participants.
	Paley et al., 2011 [123]	Cochrane review	Cancer pain	3	'There is insufficient evidence to judge whether acupuncture is effective in treating cancer pain in adults.'	?	'Acupuncture is widely used to treat cancer-related pain, but the available evidence is of low quality.'	Included studies all had arms with <100 participants.
	Peng et al., 2010 [124]	Non-Cochrane Systematic Review	Cancer pain	7	'Acupuncture is effective for pain relief.'	?	'… the poor quality of the majority of the trials reduces the reliability of the conclusion.'	Article in Chinese. Included studies all had arms with <100 participants.
	Ernst & Lee 2010 [125]	Systematic review of systematic reviews	Palliative and supportive cancer care	7 SR	'In conclusion, chemotherapy-induced nausea and vomiting is the only indication for acupuncture that is currently supported …'	?	'… SRs of acupuncture tended to be based on poor-quality primary studies. Our analysis confirms this notion.'	Short report. Only one good-quality SR on cancer pain including 7 primary studies of low quality.

Table 1. Cont.

Condition	Reference	Type of Review	Treatments Evaluated	No of RCTs in Review	Systematic Reviewers' Conclusion of Efficacy *	Our Judgement of Efficacy **	Systematic Reviewers' Conclusion of Quality of Available Evidence ***	Our Comments
	Lee et al., 2005 [126]	Non-Cochrane Systematic Review	Cancer-related pain	7 (3 RCT)	'The notion that acupuncture may be an effective analgesic adjunctive method for cancer patients is not supported by the data currently available from the majority of rigorous clinical trials.'	?	'Due to a dearth of high-quality primary studies in this field, no informative conclusion could be drawn.'	Included studies all had arms with <100 participants.
FIBROMYALGIA								
	Zhang et al., 2019 [127]	Non-Cochrane Systematic Review	Fibromyalgia	12	'… there was moderate quality evidence showing that real acupuncture was more effective than sham acupuncture in the short term.'	?	'… most of the studies had a relatively small sample size … Second, there was considerable heterogeneity in our meta-analysis.'	Included studies all had arms with <100 participants.
	Kim et al., 2019 [128]	Non-Cochrane Systematic Review	Fibromyalgia	10	'… verum acupuncture compared with sham acupuncture has a short-term efficacy on reducing pain … '	?	'… high heterogeneity downgraded the level of evidence.'	Included studies all had arms with <100 participants.
	Yang et al., 2014 [129]	Non-Cochrane Systematic Review	Fibromyalgia	9	'… there was not enough evidence to prove the efficacy of acupuncture therapy for the treatment of fibromyalgia.'	?	'… the included trials were not of high quality or had high bias risks.'	Included studies all had arms with <50 participants.
	Cao et al., 2013 [130]	Non-Cochrane Systematic Review	Fibromyalgia	16	'Acupoint stimulation appears to be effective … compared with medications.'	?	'The quality of the included studies is generally poor … '	Included studies all had arms with <50 participants.
	Deare et al., 2013 [131]	Cochrane review	Fibromyalgia	9	'Overall, there is a … moderate level of evidence that acupuncture is not better than sham controls.'	?	'The small sample size, scarcity of studies for each comparison, lack of an ideal sham acupuncture weakens the level of evidence … .'	Included studies all had arms with <100 participants. Pooled events < 500.
	Cao et al., 2010 [132]	Non-Cochrane Systematic Review	Fibromyalgia	12 (25 studies in total)	'… . acupuncture was significantly better than conventional medications for reducing pain and number of tender points … significantly better than amitriptyline for preventing relapse.'	?	'Seven trials (28%) were evaluated as having a low risk of bias and the remaining trials were identified as being as unclear or having a high risk of bias.'	Included studies all had arms with <100 participants.
	Langhorst et al, 2010 [133]	Non-Cochrane Systematic Review	Fibromyalgia	7	'… small analgesic effect of acupuncture was present … not clearly distinguishable from bias.'	?	'… great variability of the methodological quality of studies … not robust against potential methodological biases.'	Included studies all had arms with <50 participants.

Table 1. Cont.

Condition	Reference	Type of Review	Treatments Evaluated	No of RCTs in Review	Systematic Reviewers' Conclusion of Efficacy *	Our Judgement of Efficacy **	Systematic Reviewers' Conclusion of Quality of Available Evidence ***	Our Comments
	Martin-Sanchez et al., 2009 [134]	Non-Cochrane Systematic Review	Fibromyalgia	6	'This systematic review found no evidence of benefit resulting from acupuncture versus placebo, as a treatment for fibromyalgia.'	?	No specific statement on methodological quality was made but the authors stated there were reporting inconsistencies.	Included studies all had arms with <100 participants.
	Mayhew et al., 2007 [135]	Non-Cochrane Systematic Review	Fibromyalgia	5	'The notion that acupuncture is an effective symptomatic treatment … is not supported by the results from rigorous clinical trials.'	?	'… methodological quality was mixed and frequently low.'	Included studies all had arms with <100 participants.
	Berman et al., 1999 [136]	Non-Cochrane Systematic Review	Fibromyalgia (FMS)	3 (7 studies in total)	'… real acupuncture is more effective than sham acupuncture for improving symptoms of patients with FMS … this conclusion is based on a single high-quality study …'	?	'… limited amount of high-quality evidence …'	Included studies all had arms with <100 participants. Only one high quality RCT.
PELVIC PAIN								
	Qin et al., 2019 [137]	Non-Cochrane Systematic Review	Chronic prostatitis/pelvic pain	6 (4 RCT)	'Acupuncture may have clinically long-lasting benefits … However, current evidence is limited …'	?	'… insufficient quantity of studies and small sample size limited to conduct the robust evidence.'	Included studies all had arms with <100 participants.
	Zhang et al., 2019 [138]	Overview of SRs	Primary Dysmenorrhea	5 SRs	'… there are insufficient qualified evidences to determine the effectiveness of acupuncture in the treatment of PD.'	?	'All five SRs have more than one critical weakness … their methodological qualities were considered as critically low.'	Ranking of all 5 SRs was 'critically low'. No information on sample sizes in primary studies.
	Woo et al., 2018 [139]	Non-Cochrane Systematic Review	Primary Dysmenorrhea	60	'The results of this study suggest that acupuncture might reduce menstrual pain … compared to no treatment or NSAIDs.'	=	'… the quality of the included RCTs was low, and methodological restriction existed in this study.'	One study with arms including 344/173 patients. Pooled events >500 for MA vs no treatment.
	Sung et al., 2018 [140]	Non-Cochrane Systematic Review	Chronic pelvic pain in women	4	'The results of our review and meta-analysis suggest the effectiveness of AT (acupuncture) …'	?	'… most of the included studies had low methodological quality in the Cochrane ROB assessment.'	Included studies all had arms with <200 participants.
	Chang et al., 2017 [141]	Non-Cochrane Systematic Review	Chronic prostatitis/pelvic pain (CP/CPPS)	7	'Acupuncture has promising efficacy for patients with CP/CPPS. Compared to standard medical treatment, it has better efficacy.'	?	'The heterogeneous composition … contribute to the heterogeneity and possible effect modification or interactions.'	Included studies all had arms with <100 participants.

Table 1. Cont.

Condition	Reference	Type of Review	Treatments Evaluated	No of RCTs in Review	Systematic Reviewers' Conclusion of Efficacy *	Our Judgement of Efficacy **	Systematic Reviewers' Conclusion of Quality of Available Evidence ***	Our Comments
	Liu et al., 2017 [142]	Non-Cochrane Systematic Review	Primary Dysmenorrhea (PD)	23	'The available evidence suggests that acupuncture may be effective for PD and justifies future high-quality studies.'	=	'… most trials had an unclear or a high risk of bias, which may have caused an overestimation or underestimation of the true treatment effect.'	Two larger studies n = 501 and n = 600 with low risk of bias.
	Xu et al., 2017 [143]	Non-Cochrane Systematic Review	Endometriosis-related pain	10	'… acupuncture reduces pain and serum CA-125 levels, regardless of the control intervention used.'	?	'To confirm this finding, additional studies with proper controls, blinding methods, and adequate sample sizes are needed.'	Included studies all had arms with <50 participants.
	Xu et al., 2017 [144]	Non-Cochrane Systematic Review	Primary Dysmenorrhea	16	'The current evidence reveals that acupoint-stimulation in the treatment of PD has some obvious advantages compared with treatment by NSAIDs.'	?	'… sample sizes were small, leading to a low inspection efficiency … inadequate reporting of allocation concealment … the results were heterogeneous … .'	Included studies all had arms with <100 participants.
	Xu et al., 2014 [145]	Non-Cochrane Systematic Review	Primary Dysmenorrhea	20	'… acupoint therapy can relieve pain effectively for individuals with PD, and these treatments have advantages in overall efficiency.'	=	'Insufficient high-quality evidence is available in the current literature … . Hence, the findings … are by no means definitive.'	Study arms <200 but pooled events >500. However, conclusions not definitive due to quality issues
	Chen et al., 2013 [146]	Non-Cochrane Systematic Review	Primary Dysmenorrhea	4	'… insufficient high-quality evidence available… regarding the effectiveness of acupuncture … .'	?	'We were only able to determine that one of the acupuncture trials identified was free of selective reporting.'	Only studies using the SP6 acupoint were included. Included studies all had arms with <100 participants.
	Chung et al., 2012 [147]	Non-Cochrane Systematic Review	Primary Dysmenorrhea	30	'… acupoint stimulation, especially non-invasive acupoint stimulation, could have good short-term effects on the pain of primary dysmenorrhea.'	?	'… the poor quality of the methodology of the studies was indicated by a low average Jadad score, with 84%… scoring less than 3.'	Included studies all had arms with <200 participants. Most studies had Jadad scores of 1 or 2.
	Cohen et al., 2012 [148]	Non-Cochrane Systematic Review	Chronic prostatitis/chronic pelvic pain	35	'A statistically significant placebo effect was found for all outcomes and time analysis showed that efficacy of all treatments increased over time.'	?	'… there was a wide range of study quality. Several trials had questionable placebo groups and inadequate blinding. This makes interpretation of the results difficult … .'	Included studies all had arms with <200 participants. Pooled events < 500.

Table 1. Cont.

Condition	Reference	Type of Review	Treatments Evaluated	No of RCTs in Review	Systematic Reviewers' Conclusion of Efficacy *	Our Judgement of Efficacy **	Systematic Reviewers' Conclusion of Quality of Available Evidence ***	Our Comments
	Posadzki et al., 2012 [149]	Non-Cochrane Systematic Review	Chronic nonbacterial prostatitis + chronic pelvic pain syndrome	9	'The evidence … syndrome is encouraging but, because of several caveats, not conclusive …'	?	'… methodologic quality was variable; most were associated with major flaws. Only one RCT had a Jadad score of more than 3 …'	Included studies all had arms with <200 participants. Pooled events < 500
	Zhu et al., 2011 [150]	Cochrane review	Endometriosis	1	'The evidence to support the effectiveness of acupuncture for pain in endometriosis is limited …'	?	'The trial included in this review was methodologically weak.'	Only one low-quality RCT with n = 67 included in the review.
	Cho et al., 2010 [151]	Non-Cochrane Systematic Review	Primary Dysmenorrhea	27	'The review found promising evidence in the form of RCTs for the use of acupuncture ….'	?	'… the results were limited by methodological flaws.'	Included studies all had arms with <200 participants. Possible publication bias.
	Ee et al., 2008 [152]	Non-Cochrane Systematic Review	Pelvic and back pain in pregnancy	3	'We conclude that limited evidence supports acupuncture use in treating pregnancy-related pelvic and back pain.'	?	'Additional high-quality trials are needed to test the existing promising evidence for this relatively safe and popular complementary therapy.'	Based on 3 trials with insufficient sample sizes. Included studies all had arms with <200 participants.
INFLAMMATORY ARTHRITIS								
	Ramos et al., 2018 [153]	Overview of Systematic Reviews	Rheumatoid arthritis	7 SR	'The use of acupuncture probably has minimal or no impact on joint pain in rheumatoid arthritis.'	−	No formal statement of methodological quality was made but the GRADE score for the pain studies was moderate.	20 primary RCTs included. Pain data included from only 2 primary studies.
	Seca et al., 2019 [154]	Non-Cochrane Systematic Review	Rheumatoid arthritis (RA)	13	'Evidence suggests that acupuncture interventions may have a positive effect in pain relief, physical function and HRQoL (health related quality of life) in RA patients.'	?	'… due to the heterogeneity and methodological limitations of the studies included in this systematic review, evidence is not strong enough to produce a best practice guideline.'	Ten studies were published in China. No information available on sample sizes
	Lu et al., 2016 [155]	Non-Cochrane Systematic Review	Gouty arthritis	28	'… we cautiously suggest that acupuncture is an effective and safe therapy for patients with gouty arthritis.'	?	'the methodological qualities of included studies were judged to be poor; …'	Included studies all had arms with <100 participants. All were Chinese and single-site studies.
	Lee et al., 2013 [156]	Non-Cochrane Systematic Review	Gouty arthritis	10	'This study demonstrates efficacy of acupuncture treatment in decreasing VAS and uric acid in gout.'	?	'… the quality of the trials in this study is generally weak…'	Included studies all had arms with <200 participants. All studies were Chinese.

Table 1. Cont.

Condition	Reference	Type of Review	Treatments Evaluated	No of RCTs in Review	Systematic Reviewers' Conclusion of Efficacy *	Our Judgement of Efficacy **	Systematic Reviewers' Conclusion of Quality of Available Evidence ***	Our Comments
	Lee et al., 2008 [157]	Non-Cochrane Systematic Review	Rheumatoid arthritis	8	'... penetrating or non-penetrating sham-controlled RCTs failed to show specific effects of acupuncture for pain control ...'	?	'The number, size and quality of the RCTs are too low to draw firm conclusions.'	Included studies all had arms with <200 participants. Possible publication bias.
	Wang et al., 2008 [158]	Non-Cochrane Systematic Review	Rheumatoid arthritis	8	'Despite some favourable results in active-controlled trials, conflicting evidence exists in placebo-controlled trials concerning the efficacy of acupuncture for RA.'	?	'... inappropriate control interventions (non-comparable), no double-blind interventions, inadequate description of the randomization process, and scarce use of validated outcome measures.'	Included studies all had arms with <200 participants. Possible publication bias.
	Casimiro et al., 2005 [159]	Cochrane review	Rheumatoid arthritis	2	'... electroacupuncture may be beneficial ... the reviewers concluded that the poor quality of the trial, including the small sample size preclude its recommendation.'	?	'... poor quality of the trials, the high methodological variability ... and the small sample size of the included studies.'	Only 2 studies met the inclusion criteria. Sample sizes n = 64 and n = 20
	Lautenschlager 1997 [160]	Non-Cochrane Systematic Review	Inflammatory rheumatic diseases	17	'Acupuncture cannot be recommended for treatment of these diseases.'	?	'By far, the most studies examined failed to show sufficient quality.'	Written in German. No information about sample sizes.
NEUROPATHIC PAIN AND NEURALGIA								
	Pei et al., 2019 [161]	Non-Cochrane Systematic Review	Post-herpetic neuralgia	8	'... the quality of evidence was low because of the lack of blinding and the small sample sizes of the included studies.'	?	'... the quality of evidence was moderate for the assessment of pain intensity'.	Seven out of eight studies published in China. Included studies all had arms with <50 participants.
	Htu et al., 2019 [162]	Non-Cochrane Systematic Review	Trigeminal neuralgia	33	'... no statistically significant differences between the two groups for alleviating pain intensity.'	?	'... all current evidence is very limited due to the overall low methodological quality of the included RCTs.'	Only 3 small studies included with pain as an outcome measure. Included studies all had arms with <200 participants.
	Oh & Kim 2018 [163]	Non-Cochrane Systematic Review	Chemotherapy-induced peripheral neuropathy	5 (22 studies)	'... these results provide little evidence of the effectiveness of acupuncture ...'	–	Written in Korean. Insufficient high-quality data to make a judgement.	Only 5 included RCTs Acupuncture study arms had <200 participants.

Table 1. *Cont.*

Condition	Reference	Type of Review	Treatments Evaluated	No of RCTs in Review	Systematic Reviewers' Conclusion of Efficacy *	Our Judgement of Efficacy **	Systematic Reviewers' Conclusion of Quality of Available Evidence ***	Our Comments
	Choi et al., 2018 [23]	Cochrane review	Carpal tunnel syndrome	12	'… there is currently insufficient evidence to assess the effectiveness of acupuncture for symptoms of CTS.'	?	'Most studies were very small (fewer than 100 participants) and all estimates of effects suffered from imprecision.'	Included studies all had arms with <200 participants.
	Wang, et al., 2018 [164]	Non-Cochrane Systematic Review	Diabetic peripheral neuropathy	14	'ST36 injection appears … effective in reducing pain score and improving NCV compared with intramuscular injection …'	?	'… poor methodological and reporting quality reduced confidence in the findings.'	Included studies all had arms with <200 participants.
	Wang 2018 [165]	Non-Cochrane Systematic Review	Post-herpetic neuralgia	7	'… acupuncture is safe and might be effective in pain relieving for patients with PHN.'	?	'Given the low quality of included studies, the results are not conclusive …'	Included studies all had arms with <200 participants. Pooled events < 500
	Dimitrova et al., 2017 [166]	Non-Cochrane Systematic Review	Peripheral neuropathy	13 (15 studies)	'This systematic review suggests that acupuncture is effective in diabetic neuropathy, Bell's palsy, and CTS …'	?	'… various methodological issues were identified.'	Two studies reported a sample size calculation. Included studies all had arms with <200 participants.
	Ju et al., 2017 [167]	Cochrane review	Neuropathic pain	6	'… there is insufficient evidence to support or refute the use of acupuncture for neuropathic pain …'	?	'The overall quality of evidence is very low due to study limitations …'	Included studies all had arms with <200 participants.
	Franconi et al., 2013 [168]	Non-Cochrane Systematic Review	Chemotherapy-induced peripheral neuropathy	3 (6 studies)	'… although there are some indications that acupuncture may be effective … the current evidence available is limited.'	?	'All the clinical studies reviewed had important methodological limitations.'	Only 3 studies were RCTs and all had arms with <200 participants.
	Sim, et al., 2011 [169]	Non-Cochrane Systematic Review	Carpal tunnel syndrome	6	'The existing evidence is not convincing enough to suggest that acupuncture is an effective therapy for CTS.'	?	'The total number of included RCTs and their methodological quality were low.'	Included studies all had arms with <200 participants.
	Liu et al., 2010 [170]	Non-Cochrane Systematic Review	Trigeminal neuralgia	12	'The evidence reviewed previously suggests that acupuncture is of similar efficacy as CBZ but with fewer adverse effects …'	?	'… the evidence is weak because of low methodological quality of the reviewed studies.'	All studies Chinese. Included studies all had arms with <200 participants.
	Longworth et al., 1997 [171]	Non-Cochrane Systematic Review	Sciatica	7 (38 studies in total)	'The association between acupuncture (AP) and pain relief is so strong that it has tended to obscure any other … clinical results.'	?	'Although plentiful, the research is variable in quality, especially with respect to design, consistency, and follow-up.'	Included studies all had arms with <200 participants.

Table 1. Cont.

Condition	Reference	Type of Review	Treatments Evaluated	No of RCTs in Review	Systematic Reviewers' Conclusion of Efficacy *	Our Judgement of Efficacy **	Systematic Reviewers' Conclusion of Quality of Available Evidence ***	Our Comments
OTHER PAIN CONDITIONS								
	Vier et al., 2019 [172]	Non-Cochrane Systematic Review	Orofacial pain associated with temporo-mandibular joint dysfunction (TMD)	7	'To date, there is insufficient data to draw strong conclusions about DN for the treatment of orofacial pain associated with TMD.'	?	'… due the low quality of evidence and high risk of bias of some included studies, larger and low risk of bias trials are needed …'	Language restrictions. Included studies all had arms with <200 participants.
	Kim et al., 2018 [173]	Systematic review of SRs and network meta-analysis	Aromatase inhibitor induced arthralgia	2 (6 in total)	'Acupuncture … is recommended for AIA with low overall confidence based on the current evidence.'	?	'… evidence for acupuncture as an effective treatment for AIA was considered low.'	Only 2 small RCTs of acupuncture included in network analysis with total samples of 20 and 22.
	Pan et al., 2018 [174]	Non-Cochrane Systematic Review	Osteoporosis	35	'This present systematic review indicated that acupuncture could be an effective therapy for treating osteoporosis.'	?	'… nearly all Chinese studies reported positive results … and all the studies … in this meta-analysis were Chinese trials.	Publication bias. Included studies all had arms with <200 participants.
	Chau et al., 2018 [175]	Non-Cochrane Systematic Review	Shoulder pain (PSP) in stroke survivors	29	'… conventional acupuncture and electroacupuncture could be effective treatments for survivors with PSP, with regard to reducing pain …'	?	'… the very high potential for bias was prevalent in the included trials. These methodological flaws may have led to biased results in the included trials …'	All trials were conducted in China. Included studies all had arms with <200 participants.
	Luo et al., 2018 [176]	Non-Cochrane Systematic Review	Osteoporosis	9	'WNA may have beneficial effects on bone mineral density and VAS scores of patients with primary OP.'	?	'… all included trials were at high risk of bias and of low quality.'	Warm needle acupuncture (WNA). Included studies all had arms with <200 participants.
	Hall et al., 2018 [177]	Non-Cochrane Systematic Review	Upper extremity pain & dysfunction	11	'There is very low evidence to support the use of TDN (trigger point dry needling) in the shoulder region for treating patients with upper extremity pain or dysfunction.'	?	'The current evidence supporting TDN for upper extremity pain and dysfunction is very low, and future research is likely to change treatment effect estimates.'	Included studies all had arms with <200 participants.
	Chen et al., 2017 [178]	Non-Cochrane Systematic Review	Aromatase inhibitor induced arthralgia	5	'… acupuncture treatment significantly reduced Brief Pan Inventory worst pain scores and WOMAC pain scores after 6-8 weeks …'	?	'… certain trials recruited a relatively small sample size of patients per treatment group … outcomes were reported inconsistently.'	Included studies all had arms with <50 participants.

45

Table 1. Cont.

Condition	Reference	Type of Review	Treatments Evaluated	No of RCTs in Review	Systematic Reviewers' Conclusion of Efficacy *	Our Judgement of Efficacy **	Systematic Reviewers' Conclusion of Quality of Available Evidence ***	Our Comments
	Fernandes et al., 2017 [179]	Non-Cochrane Systematic Review	TMJ disorder (TMD)	4	'… acupuncture treatment appears to relieve the signs and symptoms of pain in myofascial TMD.'	?	'… the four included studies revealed two studies of good quality and two studies of weak quality.'	Included studies all had arms with <50 participants.
	Thiagarajah 2017 [180]	Non-Cochrane Systematic Review	Plantar fasciitis	4	'… acupuncture may reduce pain in the short term … insufficient evidence for a definitive conclusion regarding … the longer term.'	?	'The number of participants (range 23–53) was small in all studies and the types of controls employed varied.'	Included studies all had arms with <50 participants.
	Lee & Lim 2016 [181]	Non-Cochrane Systematic Review	Post-stroke shoulder pain	12	'Although there is some evidence for an effect of acupuncture on poststroke shoulder pain, the results are inconclusive.'	?	'… some of the included studies were of poor quality and had methodological shortcomings … .'	Included studies all had arms with <100 participants.
	Wang et al., 2016 [182]	Non-Cochrane Systematic Review	Shoulder pain	9	'Ashi point stimulation might be superior to conventional acupuncture, drug therapy and no treatment for shoulder pain.'	?	'… most of the trials suffer from many flaws …. Eight out of 9 included studies had severe methodological defects.'	Included studies all had arms with <100 participants.
	Tang et al., 2015 [183]	Non-Cochrane Systematic Review	Lateral epicondylitis	4	'For the small number of included studies … no firm conclusion can be drawn regarding the effect of acupuncture … .'	?	'The overall quality rated by GRADE was from very low to low.'	Pain was not an outcome measure. Included studies all had arms with <100 participants.
	Chang et al., 2014 [184]	Non-Cochrane Systematic Review	Lateral epicondylitis	9	'Manual acupuncture is effective in short-term pain relief … however, its long-term analgesic effect is unremarkable.'	–	'The analgesic effect of manual acupuncture on the treatment of lateral epicondylalgia is Level B'	Included studies all had arms with <100 participants.
	Lee et al., 2012 [185]	Non-Cochrane Systematic Review	Post-stroke shoulder pain	7	'It is concluded from this systematic review that acupuncture combined with exercise is effective for shoulder pain after stroke.'	?	'… there were insufficient quality assessments with respect to allocation concealment, blinding of outcome assessors, and long-term follow-up.'	All studies were Chinese. Included studies all had arms with <100 participants.
	Clark et al., 2012 [186]	Non-Cochrane Systematic Review	Plantar heel pain	5 (8 in total)	'In view of the heterogeneity of these papers, it is not possible to give a simple conclusion … .'	?	'Two studies provide good reporting of high-quality studies; six are of lesser quality.'	The included RCTs all had arms with <100 participants.

Table 1. *Cont.*

Condition	Reference	Type of Review	Treatments Evaluated	No of RCTs in Review	Systematic Reviewers' Conclusion of Efficacy *	Our Judgement of Efficacy **	Systematic Reviewers' Conclusion of Quality of Available Evidence ***	Our Comments
	Smith, et al., 2011 [187]	Cochrane review	Labour pain	13	'There are insufficient data to demonstrate whether acupuncture and acupressure are more effective than a placebo control, or whether there is additional benefit from acupuncture when used in combination with usual care.'	?	'The risk of bias was high in the majority of trials and recommendations for practice cannot be made until further high-quality research has been undertaken.'	One large study with >200 participants in the acupuncture group and >100 in the other two groups. Other studies had <200 participants in each arm and relatively high risk of bias.
	Cho et al., 2010 [188]	Non-Cochrane Systematic Review	Labour pain	10	'The evidence from RCTs does not support the use of acupuncture for controlling labour pain.'	?	'The primary studies are diverse and often flawed.'	As above—One large study. Others had <200 participants per arm
	La Touche et a, 2010 [189]	Non-Cochrane Systematic Review	TMJ disorder	9	'... acupuncture is a reasonable adjunctive treatment for producing a short-term analgesic effect...'	?	'... the relevance of these results was limited by the fact that substantial bias was present.'	Included studies all had arms with <100 participants.
	Fink et al., 2006 [190]	Non-Cochrane Systematic Review	TMJ disorder	6	'Acupuncture appears to be a suitable complementary treatment method in the management...'	?	'... results achieved must be interpreted with caution because of the methodological shortcomings identified.'	Only 3 electronic databases searched.
	Green et al., 2005 [191]	Cochrane review	Shoulder pain	9	'There is little evidence to support or refute the use of acupuncture...'	?	'This review has highlighted the paucity of methodologically rigorous, well described randomised controlled trials with adequate sample size...'	Largest study, with unclear risk of bias, had 150 participants. All others had <200 participants per arm.
	Trinh et al., 2004 [192]	Non-Cochrane Systematic Review	Lateral epicondyle pain	6	'There is strong evidence suggesting that acupuncture is effective in the short-term relief of lateral epicondyle pain.'	?	'The six studies being assessed were considered consistent high-quality... because they were all within the 3–5 range on the Jadad scale.'	In spite of the relatively high Jadad score the studies all had small sample sizes, ranging from 17–82.
	Lee & Ernst 2004 [193]	Non-Cochrane Systematic Review	Labour pain management	3	'Overall, the evidence of acupuncture for pain management during labour is encouraging...'	?	'The methodologic quality of the primary studies is generally good...'	Conclusions based on 3 studies with trials arms <200 participants.
	Green et al., 2002 [194]	Cochrane review	Lateral elbow pain	4	'There is insufficient evidence to either support or refute the use of acupuncture...'	?	'Due to ... problems with methodology of the included trials... the results of this review are inconclusive.'	Included studies all had arms with <100 participants.

Table 1. Cont.

Condition	Reference	Type of Review	Treatments Evaluated	No of RCTs in Review	Systematic Reviewers' Conclusion of Efficacy *	Our Judgement of Efficacy **	Systematic Reviewers' Conclusion of Quality of Available Evidence ***	Our Comments
	Rosted 2001 [195]	Non-Cochrane Systematic Review	TMJ disorder	3	'Acupuncture has in three out of three randomised controlled trials (RCT) proved effective for the treatment of TMD.'	?	'… publications … fulfilled the list of predefined methodological criteria with a score between 77% and 84%.'	Trial arms included <100 participants. However, the purpose of this review was to present standard acupuncture procedure.
	Ernst & White 1999 [196]	Non-Cochrane Systematic Review	TMJ dysfunction	3	'Even though all studies are in accordance with the notion that acupuncture is effective for temporomandibular joint dysfunction, this hypothesis requires confirmation….'	?	'None of the trials was performed with blinded evaluators, details of randomization are not given, and therefore all studies are subject to important bias.'	Studies as in Rosted 2001 above. All 3 studies from Scandinavia.
	Rosted 1998 [197]	Non-Cochrane Systematic Review	Dentistry	15	'Acupuncture in 11 out of 15 studies proved effective … as analgesia.'	?	No definitive statement on quality but authors report that 6 studies were of 'excellent' or 'good' quality.	Insufficient sample sizes.
	Ter Riet et al., 1989 [21]	Non-Cochrane Systematic Review	Facial pain	2	'The effectiveness of acupuncture on facial pain may not be accepted as proven.'	?	'The shortcomings of the studies are clear from the table. The big spread in the score of the study [by] Lewith et al. is mainly due to the poor reporting.'	Only two small RCTs included.

Key: * Systematic reviewers' conclusion about efficacy: Direct quote taken from the conclusion of the article (from either Abstract or Discussion section). ** Our judgement of efficacy within the review: Determined by the following criteria: + means sufficient evidence and in favour of acupuncture; − means sufficient evidence in favour of control/placebo; = means sufficient evidence but inconclusive; ? means insufficient evidence to make a judgement. Sufficient evidence = pooled analysis of 500 events or >200 participants in each arm of at least one RCT. *** Systematic reviewers' conclusion of quality of available evidence: Direct quote taken from the conclusion of the article (from either Abstract or Discussion section).

3.2. Headache (Including Migraine)

We found one overview of Cochrane reviews of acupuncture for various pain conditions [28] (described above) that claimed there to be evidence that acupuncture was effective for tension-type headache (1 Cochrane review [45]) and migraine (1 Cochrane review [51]).

The earliest SR was published in 1999 and judged there to be too few RCTs of sufficient methodological quality to determine efficacy of acupuncture for recurrent headache (22 randomised or 'quasi' randomised trials, Melchart [54]) or tension-type and cervicogenic headache (8 RCTs [47]). A similar pattern of 'promising' but not definitive evidence continued through the next decade (27 RCTs [53]; 8 RCTs [46]), including a Cochrane review of 26 RCTs of acupuncture for idiopathic headache [52]. Nevertheless, some reviewers have claimed that there is evidence that acupuncture is superior to sham for chronic headache (31 RCTs, only 2 RCTs were of high quality and adequately powered, Sun [48]), and a recent Cochrane review providing evidence of superiority of acupuncture over placebo for the prevention of tension-type headache ([44] 12 RCTs, including two adequately powered RCTs) and episodic migraine ([49], 22 RCTs, including two adequately powered RCTs). A systematic review published in 2016 is consistent with the latter finding that acupuncture was superior to sham acupuncture for migraine (10 RCTs [50]).

Evidence from the SRs suggests that acupuncture prevents episodic or chronic tension-type headaches and episodic migraine, although long-term studies and studies comparing acupuncture with other treatment options are still required. The current NICE guidance (clinical guideline CG150) is that a course of up to 10 sessions of acupuncture over 5–8 weeks is recommended for tension-type headache and migraine [12].

3.3. Osteoarthritis (OA)

The overview of eight Cochrane reviews of acupuncture for various pain conditions described previously [28], judged there to be evidence that acupuncture produced short-term improvements in pain based on a SR of 16 RCTs on peripheral joint osteoarthritis [69]). In 2019, an overview of non-Cochrane SRs that included a meta-analysis concluded that acupuncture was beneficial for alleviating pain associated with OAK, although RCT outcomes assessed using the Grades of Recommendation, Assessment, Development and Evaluation (GRADE) indicated that the SR evidence was of mixed quality (12 SRs [55]).

We found that the earliest SR on acupuncture for OA was published in 1997 and found studies to be contradictory with no evidence that acupuncture was more effective than sham (9 RCTs [71]). SRs on acupuncture for peripheral joint OA were inconclusive in 2006 (18 RCTs [70]), superior to waiting list controls in 2010 ([69], Cochrane review of 16 RCTs) and associated with reductions in pain intensity, improvement in functional mobility and quality of life in 2014 (12 RCTs [68]). In 2018, a Cochrane review by Manheimer et al. found little evidence that acupuncture significantly reduced pain associated with OA of the hip [67]. To date, the majority of SRs have evaluated the clinical efficacy of acupuncture for OA of the knee (OAK).

We found that the earliest SR on acupuncture for OAK was published in 2001 and was inconclusive (7 RCTs, with 4 of low methodological quality [66]). Chronologically, SRs in 2002 (4 RCTs, [65]) and 2007 (11 RCTs [64]) were inconclusive, whereas a SR by Bjordal et al. in 2007 found statistically significant and clinically relevant short-term pain relief from two to four weeks of intensive electroacupuncture (7 RCTs [63]). In 2008 and 2012, two further SRs (10 RCTs [62]; 14 RCTs, [61] respectively) reported superiority over sham acupuncture. More recently, SRs in 2016 (10 RCTs [59]), 2017 (17 RCTs [72], 11 RCTs [58]), 2018 (16 RCTs [57]) and 2019 (8 RCTs [56]) judged there to be evidence that acupuncture provides relief of pain associated with OAK when administered alone or in combination with other treatments.

These positive findings are supported by a network meta-analysis published in 2013 that evaluated 22 treatments, including acupuncture (11 RCTs [60]), and judged there to be evidence of short-term efficacy. This finding was confirmed in another network meta-analysis published in 2018, which found that needle or electro-acupuncture decreased pain compared with other treatments (16 RCTs [57]). Nevertheless, reviewers consistently mitigate these positive findings by describing RCTs as having low methodological quality, thus reducing confidence in judgements.

The most recent evidence from a Cochrane review of 16 RCTs suggests that acupuncture is not superior to sham acupuncture for OA of the hip [67], although in contrast, evidence from non-Cochrane reviews suggests that there is moderate-quality evidence that acupuncture may be effective in the symptomatic relief of pain from OA of the knee. Why there should be a difference in evidence between the knee and the hip is not known. Interestingly, guidance from NICE (CG177) states: "Do not offer acupuncture for the management of osteoarthritis" Section 1.4.6. [198].

3.4. Chronic Low Back Pain and/or Neck Pain

The overview of eight Cochrane reviews of acupuncture for various pain conditions described previously [28] included one Cochrane review on low back pain [88] and judged there to be evidence that acupuncture might be an effective adjunctive intervention for low back pain. However, the quality of the primary studies was low. An overview of 16 SRs on acupuncture for low back pain published in 2015 judged that acupuncture either in isolation or as an adjunct to conventional treatment had short-term benefits but again, the quality of the included reviews was variable [78].

We found that the earliest SR on acupuncture chronic low back pain was published in 1989 and evaluated the clinical efficacy of acupuncture for neck and/or back pain (22 studies including 16 RCTs [19]) but the findings were inconclusive. The earliest SR that evaluated the clinical efficacy of acupuncture specifically for chronic low back pain was published in 1998 by Ernst et al. (12 RCTs [94]), and found evidence that acupuncture was superior to various control interventions, but insufficient evidence to judge whether it was superior to placebo. The included studies were mostly of high-quality, but sample sizes were inadequate. In 2000, Smith et al. published a SR that found no evidence that acupuncture was effective for either chronic neck or low back pain (13 RCTs [99]).

Throughout the following decade, SRs reported insufficient high-quality evidence to make any judgement on efficacy of acupuncture in treating low back pain (4 RCTs [93], 11 RCTs [22], 5 RCTs [91], 6 RCTs [95], 33 RCTs [89], 35 RCTs [88] and 10 RCTs [90]). In 2010, Trigkilidas published a SR that evaluated the clinical efficacy of acupuncture for low back pain (4 RCTs [85]) that judged there to be evidence of superiority of acupuncture compared with usual care in treating chronic low back pain, especially when patients have positive expectations about the intervention. Between 2011 and 2017, none of the published SRs provided compelling evidence to support the efficacy of acupuncture for chronic low back pain (2 RCTs [84], 7 RCTs [83], 13 RCTs [82], 32 RCTs [81], 8 RCTs [79] and 7 RCTs [77]), or lumbar spinal stenosis (12 studies, 6 RCTs [80]).

In 2018, Hu et al. published a SR that evaluated the clinical efficacy of acupuncture for low back pain (16 RCTs [75]) and found evidence that dry needling was more effective for low back pain than conventional acupuncture or sham immediately post treatment, but at follow-up, was equal to acupuncture. In 2018, Tang et al. published a SR that evaluated the clinical efficacy of acupuncture for the relief of pain associated with lumbar disc herniation (30 RCTs [76]), which found insufficient robust evidence to draw firm conclusions because of methodological shortcomings in primary RCTs. However, there was tentative evidence that dry needling was more beneficial than lumbar traction, drug therapy or Chinese herbal medicine. In 2019, Xiang et al. published a SR on acupuncture for non-specific low back pain (14 RCTs [74]). There was moderate evidence of benefit but confidence in the results was diminished due to heterogeneity and small sample sizes in the included studies.

Evidence suggests that there are insufficient high-quality RCTs to judge the efficacy of acupuncture for low back pain. In 2009, NICE published guidance for the management of non-specific low back pain that recommended a course of acupuncture as part of first line treatment [10]. This guidance produced much debate. Subsequently, NICE have updated guidance for the management of low back pain and sciatica in people over 16 (NG59) and currently recommend in Section 1.2.8 "Do not offer acupuncture for managing low back pain with or without sciatica", even though the evidence had not significantly changed [9].

3.5. Myofascial Pain Syndrome and Myofascial Trigger Points

We found that the earliest SR on acupuncture (dry needling) to alleviate pain associated with myofascial trigger points (MTPs) was published in 2001 (23 RCTs [116]) and found no evidence to demonstrate the efficacy of any needling technique beyond placebo. In 2009, Tough et al. published a SR that evaluated the efficacy of dry needling acupuncture (7 RCTs [115]) which produced insufficient evidence to determine efficacy. A further systematic review by Tough et al. published in 2011 (3 RCTs [113]) had similar conclusions. In 2013, a SR found that acupuncture was superior to sham or placebo in reducing pain associated with upper quadrant myofascial pain immediately post-treatment and at four weeks, although the quality of the primary studies was low (12 RCTs [112]). In 2014, Ong and Claydon published a SR that evaluated the clinical efficacy of dry needling to alleviate pain associated with MTPs in the neck and shoulders (5 RCTs [111]) and found that there was no significant difference between dry needling and lidocaine.

In 2017, Espejo-Antúnez et al. published a SR that evaluated the clinical efficacy of dry needling to alleviate pain associated with myofascial trigger points (15 RCTs [106]) and found a possible short-term benefit following dry needling. In 2017, SRs have found tentative evidence that acupuncture alone or combined with other therapies improved outcomes associated with myofascial pain syndrome (10 RCTs [108]; 33 RCTs [107]), although substantial heterogeneity and a high risk of bias, including inadequate sample sizes in the primary RCTs, undermined confidence in the findings.

Evidence from SRs suggests that dry needling acupuncture might be effective in alleviating pain associated with myofascial trigger points, at least in the short-term, although there are insufficient high-quality RCTs to judge the efficacy with any degree of certainty. There is no guidance from NICE on the management of myofascial pain syndrome.

3.6. Cancer Pain

We found one overview of SRs of acupuncture for palliative and supportive cancer care that included 7 SRs [125], but only one systematic review on cancer-related pain [126]. We found that the earliest SR on acupuncture for pain associated with cancer and/or its treatment (7 studies with 3 RCTs [126]) concluded that there was evidence of efficacy for chemotherapy-induced nausea and vomiting, but insufficient evidence to judge efficacy for cancer-related pain. In 2010, a SR of 7 RCTs provided tentative evidence that that acupuncture alleviated cancer-related pain [124], and in 2011, the first Cochrane review on acupuncture for cancer pain judged there to be insufficient evidence to determine the efficacy (3 RCTs [123]), and this was confirmed in an update in 2015 (5 RCTs [119]). Subsequently, non-Cochrane SRs in 2012 (15 RCTs [122]), 2013 (11 RCT [121]), 2014 (33 studies, 6 RCTs [120]) and 2016 (20 RCTs [120]) provide promising but inconclusive evidence of efficacy. In 2017, Chiu et al. published a Cochrane review that evaluated the clinical efficacy of acupuncture for cancer-related pain, which included treatment-related or surgery-related pain, and judged there to be evidence that acupuncture alleviated pain associated with malignancy (29 RCTs [117]), but there was a high risk of bias due to inadequate sample sizes.

Evidence from the SRs suggests that there are insufficient high-quality RCTs to judge the efficacy of acupuncture for cancer-related pain and more high-quality, appropriately designed and adequately powered studies are needed. The most recent guidance from NICE (CSG4) recognises that patients who are receiving palliative care often seek complementary therapies, but it does not specifically recommend acupuncture. It recognises that "Many studies have a considerable number of methodological limitations, making it difficult to draw definitive conclusions" (Section 11.27) [199].

3.7. Fibromyalgia

We found that the earliest SR on acupuncture for fibromyalgia was published in 1999 (7 studies, 3 RCTs [136]) and concluded that there was limited evidence supporting the use of acupuncture for fibromyalgia but this was based on only one high-quality study. Subsequently, SRs published in 2007 (5 RCTs [135]) and 2009 (6 RCTs [134]) concluded that acupuncture had no symptomatic benefit, and in 2010 were inconclusive (7 RCTs [133], and 25 studies, 12 RCTs [132] respectively).

In 2013, a Cochrane review conducted by Deare et al. (9 RCTs [131]) found low-quality evidence that acupuncture might be superior to no acupuncture or medication, and moderate-quality evidence that acupuncture was not superior to sham. Non-Cochrane SRs published in 2013 (16 RCTs [130]) and 2014 (9 RCTs [129]) were inconclusive. In 2019, two SRs have produced evidence that acupuncture was superior to sham but the evidence status was downgraded due to high levels of heterogeneity and inadequate sample sizes (10 RCTs [128]; 12 RCT [127]).

Evidence from SRs suggests that there are insufficient high-quality RCTs to judge the efficacy of acupuncture for fibromyalgia pain. There is no NICE guidance on the treatment of fibromyalgia.

3.8. Pelvic Pain

We found one overview of SRs on acupuncture for primary dysmenorrhoea which was published in 2018 and concluded that the evidence was inconclusive (5 SRs [138]). We found a number of SRs on acupuncture and associated therapies for primary dysmenorrhea, although all report a high-risk of bias leading to evidence that is inconclusive (30 RCTs [147]; 4 RCTs [146]; 16 RCTs [144]; 20 RCTs [145]; 23 RCTs [142]; 60 RCTs [139]). In 2008, a SR investigating acupuncture for pelvic and back pain during pregnancy was inconclusive (3 RCTs [152]), and in 2010, a SR described RCTs findings as 'promising' but inconclusive for primary dysmenorrhea (27 RCTs [151]). A Cochrane review by Zhu et al. in 2011 on acupuncture for endometriosis included one low-quality RCT and was inconclusive [150]. A follow-up non-Cochrane review in 2017 including 10 RCTs was still inconclusive [143].

We found five SRs on acupuncture for chronic prostatitis and/or chronic pelvic pain, and despite promising RCT findings, all reviewers concluded that the evidence was inconclusive (9 RCTs [149]; 35 RCTs [148]; 7 RCTs [141]; 4 RCTs [140]; 4 RCTs [137]).

Evidence from the SRs suggests that there are insufficient high-quality RCTs to judge the efficacy of acupuncture for primary dysmenorrhea or chronic pelvic pain. There is NICE guidance on endometriosis (NG73) [200] but this does not recommend any form of Chinese medicine for this type of pelvic pain, although acupuncture is not specifically mentioned.

3.9. Inflammatory Arthritis

In 2018, an overview of SRs concluded that acupuncture has minimal or no impact on joint pain associated with rheumatoid arthritis (7 SRs, 20 RCTs [153]). We found that the earliest SR on acupuncture for pain associated with inflammatory rheumatic diseases was published in 1997 and found insufficient high-quality evidence to make a judgement on efficacy. Subsequently, a Cochrane review published in 2005 (2 RCTs [159]) and various non-Cochrane SRs published in 2008 (8 RCTs [158]; 8 RCTs [157]), 2013 (10 RCTs [156]) and 2016 (28 RCTs [155]) have been inconclusive. The most recent SR on acupuncture for rheumatoid arthritis reported that RCT findings were tentatively positive but inconclusive (13 RCTs [154]).

Evidence from the SRs suggests that there are insufficient high-quality RCTs to judge the efficacy of acupuncture for pain in inflammatory arthritis. There is a NICE guideline (NG100) [201] for the treatment of rheumatoid arthritis but this does not recommend acupuncture.

3.10. Neuropathic Pain/Neuralgia

The earliest SR on acupuncture for neurological symptoms was published in 1997 and reported that findings were positive for alleviation of symptoms associated with lumbar disk herniation (38 studies, 7 RCTs [171]).

The majority of SRs have been conducted on peripheral neuropathy of various aetiologies, but all had methodological shortcomings resulting in inconclusive evidence (chemotherapy-induced peripheral neuropathy, 6 studies, 3 RCTs [168]; various peripheral neuropathies, 15 studies, 13 RCTs [166]; and diabetic peripheral neuropathy, 14 RCTs [164]).

There are two SRs on acupuncture for trigeminal neuralgia (12 RCTs [170]; 33 RCTs [162]), two SRs on acupuncture for carpal tunnel syndrome (6 RCTs [169]; 12 RCTs [23]) and one SR on acupuncture for post-herpetic neuralgia (7 RCTs [165]). None were able to judge efficacy with any degree of confidence due to insufficient high-quality RCTs.

Evidence from the SRs suggests that there are insufficient high-quality RCTs to judge the efficacy of acupuncture for neuropathic pain or neuralgia. There is NICE guidance (CG173) [202] on the management of neuropathic pain, but acupuncture is not included in the list of recommended/not recommended treatments.

3.11. Other Pain Conditions

In 2002, a Cochrane review found insufficient high-quality RCTs to determine the efficacy of acupuncture for lateral elbow pain (4 RCTs [194]). In 2005, a Cochrane review found insufficient high-quality RCTs to judge the efficacy of acupuncture for shoulder pain. In 2011, a Cochrane review by Smith et al. found insufficient evidence to judge the efficacy of acupuncture or acupressure for labour pain (13 RCTs [187]).

Our search found an additional 27 reviews for a variety of other pain conditions, including dental/facial pain, osteoporosis and upper extremity pain of various aetiologies, although none of these reviews provides sufficient high-quality evidence to make a judgement about the efficacy of acupuncture (Table 1) [21,172–197].

Evidence from SRs suggests that there are insufficient high-quality RCTs to judge the efficacy of acupuncture for a variety of other painful conditions, including lateral elbow pain, shoulder pain and labour pain. There is no guidance available from NICE on the treatment of any of these conditions.

4. Discussion

Our evidence synthesis reveals long-standing and continued uncertainty about the clinical efficacy of acupuncture to alleviate pain, despite a high volume of published research. We have revealed a raft of SRs with inconclusive findings due to persistent methodological shortcomings in RCTs contributing to a high risk of bias and downgrading of evidence. These shortcomings include inadequate statistical power, uncertainty about adequacy of acupuncture technique and dose, and inappropriate design of 'placebo' acupuncture controls. These contribute to methodological and clinical heterogeneity, deterring systematic reviewers from pooling data for meta-analyses. When meta-analyses are conducted, substantial statistical heterogeneity results, markedly reducing confidence in findings and inferences [18,203,204]. The high financial cost of continuing to undertake research that produces inconclusive evidence is of concern and demands reconsideration of the methodological design and delivery of future RCT design. We will discuss three common challenges to the design of RCTs of acupuncture that emerge from our evidence synthesis: adequate sample sizes, adequate acupuncture intervention, and adequate placebo controls.

4.1. The Challenge of Inadequate Sample Sizes

RCTs with small sample sizes are associated with an overestimation of treatment effects. Dechartres et al. [18] found that treatment effects were, on average, 48% larger in trials with fewer than 50 patients.

Overestimation of treatment effects occurs in studies with sample sizes of 100–200 participants per treatment arm, suggesting that at least 200 participants per treatment arm is necessary to achieve a low risk of bias. Roberts [205] argued that the production of fewer but broader reviews that exclude underpowered trials would increase the validity of review findings and create a more trustworthy evidence base. Turner et al. [203] examined the distribution of statistical power within meta-analyses published as part of Cochrane reviews and argued that the results of meta-analyses that contain at least two adequately powered studies are not influenced to any significant degree when underpowered studies are omitted. At present, the inclusion of underpowered studies in meta-analyses is at the discretion of reviewers.

Funding constraints that prevent the use of larger sample sizes in RCTs is likely to continue into the future. Thus, strategies to reduce statistical heterogeneity associated with high variance in pain data in RCTs need consideration. Often, pain data used as the primary outcome within RCTs is a continuous variable, such as pain intensity measured on a visual analogue scale (VAS) and expressed as an average. Averages of pain intensity data from VAS can be misleading because averages may obscure good and poor responders to acupuncture [206,207]. There is a likelihood that scores of pain intensity produce U-shaped rather than bell-shaped distributions, with some participants experiencing large reductions in pain and others not. Thus, pain intensity data from acupuncture responders may be diluted by data from non-responders [208]. For this reason, the Pain and Palliative Support and Care group of the Cochrane collaboration recommends the use of primary outcome responder rates of participants reporting relief of 30% or greater (i.e., at least moderate pain relief) or 50% or greater (i.e., significant pain relief) expressed as frequency (dichotomous) data.

4.2. The Challenge of Appropriate Controls

Acupuncture RCTs can assess two aspects of the active ingredient of treatment: effects associated with needling acupuncture points and effects associated with needles piercing the skin. Thus, two common controls used in RCTs of acupuncture are: inserting real needles into the skin at non-acupuncture points and using 'sham' needles which touch but do not penetrate the skin. It is important that SRs and RCTs emphasise exactly which outcome is being assessed at the outset, and ideally include this in the title and aim of the report.

Controls that involve inserting needles into the skin at non-acupuncture points can be used to determine the influence of needling discrete points of the skin on outcome. If administering treatment at any point on the skin produced equivalent benefits and harms when compared with needling specific points, this would challenge the need for anatomical acupuncture charts and prescribed acupuncture practitioner training.

Controls that use 'sham' needles which touch but don't penetrate the skin are often labelled as placebo controls. The purpose of a placebo control comparison is to isolate the effect of the act of receiving a treatment from the active ingredient of the treatment. Placebo controls are usually operationalised using fake or sham interventions and enable measurement of non-specific treatment effects associated with expectations, conditioning, anxiety and social context (i.e., therapist/patient interaction and theatrical elements of the treatment) [209,210]. It has been argued that the reason why some RCTs fail to detect differences in treatment effects between real and sham acupuncture is that sham needling techniques are not physiologically inert, and this may have contributed to an underestimation of acupuncture effects in the evidence base [211]. This argument is valid but can be misleading if taken at face value. The purpose of a control intervention is not to be physiologically inert but rather to control for outcomes associated with non-specific effects of the act (theatre) of receiving the treatment. No placebo control (including a sham needling) is ever physiologically inert because it instigates changes in physiological (and psychological) state. The human body evolved to detect and respond to disturbances in the internal and/or external environment (i.e., stimuli) from physical, physiological, social and/or environmental change. This is the premise of homeostasis.

Placebo controls are research tools that enable isolation of effects associated with the active ingredient(s) of the treatment. Thus, a comparison of effects during real needling versus sham needling, whereby needles touch but do not penetrate the skin, enable investigators to isolate the magnitude and incidence of effects associated with needles piercing the skin per se (i.e., the 'acu' and 'puncture'). If puncturing the skin with needles produces equivalent benefits to touching without puncturing the skin, then it may be safer not to puncture the skin in clinical practice, providing that the sham needles do less harm. Interestingly, a system of evaluating the physiological effects of sham needling has been proposed to assist researchers [212].

The term 'placebo' is used extensively in research and clinical literature, although it lacks scientific precision and has become emotive. We would prefer precise statements of purpose and method when describing control interventions. For example, a control group that uses fake needles that do not puncture the skin would be used to isolate effects associated with needles puncturing the skin. We would also encourage a shift away from assessing patient 'blinding' using questions such as 'Do you think the intervention was a placebo?' to questions assessing the 'credibility' and 'functioning' of interventions using questions such as 'Do you think the intervention was credible?' and 'Do you think the intervention was functioning correctly?', as has been suggested for other non-pharmacological interventions such as transcutaneous electrical nerve stimulation (TENS) [213].

4.3. The Challenge of Adequacy of Dose

Acupuncture practitioners argue that acupuncture is a complex intervention that should not be standardised but instead tailored to each individual patient, based on principles of practice and the experience of the clinician. Components of needling include type, number, and location of needles, needling technique (e.g., thrusting, rotation, flicking, pecking), duration of needle insertion, regimen of treatment and philosophical paradigm. Debates about optimal technique are long-standing and there are evidence-based principles underpinning optimisation of technique for acupuncture treatment [214]. Delivering identical acupuncture prescription to all participants runs the risk of some participants receiving sub-optimal dose. Often, acupuncture interventions used in RCTs are grounded in principles of Western acupuncture with flexibility to individualise treatment at the discretion of individual practitioners. Individualising acupuncture treatment increases between-subject variability in treatment (e.g., needling number, location, technique, duration). At face value, this may appear to conflict with classical RCT methodology that aims to standardise methodology and treatment intervention under strictly controlled conditions. However, standardisation can be based on the principles of optimising treatment per individual, as is the case when titrating drug dosage to therapeutic window. What constitutes adequacy of acupuncture technique and dose has been a matter of much debate [56,214–216].

In trials of pharmacological agents, dose is crucial, and it should be no different in studies investigating the efficacy of acupuncture. The Standards for Reporting Interventions in Controlled Trials of Acupuncture (STRICTA) were developed from the consolidated standards for reporting trials (CONSORT) [217] to encourage accurate reporting of the acupuncture intervention [218]. STRICTA recommend that six items should be included: rationale, details of needling (e.g., points used, depth, angle, needle thickness, number of needles), treatment regimen, co-intervention, practitioner background and control interventions [219]. The impact of using STRICTA has been positive with improvements in reporting quality of RCTs on acupuncture [220–223]. In 2008, White et al. published a meta-analysis that provided evidence that better outcomes in comparisons of acupuncture with non-acupuncture controls were achieved when noted that greater numbers of needles and treatment sessions were used [214]. In 2019, Sun et al. conducted a systematic review of eight RCTs (2106 participants) to determine whether the effect of acupuncture is dose-dependent for symptom management in knee osteoarthritis [56]. Sun et al. proposed a scoring system whereby +1 score was awarded if ≥9 points needled, if de qi was present, if ≥2 treatment sessions a week and if ≥8 treatment sessions in total. A score of −1 was awarded to each of these parameters if they were below these thresholds. The sum of scores was taken and high dosage categorised for total between 1 and

4, medium dosage for a score of 0 and low dosage for scores from −4 to −1. Sun et al. categorised one RCT as low dose, one RCT as medium dose and 6 RCTs as high dose and concluded that higher dosage of acupuncture was associated with better pain relief and functional improvements. It is becoming common for journal editors to require STRICTA in RCTs of acupuncture and this will improve comparison and assessment of adequacy of acupuncture dose in systematic reviews. What is less common, however, is the inclusion and reporting of 'run-in phases' in RCTs, whereby optimisation of technique and dosage is titrated over a period of weeks prior to randomisation into real and placebo acupuncture.

4.4. Design of Future Randomised Controlled Trials (RCTS)

It has been argued that enriched enrolment with randomised withdrawal (EERW) study designs are of value for treatments influencing symptoms but not necessarily the course of the underlying disease or pathology, as is the case for acupuncture in the management of chronic pain [224]. The potential for using such designs in the assessment of pharmacological agents has been recognised [225], although EERW designs are rarely used to assess non-pharmacological interventions. The EERW trials consist of (i) an observational 'open-label' phase with all participants receiving active treatment (acupuncture), during which treatment technique and dosage would be titrated and optimized, followed by (ii) a RCT phase, whereby participants who had potential for response were enrolled (i.e., an enriched sample) and randomised to receive either experimental (real needling) or control interventions (sham needling). Selection of participants for the enriched sample of the RCT is based on the findings from phase one and would exclude participants who did not wish to continue treatment or experienced non-manageable adverse events, although their data from phase one would be analysed. Trials with EERW designs increase sensitivity to detect treatment effects by enriching the sample of participants enrolling into the randomised controlled phase of the trial, thus reducing the need for large sample sizes [207].

To our knowledge, there have not been any published studies of acupuncture using the EERW design, although it has been used to determine the efficacy of drugs for chronic pain conditions. Given the shortcomings in classically design RCTs on acupuncture, it would be interesting to observe the results of studies using an EERW design.

4.5. Limitations of This Review

A limitation of this synthesis is that it does not contain granular quantitative analyses. It could be argued that there is a case for an all-encompassing SR and meta-analysis of all RCTs on acupuncture for pain conditions, but this would be a considerable undertaking with the possibility that it not produce any meaningful information due to the relatively poor quality of RCTs resulting in amplification of heterogeneity.

5. Conclusions

We hope that our evidence synthesis of systematic reviews and meta-analyses of RCTs of acupuncture for chronic pain conditions serves as a reference tool for practitioners, researchers and commissioners. Our evidence synthesis reveals a long-standing unresolved debate about the clinical efficacy of acupuncture to alleviate pain that is grounded in a high volume of inconclusive RCT evidence. If healthcare providers and commissioners are to be able to make informed choices on the role of acupuncture for chronic pain, it is essential that the quality of clinical trials of acupuncture is improved. Our evidence synthesis has revealed three methodological challenges that have faced investigators of RCT of acupuncture for decades. We have argued that enriched enrolment with randomised withdrawal trial designs may provide a way forward. We hope that our review catalyses further debate on this issue.

Author Contributions: Conceptualization, C.A.P. and M.I.J.; methodology, C.A.P.; formal analysis, C.A.P. and M.I.J.; writing—Original draft preparation, C.A.P.; writing—Review and editing, C.A.P. and M.I.J. All authors have read and agreed to the published version of the manuscript.

Funding: This research received no external funding.

Conflicts of Interest: C.A.P. declares no conflict of interest. M.I.J.'s institution has received research and consultancy funding for work that he has undertaken for GlaxoSmithKline.

References

1. Treede, R.D.; Rief, W.; Barke, A.; Aziz, Q.; Bennett, M.I.; Benoliel, R.; Cohen, M.; Evers, S.; Finnerup, N.B.; First, M.B.; et al. Chronic pain as a symptom or a disease: The IASP Classification of Chronic Pain for the International Classification of Diseases (ICD-11). *Pain* **2019**, *160*, 19–27. [CrossRef]
2. Fayaz, A.; Croft, P.; Langford, R.M.; Donaldson, L.J.; Jones, G.T. Prevalence of chronic pain in the US: A systematic review and meta-analysis of population studies. *BMJ Open* **2016**, *6*, e010364. [CrossRef] [PubMed]
3. Hadi, M.A.; McHugh, G.A.; Closs, S.J. Impact of Chronic Pain on Patients' Quality of Life: A Comparative Mixed-Methods Study. *J. Patient Exp.* **2019**, *6*, 133–141. [CrossRef] [PubMed]
4. IASP. Musculoskeletal Pain Fact Sheet. Fact Sheet No. 5. Available online: https://www.iasp-pain.org/Advocacy/Content.aspx?ItemNumber=1101 (accessed on 24 December 2019).
5. White, A.; Ernst, E. A brief history of acupuncture. *Rheumatology* **2004**, *43*, 662–663. [CrossRef] [PubMed]
6. Han, J.; Terenius, L. Neurochemical basis of acupuncture analgesia. *Annu. Rev. Pharmacol. Toxicol.* **1982**, *22*, 193–220. [CrossRef]
7. Johnson, M.I. The clinical effectiveness of acupuncture for pain relief-you can be certain of uncertainty. *Acupunct. Med.* **2006**, *24*, 71–79. [CrossRef]
8. Colquhoun, D.; Novella, S.P. Acupuncture Is Theatrical Placebo. *Anesth. Analg.* **2013**, *116*, 1360–1363. [CrossRef]
9. NICE. Low Back Pain and Sciatica in over 16s. Assessment and Management. Available online: http//www.nice.org.uk/guidance/ng59 (accessed on 26 May 2019).
10. NICE. Low Back Pain in Adults Early Management. Available online: https//www.nice.org.uk/guidance/cg88 (accessed on 25 June 2019).
11. Savigny, P.; Kuntze, S.; Watson, P.; Underwood, M.; Ritchie, G.; Cotterell, M.; Hill, D.; Browne, N.; Buchanan, E.; Coffey, P.; et al. Low back pain. Early management of persistent non-specific low back pain. In *NICE Guideline CG88*; National Collaborating Centre for Primary Care and Royal College of General Practitioners: London, UK, 2009.
12. NICE. Headaches in over 12: Diagnosis and Management. Available online: http//www.nice.org.uk/guidance/cg150/chapter/recommendations#management-2 (accessed on 26 May 2019).
13. NHS. Acupuncture. Available online: https://www.nhs.uk/conditions/acupuncture/ (accessed on 30 September 2019).
14. Singh, S.; Ernst, E. The Truth About Acupuncture. In *Trick or Treatment? Alternative Medicine on Trial*; Bantam Press: London, UK, 2009; p. 410.
15. Murad, M.H.; Asi, N.; Alsawas, M.; Alahdab, F. New evidence pyramid. *Evid. Based Med.* **2016**, *21*, 125–127. [CrossRef]
16. Moore, A.R.; Straube, S.; Eccleston, C.; Derry, S.; Aldington, D.; Wiffen, P.; Bell, R.F.; Hamunen, K.; Phillips, C.; McQuay, H. Evidence in chronic pain-establishing best practice in the reporting of systematic reviews. *Pain* **2010**, *150*, 386–389. [CrossRef]
17. Moore, R.A.; Gavaghan, D.; Tramer, M.R.; Collins, S.L.; McQuay, H.J. Size is everything—Large amounts of information are needed to overcome random: Effects in estimating direction and magnitude of treatment effects. *Pain* **1998**, *78*, 209–216. [CrossRef]
18. Dechartres, A.; Trinquart, L.; Boutron, I.; Ravaud, P. Influence of trial sample size on treatment effect estimate. Meta-epidemiological study. *BMJ (Clin. Res. Ed.)* **2013**, *346*, f2304. [CrossRef] [PubMed]
19. Ter Riet, G.; Kleijnen, J.; Knipschild, P. [Acupuncture and neck pain/back pain]. *Huisarts Wet.* **1989**, *32*, 223–227.
20. Ter Riet, G.; Kleijnen, J.; Knipschild, P. Acupunctuur bij migraine en spanningshoofdpijn. *Huisarts Wet.* **1989**, *32*, 258–263.

21. Ter Riet, G.; Kleijnen, J.; Knipschild, P. Acupuncture and facial pain. *Huisarts Wet.* **1989**, *32*, 264–266.
22. Van Tulder, M.W.; Cherkin, D.C.; Berman, B.; Lao, L.; Koes, B.W. Acupuncture for low back pain. *Cochrane Database Syst. Rev.* **2000**, *2*, CD001351.
23. Choi, G.-H.; Wieland, L.S.; Lee, H.; Sim, H.; Lee, M.S.; Shin, B.-C. Acupuncture and related interventions for the treatment of symptoms associated with carpal tunnel syndrome. *Cochrane Database Syst. Rev.* **2018**, *12*, CD011215. [CrossRef]
24. Ezzo, J.; Berman, B.; Hadhazy, V.A.; Jadad, A.R.; Lao, L.; Singh, B.B. Is acupuncture effective for the treatment of chronic pain? A systematic review. *Pain* **2000**, *86*, 217–225. [CrossRef]
25. Derry, C.J.; Derry, S.; McQuay, H.J.; Moore, R.A. Systematic review of systematic reviews of acupuncture published 1996–2005. *Clin. Med.* **2006**, *6*, 381–386. [CrossRef]
26. Ernst, E.; Lee, M.S. Acupuncture for rheumatic condition? An overview of systematic reviews. *Rheumatology* **2010**, *49*, 1957–1961. [CrossRef]
27. Hopton, A.; MacPherson, H. Acupuncture for Chronic Pai? Is Acupuncture More than an Effective Placebo? A Systematic Review of Pooled Data from Meta-analyses. *Pain Pract.* **2010**, *10*, 94–102. [CrossRef]
28. Lee, M.S.; Ernst, E. Acupuncture for pain: An overview of Cochrane reviews. *Chin. J. Integr. Med.* **2011**, *17*, 187–189. [CrossRef] [PubMed]
29. Ernst, E.; Lee, M.S.; Choi, T.-Y. Acupuncture: Does it alleviate pain and are there serious risks? A review of reviews. *Pain* **2011**, *152*, 755–764. [CrossRef] [PubMed]
30. Zhu, L.B.; Chan, W.C.; Lo, K.C.; Yum, T.P.; Li, L. Wrist-ankle acupuncture for the treatment of pain symptoms: A systematic review and meta-analysis. *Evid.-Based Complement. Altern. Med. Ecam* **2014**, *2014*, 261709. [CrossRef] [PubMed]
31. Yeh, C.H.; Chiang, Y.C.; Hoffman, S.L.; Liang, Z.; Klem, M.L.; Tam, W.W.S.; Chien, L.-C.; Suen, L.K.-P. Efficacy of auricular therapy for pain management: A systematic review and meta-analysis. *Evid.-Based Complement. Altern. Med. Ecam* **2014**, *2014*, 934670. [CrossRef] [PubMed]
32. Cox, J.; Varatharajan, S.; Côté, P.; Optima, C. Effectiveness of Acupuncture Therapies to Manage Musculoskeletal Disorders of the Extremities: A Systematic Review. *J. Orthop. Sports Phys. Ther.* **2016**, *46*, 409–429. [CrossRef] [PubMed]
33. Yuan, Q.-L.; Wang, P.; Liu, L.; Sun, F.; Cai, Y.-S.; Wu, W.-T.; Ye, M.-L.; Ma, J.-T.; Xu, B.-B.; Zhang, Y.-G. Acupuncture for musculoskeletal pain: A meta-analysis and meta-regression of sham-controlled randomized clinical trials. *Sci. Rep.* **2016**, *6*, 30675. [CrossRef]
34. Wong Lit Wan, D.; Wang, Y.; Xue, C.C.L.; Wang, L.P.; Liang, F.R.; Zheng, Z. Local and distant acupuncture points stimulation for chronic musculoskeletal pain: A systematic review on the comparative effects. *Eur. J. Pain (Lond. Engl.)* **2015**, *19*, 1232–1247. [CrossRef]
35. Zhao, H.-J.; Tan, J.-Y.; Wang, T.; Jin, L. Auricular therapy for chronic pain management in adult: A synthesis of evidence. *Complement. Ther. Clin. Pract.* **2015**, *21*, 68–78. [CrossRef]
36. Gattie, E.; Cleland, J.A.; Snodgrass, S. The Effectiveness of Trigger Point Dry Needling for Musculoskeletal Conditions by Physical Therapist: A Systematic Review and Meta-analysis. *J. Orthop. Sports Phys. Ther.* **2017**, *47*, 133–149. [CrossRef]
37. Vickers, A.J.; Vertosick, E.A.; Lewith, G.; MacPherson, H.; Foster, N.E.; Sherman, K.J.; Irnich, D.; Witt, C.M.; Linde, K. Acupuncture for Chronic Pain: Update of an Individual Patient Data Meta-Analysis. *J. Pain* **2018**, *19*, 455–474. [CrossRef]
38. MacPherson, H.; Vertosick, E.A.; Foster, N.E.; Lewith, G.; Linde, K.; Sherman, K.J.; Witt, C.M.; Vickers, A.J. The persistence of the effects of acupuncture after a course of treatment: A meta-analysis of patients with chronic pain. *Pain* **2017**, *158*, 784–793. [CrossRef] [PubMed]
39. Zhang, Y.-J.; Cao, H.-J.; Li, X.-L.; Yang, X.-Y.; Lai, B.-Y.; Yang, G.-Y.; Liu, J.-P. Cupping therapy versus acupuncture for pain-related conditions: A systematic review of randomized controlled trials and trial sequential analysis. *Chin. Med.* **2017**, *12*, 21. [CrossRef] [PubMed]
40. Vickers, A.J.; Cronin, A.M.; Maschino, A.C.; Lewith, G.; MacPherson, H.; Foster, N.E.; Sherman, K.J.; Witt, C.M.; Linde, K. Acupuncture for chronic pain: Individual patient data meta-analysis. *Arch. Intern. Med.* **2012**, *172*, 1444–1453. [CrossRef] [PubMed]
41. Asher, G.N.; Jonas, D.E.; Coeytaux, R.R.; Reilly, A.C.; Loh, Y.L.; Motsinger-Reif, A.A.; Winham, S.J. Auriculotherapy for pain management: A systematic review and meta-analysis of randoiized controlled trials. *J. Altern. Complement. Med. (N. Y.)* **2010**, *16*, 1097–1108. [CrossRef]

42. Madsen, M.V.; Gotsche, P.C.; Hróbjartsson, A. Acupuncture treatment for pain. Systematic review of randomised clinical trials with acupuncture, placebo acupuncture, and no acupuncture groups. *BMJ Online First* **2009**, *338*. [CrossRef]
43. Ernst, E. Acupuncture: What Does the Most Reliable Evidence Tell Us? *J. Pain Sympt. Man.* **2009**, *37*, 709–714. [CrossRef]
44. Linde, K.; Allais, G.; Brinkhaus, B.; Fei, Y.; Mehring, M.; Shin, B.-C.; Vickers, A.; White, A.R. Acupuncture for the prevention of tension-type headache. *Cochrane Database Syst. Rev.* **2016**, CD007587. [CrossRef]
45. Linde, K.; Allais, G.; Brinkhaus, B.; Manheimer, E.; Vickers, A.; White, A.R. Acupuncture for tension-type headache. *Cochrane Database Syst. Rev.* **2009**, *20*, CD007587.
46. Davis, M.A.; Kononowech, R.W.; Rolin, S.A.; Spierings, E.L. Acupuncture for tension-type headache: A meta-analysis of randomized, controlled trials. *Pain* **2008**, *9*, 667–677. [CrossRef]
47. Vernon, H.; McDermaid, C.; Hagino, C. Systematic review of randomised clinical trials of complementary/alternative therapies in the treatment of tension-type and cervicogenic headache. *Complement. Ther. Med.* **1999**, *7*, 142–155.
48. Sun, Y.; Gan, T.J. Acupuncture for the management of chronic headache. A systematic review. *Anesth. Analg.* **2008**, *107*, 2038–2047. [CrossRef] [PubMed]
49. Linde, K.; Allais, G.; Brinkhaus, B.; Fei, Y.; Mehring, M.; Vertosick, E.A.; Vickers, A.; White, A.R. Acupuncture for the prevention of episodic migraine. *Cochrane Database Syst. Rev.* **2016**, CD001218. [CrossRef] [PubMed]
50. Yang, Y.; Que, Q.; Ye, X.; Zheng, G.H. Verum versus sham manual acupuncture for migraine A systematic review of randomized controlled trials. *Acupunct. Med. J. Br. Med. Acupunct. Soc.* **2016**, *34*, 76–83. [CrossRef] [PubMed]
51. Linde, K.; Allais, G.; Brinkhaus, B.; Manheimer, E.; Vickers, A.; White, A.R. Acupuncture for migraine prophylaxis. *Cochrane Database Syst. Rev.* **2009**, *21*, CD001218.
52. Melchart, D.; Linde, K.; Fischer, P.; Berman, B.; White, A.; Vickers, A.; Allais, G. Acupuncture for idiopathic headache. *Cochrane Database Syst. Rev.* **2001**, *19*, 779–786.
53. Manias, P.; Tagaris, G.; Karageorgiou, K. Acupuncture in headache: A critical review. *Clin. J. Pain* **2000**, *16*, 334–339. [CrossRef]
54. Melchart, D.; Linde, K.; Fischer, P. Acupuncture for recurrent headache. A systematic review of randomized controlled trials. *Cephalagia* **1999**, *19*, 776–786. [CrossRef]
55. Li, J.; Li, Y.-X.; Luo, L.-J.; Ye, J.; Zhong, D.-L.; Xiao, Q.-W.; Zheng, H.; Geng, C.-M.; Jin, R.-J.; Liang, F.-R. The effectiveness and safety of acupuncture for knee osteoarthritis: An overview of systematic reviews. *Medicine* **2019**, *98*, e16301. [CrossRef]
56. Sun, N.; Tu, J.F.; Lin, L.L.; Li, Y.T.; Yang, J.W.; Shi, G.X.; Lao, L.X.; Liu, C.Z. Correlation between acupuncture dose and effectiveness in the treatment of knee osteoarthritis: A systematic review. *Acupunct. Med.* **2019**, *37*, 261–267. [CrossRef]
57. Li, S.; Xie, P.; Liang, Z.; Huang, W.; Huang, Z.; Ou, J.; Lin, Z.; Chai, S. Efficacy Comparison of Five Different Acupuncture Methods on Pain, Stiffness, and Function in Osteoarthritis of the Knee: A Network Meta-Analysis. *Evid.-Based Complement. Altern. Med.* **2018**, *2018*, 1638904. [CrossRef]
58. Chen, N.; Wang, J.; Mucelli, A.; Zhang, X.; Wang, C. Electro-Acupuncture is Beneficial for Knee Osteoarthritis: The Evidence from Meta-Analysis of Randomized Controlled Trials. *Am. J. Chin. Med.* **2017**, *45*, 965–985. [CrossRef] [PubMed]
59. Lin, X.; Huang, K.; Zhu, G.; Huang, Z.; Qin, A.; Fan, S. The Effects of Acupuncture on Chronic Knee Pain Due to Osteoarthritis: A Meta-Analysis. *J. Bone Jt. Surg. Am. Vol.* **2016**, *98*, 1578–1585. [CrossRef] [PubMed]
60. Corbett, M.S.; Rice, S.J.C.; Madurasinghe, V.; Slack, R.; Fayter, D.A.; Harden, M.; Sutton, A.J.; Macpherson, H.; Woolacott, N.F. Acupuncture and other physical treatments for the relief of pain due to osteoarthritis of the knee: Network meta-analysis. *Osteoarthr. Cartil.* **2013**, *21*, 1290–1298. [CrossRef] [PubMed]
61. Cao, L.; Zhang, X.-L.; Gao, Y.-S.; Jiang, Y. Needle acupuncture for osteoarthritis of the knee. A systematic review and updated meta-analysis. *Saudi Med. J.* **2012**, *33*, 526–532. [PubMed]
62. Selfe, T.K.; Taylor, A.G. Acupuncture and osteoarthritis of the knee: A review of randomized, controlled trials. *Fam. Community Health* **2008**, *31*, 247–254. [CrossRef]
63. Bjordal, J.M.; Johnson, M.I.; Lopes-Martins, R.A.B.; Bogen, B.; Chow, R.; Ljunggren, A.E. Short-term efficacy of physical interventions in osteoarthritic knee pain. A systematic review and meta-analysis of randomised placebo-controlled trials. *BMC Musculoskelet. Disord.* **2007**, *8*, 51. [CrossRef]

64. Manheimer, E.; Linde, K.; Lao, L.; Bouter, L.M.; Berman, B.M. Meta-analysis: Acupuncture for Osteoarthritis of the Knee. *Ann. Intern. Med.* **2007**, *146*, 868–877. [CrossRef]
65. Ferrández Infante, A.; García Olmos, L.; González Gamarra, A.; Meis Meis, M.J.; Sánchez Rodríguez, B.M. Effectiveness of acupuncture in the treatment of pain from osteoarthritis of the knee. *Aten. Primaria/Soc. Española De Med. De Fam. Y Comunitaria* **2002**, *30*, 602–608. [CrossRef]
66. Ezzo, J.; Hadhazy, V.; Birch, S.; Lao, L.; Kaplan, G.; Hochberg, M.; Berman, B. Acupuncture for osteoarthritis of the knee: A systematic review. *Arthr. Rheum.* **2001**, *44*, 819–825. [CrossRef]
67. Manheimer, E.; Cheng, K.; Wieland, L.S.; Shen, X.; Lao, L.; Guo, M.; Berman, B.M. Acupuncture for hip osteoarthritis. *Cochrane Database Syst. Rev.* **2018**. [CrossRef]
68. Manyanga, T.; Froese, M.; Zarychanski, R.; Abou-Setta, A.; Friesen, C.; Tennenhouse, M.; Shay, B.L. Pain management with acupuncture in osteoarthritis: A systematic review and meta-analysis. *BMC Complement. Altern. Med.* **2014**, *14*, 312. [CrossRef] [PubMed]
69. Manheimer, E.; Cheng, K.; Linde, K.; Lao, L.; Yoo, J.; Wieland, S.; van der Windt, D.A.; Berman, B.M.; Bouter, L.M. Acupuncture for peripheral joint osteoarthritis. *Cochrane Database Syst. Rev.* **2010**, *20*, CD001977. [CrossRef] [PubMed]
70. Kwon, Y.D.; Pittler, M.H.; Ernst, E. Acupuncture for peripheral joint osteoarthritis: A systematic review and meta-analysis. *Rheumatology* **2006**, *45*, 1331–1337. [CrossRef] [PubMed]
71. Ernst, E. Acupuncture as a symptomatic treatment of osteoarthritis. *Scand. J. Rheumatol.* **1997**, *26*, 444–447. [CrossRef] [PubMed]
72. Zhang, Q.; Yue, J.; Golianu, B.; Sun, Z.; Lu, Y. Updated systematic review and meta-analysis of acupuncture for chronic knee pain. *Acupunct. Med. J. Br. Med. Acupunct. Soc.* **2017**, *35*, 392–403. [CrossRef] [PubMed]
73. White, A.; Foster, N.E.; Cummings, M.; Barlas, P. Acupuncture treatment for chronic knee pain. A systematic review. *Rheumatology* **2007**, *46*, 384–390. [CrossRef] [PubMed]
74. Xiang, Y.; He, J.-Y.; Tian, H.-H.; Cao, B.-Y.; Li, R. Evidence of efficacy of acupuncture in the management of low back pain: A systematic review and meta-analysis of randomised placebo- or sham-controlled trials. *Acupunct. Med. J. Br. Med. Acupunct. Soc.* **2019**. [CrossRef]
75. Hu, H.-T.; Gao, H.; Ma, R.-J.; Zhao, X.-F.; Tian, H.-F.; Li, L. Is dry needling effective for low back pain: A systematic review and PRISMA-compliant meta-analysis. *Medicine* **2018**, *97*, e11225. [CrossRef]
76. Tang, S.; Mo, Z.; Zhang, R. Acupuncture for lumbar disc herniation: A systematic review and meta-analysis. *Acupunct. Med. J. Br. Med. Acupunct. Soc.* **2018**, *36*, 62–70. [CrossRef]
77. Yeganeh, M.; Baradaran, H.R.; Qorbani, M.; Moradi, Y.; Dastgiri, S. The effectiveness of acupuncture, acupressure and chiropractic interventions on treatment of chronic nonspecific low back pain in Iran: A systematic review and meta-analysis. *Complement. Ther. Clin. Pract.* **2017**, *27*, 11–18. [CrossRef]
78. Liu, L.; Skinner, M.; McDonough, S.; Mabire, L.; Baxter, G.D. Acupuncture for low back pain: An overview of systematic reviews. *Evid.-Based Complement. Altern. Med.* **2015**, *2015*, 328196. [CrossRef] [PubMed]
79. Close, C.; Sinclair, M.; Liddle, S.D.; Madden, E.; McCullough, J.E.M.; Hughes, C. A systematic review investigating the effectiveness of Complementary and Alternative Medicine (CAM) for the management of low back and/or pelvic pain (LBPP) in pregnancy. *J. Adv. Nurs.* **2014**, *70*, 1702–1716. [CrossRef] [PubMed]
80. Kim, K.H.; Kim, T.-H.; Lee, B.R.; Kim, J.K.; Son, D.W.; Lee, S.W.; Yang, G.Y. Acupuncture for lumbar spinal stenosis: A systematic review and meta-analysis. *Complement. Ther. Med.* **2013**, *21*, 535–556. [CrossRef] [PubMed]
81. Lam, M.; Galvin, R.; Curry, P. Effectiveness of acupuncture for nonspecific chronic low back pain: A systematic review and meta-analysis. *Spine* **2013**, *38*, 2124–2138. [CrossRef] [PubMed]
82. Xu, M.; Yan, S.; Yin, X.; Li, X.; Gao, S.; Han, R.; Wei, L.; Luo, W.; Lei, G. Acupuncture for chronic low back pain in long-term follow-up: A meta-analysis of 13 randomized controlled trials. *Am. J. Chin. Med.* **2013**, *41*, 1–19. [CrossRef]
83. Hutchinson, A.J.P.; Ball, S.; Andrews, J.C.H.; Jones, G.G. The effectiveness of acupuncture in treating chronic non-specific low back pain: A systematic review of the literature. *J. Orthop. Surg. Res.* **2012**, *7*, 36. [CrossRef]
84. Standaert, C.J.; Friedly, J.; Erwin, M.W.; Lee, M.J.; Rechtine, G.; Henrikson, N.B.; Norvell, D.C. Comparative Effectiveness of Exercise, Acupuncture, and Spinal Manipulation for Low Back Pain. *Spine* **2011**, *36*, S120–S130. [CrossRef]
85. Trigkilidas, D. Acupuncture therapy for chronic lower back pain: A systematic review. *Ann. R. Coll. Surg. Engl.* **2010**, *92*, 595–598. [CrossRef]

86. Yuan, J.; Kerr, D.; Park, J.; Liu, X.H.; McDonough, S. Treatment regimens of acupuncture for low back pain-A systematic review. *Complement. Ther. Med.* **2008**, *16*, 295–304. [CrossRef]
87. Yuan, J.; Purepong, N.; Kerr, D.P.; Park, J.; Bradbury, I.; McDonough, S. Effectiveness of acupuncture for low back pain: A systematic review. *Spine* **2008**, *33*, E887–E900. [CrossRef]
88. Furlan, A.D.; van Tulder, M.W.; Cherkin, D.C.; Tsukayama, H.; Lao, L.; Koes, B.W.; Berman, B.M. Acupuncture and dry-needling for low back pain. *Cochrane Database Syst. Rev.* **2005**, *25*, CD001351. [CrossRef] [PubMed]
89. Manheimer, E.; White, A.; Berman, B.; Forys, K.; Ernst, E. Meta-analysis: Acupuncture for low back pain. *Ann. Intern. Med.* **2005**, *142*, 651–663. [CrossRef] [PubMed]
90. Yuan, J.; Purepong, N.; Kerr, D.; McDonough, S. Acupuncture for non-specific low back pain. A systematic review of RCTs. *Focus Altern Complement.* **2004**, *9* (Suppl. 1), 61. [CrossRef]
91. Henderson, H. Acupuncture: Evidence for its use in chronic low back pain. *Br. J. Nurs.* **2002**, *11*, 1395–1403. [CrossRef]
92. Van Tulder, M.W.; Cherkin, D.C.; Berman, B.; Lao, L.; Koes, B.W.; van Tulder, M.W. Acupuncture for low back pain. *Cochrane Database Syst. Rev.* **1999**. [CrossRef]
93. Strauss, A. Acupuncture and the treatment of chronic low back pain: A review of the literature. *Chiro J. Austral.* **1999**, *29*, 213–218.
94. Ernst, E.; White, A. Acupuncture for back pain: A meta-analysis of randomized controlled trials. *Arch. Intern. Med.* **1998**, *158*, 2235–2241. [CrossRef]
95. Cherkin, D.C.; Sherman, K.; Deyo, R.; Shekelle, P. A review of the evidence for the effectiveness, safety and cost of acupuncture, massage therapy and manipulation for back pain. *Ann. Intern. Med.* **2003**, *138*, 898–906. [CrossRef]
96. van Tulder, M.W.; Cherkin, D.C.; Berman, B.; Lao, L.X.; Koes, B.W. The effectiveness of acupuncture in the management of acute and chronic low back pain-A systematic review within the framework of the Cochrane Collaboration back review group. *Spine* **1999**, *24*, 1113–1123. [CrossRef]
97. Griswold, D.; Wilhelm, M.; Donaldson, M.; Learman, K.; Cleland, J. The effectiveness of superficial versus deep dry needling or acupuncture for reducing pain and disability in individuals with spine-related painful condition. A systematic review with meta-analysis. *J. Man. Manip. Ther.* **2019**, *27*, 128–140. [CrossRef]
98. Yuan, Q.-L.; Guo, T.-M.; Liu, L.; Sun, F.; Zhang, Y.-G. Traditional Chinese medicine for neck pain and low back pain. A systematic review and meta-analysis. *PLoS ONE* **2015**, *10*, e0117146. [CrossRef]
99. Smith, L.A.; Oldman, A.D.; McQuay, H.J.; Moore, R.A. Teasing apart quality and validity in systematic review: An example from acupuncture trials in chronic neck and back pain. *Pain* **2000**, *86*, 119–132. [CrossRef]
100. Seo, S.Y.; Lee, K.-B.; Shin, J.-S.; Lee, J.; Kim, M.-R.; Ha, I.-H.; Ko, Y.; Lee, Y.J. Effectiveness of Acupuncture and Electroacupuncture for Chronic Neck Pain. A Systematic Review and Meta-Analysis. *Am. J. Chin. Med.* **2017**, *45*, 1573–1595. [CrossRef] [PubMed]
101. Moon, T.-W.; Posadzki, P.; Choi, T.-Y.; Park, T.-Y.; Kim, H.-J.; Lee, M.S.; Ernst, E. Acupuncture for treating whiplash associated disorder: A systematic review of randomised clinical trials. *Evid.-Based Complement. Altern. Med.* **2014**, *2014*, 870271. [CrossRef] [PubMed]
102. Wang, Y.-W.; Fu, W.-B.; Ou, A.-H.; Fan, L.; Huang, Y.-F. A systematic review of randomized controlled clinical trials of abdominal acupuncture treatment of cervical spondylosis. *Zhen Ci Yan Jiu = Acupunct. Res.* **2011**, *36*, 137–144.
103. Fu, L.-M.; Li, J.-T.; Wu, W.-S. Randomized controlled trials of acupuncture for neck pain. Systematic review and meta-analysis. *J. Altern. Complement. Med. (N. Y.)* **2009**, *15*, 133–145. [CrossRef]
104. Trinh, K.V.; Graham, N.; Gross, A.R.; Goldsmith, C.H.; Wang, E.; Cameron, I.D.; Kay, T. Acupuncture for neck disorders. *Cochrane Database Syst. Rev.* **2006**, *3*, CD004870.
105. White, A.R.; Ernst, E. A systematic review of randomized controlled trials of acupuncture for neck pain. *Rheumatology* **1999**, *38*, 143–147. [CrossRef]
106. Espejo-Antúnez, L.; Tejeda, J.F.-H.; Albornoz-Cabello, M.; Rodríguez-Mansilla, J.; de la Cruz-Torres, B.; Ribeiro, F.; Silva, A.G. Dry needling in the management of myofascial trigger points: A systematic review of randomized controlled trials. *Complement. Ther. Med.* **2017**, *33*, 46–57. [CrossRef]
107. Li, X.; Wang, R.; Xing, X.; Shi, X.; Tian, J.; Zhang, J.; Ge, L.; Zhang, J.; Li, L.; Yang, K. Acupuncture for Myofascial Pain Syndrome: A Network Meta-Analysis of 33 Randomized Controlled Trials. *Pain Physician* **2017**, *20*, E883–E902.

108. Wang, R.; Li, X.; Zhou, S.; Zhang, X.; Yang, K.; Li, X. Manual acupuncture for myofascial pain syndrome: A systematic review and meta-analysis. *Acupunct. Med. J. Br. Med. Acupunct. Soc.* **2017**, *35*, 241–250. [CrossRef] [PubMed]
109. Rodríguez-Mansilla, J.; González-Sánchez, B.; De Toro García, Á.; Valera-Donoso, E.; Garrido-Ardila, E.M.; Jiménez-Palomares, M.; González López-Arza, M.V. Effectiveness of dry needling on reducing pain intensity in patients with myofascial pain syndrome. A Meta-analysis. *J. Tradit. Chin. Med. = Chung I Tsa Chih Ying Wen Pan* **2016**, *36*, 1–13. [CrossRef]
110. Cagnie, B.; Castelein, B.; Pollie, F.; Steelant, L.; Verhoeyen, H.; Cools, A. Evidence for the Use of Ischemic Compression and Dry Needling in the Management of Trigger Points of the Upper Trapezius in Patients with Neck Pain: A Systematic Review. *Am. J. Phys. Med. Rehabil.* **2015**, *94*, 573–583. [CrossRef] [PubMed]
111. Ong, J.; Claydon, L.S. The effect of dry needling for myofascial trigger points in the neck and shoulder: A systematic review and meta-analysis. *J. Bodyw. Mov. Ther.* **2014**, *18*, 390–398. [CrossRef] [PubMed]
112. Kietrys, D.M.; Palombaro, K.M.; Azzaretto, E.; Hubler, R.; Schaller, B.; Schlussel, J.M.; Tucker, M. Effectiveness of dry needling for upper-quarter myofascial pain: A systematic review and meta-analysis. *J. Orthop. Sports Phys. Ther.* **2013**, *43*, 620–634. [CrossRef] [PubMed]
113. Tough, E.A.; White, A.R. Effectiveness of acupuncture/dry needling for myofascial trigger point pain. *Phys. Ther. Rev.* **2011**, *16*, 147–154. [CrossRef]
114. Cotchett, M.P.; Landorf, K.B.; Munteanu, S.E. Effectiveness of dry needling and injections of myofascial trigger points associated with plantar heel pain. A systematic review. *J. Foot Ankle Res.* **2010**, *3*, 18. [CrossRef]
115. Tough, E.A.; White, A.R.; Cummings, T.M.; Richards, S.H.; Campbell, J.L. Acupuncture and dry needling in the management of myofascial trigger point pain: A systematic review and meta-analysis of randomised controlled trials. *Eur. J. Pain* **2009**, *13*, 3–10. [CrossRef]
116. Cummings, T.M.; White, A.R. Needling therapies in the management of myofascial trigger point pain: A systematic review. *Arch. Phys. Med. Rehabil.* **2001**, *82*, 986–992. [CrossRef]
117. Chiu, H.Y.; Hsieh, Y.J.; Tsai, P.S. Systematic review and meta-analysis of acupuncture to reduce cancer-related pain. *Eur. J. Cancer Care* **2017**, *26*. [CrossRef]
118. Hu, C.; Zhang, H.; Wu, W.; Yu, W.; Li, Y.; Bai, J.; Luo, B.; Li, S. Acupuncture for Pain Management in Cancer: A Systematic Review and Meta-Analysis. *Evid.-Based Complement. Altern. Med.* **2016**, *2016*, 1720239. [CrossRef] [PubMed]
119. Paley, C.A.; Johnson, M.I.; Tashani, O.A.; Bagnall, A.-M. Acupuncture for cancer pain in adults. *Cochrane Database Syst. Rev.* **2015**. [CrossRef] [PubMed]
120. Lian, W.-L.; Pan, M.-Q.; Zhou, D.-H.; Zhang, Z.-J. Effectiveness of acupuncture for palliative care in cancer patients: A systematic review. *Chin. J. Integr. Med.* **2014**, *20*, 136–147. [CrossRef] [PubMed]
121. Garcia, M.K.; McQuade, J.; Haddad, R.; Patel, S.; Lee, R.; Yang, P.; Palmer, J.L.; Cohen, L. Systematic review of acupuncture in cancer care: A synthesis of the evidence. *J. Clin. Oncol.* **2013**, *31*, 952–960. [CrossRef] [PubMed]
122. Choi, T.-Y.; Lee, M.; Kim, T.-H.; Zaslawski, C.; Ernst, E. Acupuncture for the treatment of cancer pain: A systematic review of randomised clinical trials. *Support. Care Cancer* **2012**, *20*, 1147–1158. [CrossRef] [PubMed]
123. Paley, C.; Johnson, M.; Tashani, O.; Bagnall, A.-M. Acupuncture for cancer pain in adults. *Cochrane Database Syst. Rev.* **2011**. [CrossRef]
124. Peng, H.; Peng, H.; Xu, L.; Lao, L. Efficacy of acupuncture in treatment of cancer pain: A systematic review. *J. Chin. Integr. Med.* **2010**, *8*, 501–509. [CrossRef]
125. Ernst, E.; Lee, M.S. Acupuncture for Palliative and Supportive Cancer Care: A Systematic Review of Systematic Reviews. *J. Pain Sympt. Man.* **2010**, *40*, e3–e5. [CrossRef]
126. Lee, H.; Schmidt, K.; Ernst, E. Acupuncture for the relief of cancer-related pain—A systematic review. *Eur. J. Pain* **2005**, *9*, 437–444. [CrossRef]
127. Zhang, X.-C.; Chen, H.; Xu, W.-T.; Song, Y.-Y.; Gu, Y.-H.; Ni, G.-X. Acupuncture therapy for fibromyalgia. A systematic review and meta-analysis of randomized controlled trials. *J. Pain Res.* **2019**, *12*, 527–542. [CrossRef]
128. Kim, J.; Kim, S.-R.; Lee, H.; Nam, D.-H. Comparing Verum and Sham Acupuncture in Fibromyalgia Syndrome. A Systematic Review and Meta-Analysis. *Evid.-Based Complement. Altern. Med.* **2019**, *2019*, 13. [CrossRef] [PubMed]

129. Yang, B.; Yi, G.; Hong, W.; Bo, C.; Wang, Z.; Liu, Y.; Xue, Z.; Li, Y. Efficacy of acupuncture on fibromyalgia syndrome: A meta-analysis. *J. Tradit. Chin. Med.* **2014**, *34*, 381–391. [PubMed]
130. Cao, H.; Li, X.; Han, M.; Liu, J. Acupoint stimulation for fibromyalgia. A systematic review of randomized controlled trials. *Evid.-Based Complement. Altern. Med.* **2013**, *2013*, 362831. [CrossRef] [PubMed]
131. Deare, J.C.; Zheng, Z.; Xue, C.C.L.; Liu, J.P.; Shang, J.; Scott, S.W.; Littlejohn, G. Acupuncture for treating fibromyalgia. *Cochrane Database Syst. Rev.* **2013**. [CrossRef] [PubMed]
132. Cao, H.; Liu, J.; Lewith, G.T. Traditional Chinese Medicine for treatment of fibromyalgia: A systematic review of randomized controlled trials. *J. Altern. Complement. Med. (N. Y.)* **2010**, *16*, 397–409. [CrossRef] [PubMed]
133. Langhorst, J.; Klose, P.; Musial, F.; Irnich, D.; Häuser, W. Efficacy of acupuncture in fibromyalgia syndrome—A systematic review with a meta-analysis of controlled clinical trials. *Rheumatology* **2010**, *49*, 778–788. [CrossRef]
134. Martin-Sanchez, E.; Torralba, E.; Díaz-Domínguez, E.; Barriga, A.; Martin, J.L.R. Efficacy of Acupuncture for the Treatment of Fibromyalgia: Systematic Review and Meta-Analysis of Randomized Trials. *Open Rheumatol. J.* **2009**, *3*, 25–29. [CrossRef]
135. Mayhew, E.; Ernst, E. Acupuncture for fibromyalgia–a systematic review of randomized clinical trials. *Rheumatology* **2007**, *46*, 801–804. [CrossRef]
136. Berman, B.; Ezzo, J.; Hadhazy, V.; Swyers, J. Is acupuncture effective in the treatment of fibromyalgia. *J. Fam. Pract.* **1999**, *48*, 213–218.
137. Qin, Z.; Wu, J.; Xu, C.; Sang, X.; Li, X.; Huang, G.; Liu, Z. Long-term effects of acupuncture for chronic prostatitis/chronic pelvic pain syndrome. Systematic review and single-arm meta-analyses. *Ann. Transl. Med.* **2019**, *7*, 113. [CrossRef]
138. Zhang, F.; Sun, M.; Han, S.; Shen, X.; Luo, Y.; Zhong, D.; Zhou, X.; Liang, F.; Jin, R. Acupuncture for Primary Dysmenorrhea. An Overview of Systematic Reviews. *Evid.-Based Complement. Altern. Med.* **2018**, *2018*, 8791538. [CrossRef] [PubMed]
139. Woo, H.L.; Ji, H.R.; Pak, Y.K.; Lee, H.; Heo, S.J.; Lee, J.M.; Park, K.S. The efficacy and safety of acupuncture in women with primary dysmenorrhea. A systematic review and meta-analysis. *Medicine* **2018**, *97*, e11007. [CrossRef] [PubMed]
140. Sung, S.-H.; Sung, A.-D.-M.; Sung, H.-K.; An, T.-E.B.; Kim, K.H.; Park, J.-K. Acupuncture Treatment for Chronic Pelvic Pain in Women. A Systematic Review and Meta-Analysis of Randomized Controlled Trials. *Evid.-Based Complement. Altern. Med.* **2018**, *2018*, 9415897. [CrossRef] [PubMed]
141. Chang, S.-C.; Hsu, C.-H.; Hsu, C.-K.; Yang, S.S.-D.; Chang, S.-J. The efficacy of acupuncture in managing patients with chronic prostatitis/chronic pelvic pain syndrome. A systemic review and meta-analysis. *Neurourol. Urodyn.* **2017**, *36*, 474–481. [CrossRef] [PubMed]
142. Liu, T.; Yu, J.-N.; Cao, B.-Y.; Peng, Y.-Y.; Chen, Y.-P.; Zhang, L. Acupuncture for Primary Dysmenorrhea: A Meta-analysis of Randomized Controlled Trials. *Altern. Ther. Health Med.* **2017**, *23*, AT5435.
143. Xu, Y.; Zhao, W.; Li, T.; Zhao, Y.; Bu, H.; Song, S. Effects of acupuncture for the treatment of endometriosis-related pain. A systematic review and meta-analysis. *PLoS ONE* **2017**, *12*, e0186616. [CrossRef]
144. Xu, Y.; Zhao, W.; Li, T.; Bu, H.; Zhao, Z.; Zhao, Y.; Song, S. Effects of acupoint-stimulation for the treatment of primary dysmenorrhoea compared with NSAID. A systematic review and meta-analysis of 19 RCTs. *BMC Complement. Altern. Med.* **2017**, *17*, 436. [CrossRef]
145. Xu, T.; Hui, L.; Juan, Y.L.; Min, S.G.; Hua, W.T. Effects of moxibustion or acupoint therapy for the treatment of primary dysmenorrhea. A meta-analysis. *Altern. Ther. Health Med.* **2014**, *20*, 33–42.
146. Chen, M.-N.; Chien, L.-W.; Liu, C.-F. Acupuncture or Acupressure at the Sanyinjiao (SP6) Acupoint for the Treatment of Primary Dysmenorrhea. A Meta-Analysis. *Evid.-Based Complement. Altern. Med.* **2013**, *2013*, 493038. [CrossRef]
147. Chung, Y.-C.; Chen, H.-H.; Yeh, M.-L. Acupoint stimulation intervention for people with primary dysmenorrhea: Systematic review and meta-analysis of randomized trials. *Complement. Ther. Med.* **2012**, *20*, 353–363. [CrossRef]
148. Cohen, J.M.; Fagin, A.P.; Hariton, E.; Niska, J.R.; Pierce, M.W.; Kuriyama, A.; Whelan, J.S.; Jackson, J.L.; Dimitrakoff, J.D. Therapeutic intervention for chronic prostatitis/chronic pelvic pain syndrome (CP/CPPS) A systematic review and meta-analysis. *PLoS ONE* **2012**, *7*, e41941. [CrossRef] [PubMed]
149. Posadzki, P.; Zhang, J.; Lee, M.S.; Ernst, E. Acupuncture for Chronic Nonbacterial Prostatitis/Chronic Pelvic Pain Syndrome: A Systematic Review. *J. Androl.* **2012**, *33*, 15–21. [CrossRef] [PubMed]

150. Zhu, X.; Hamilton, K.D.; McNicol, E.D. Acupuncture for pain in endometriosis. *Cochrane Database Syst. Rev.* **2011**. [CrossRef] [PubMed]
151. Cho, S.H.; Hwang, E.W. Acupuncture for primary dysmenorrhoea: A systematic review. *BJOJ Int. J. Obstet. Gynaecol.* **2010**, *117*, 509–521. [CrossRef] [PubMed]
152. Ee, C.C.; Manheimer, E.; Pirotta, M.V.; White, A.R. Acupuncture for pelvic and back pain in pregnancy: A systematic review. *Am. J. Obstet. Gynecol.* **2008**, *198*, 254–259. [CrossRef] [PubMed]
153. Ramos, A.; Domínguez, J.; Gutiérrez, S. Acupuncture for rheumatoid arthritis. *Medwave* **2018**, *18*, e7284. [CrossRef] [PubMed]
154. Seca, S.; Miranda, D.; Cardoio, D.; Nogueira, B.; Greten, H.J.; Cabrita, A.; Alves, M. Effectiveness of Acupuncture on Pain, Physical Function and Health-Related Quality of Life in Patients with Rheumatoid Arthritis. A Systematic Review of Quantitative Evidence. *Chin. J. Integr. Med.* **2019**, *25*, 704–709. [CrossRef]
155. Lu, W.-W.; Zhang, J.-M.; Lv, Z.-T.; Chen, A.-M. Update on the Clinical Effect of Acupuncture Therapy in Patients with Gouty Arthritis: Systematic Review and Meta-Analysis. *Evid.-Based Complement. Altern. Med. ECAM* **2016**, *2016*, 9451670. [CrossRef]
156. Lee, W.B.; Woo, S.H.; Min, B.-I.; Cho, S.-H. Acupuncture for gouty arthritis: A concise report of a systematic and meta-analysis approach. *Rheumatology* **2013**, *52*, 1225–1232. [CrossRef]
157. Lee, M.S.; Shin, B.C.; Ernst, E. Acupuncture for rheumatoid arthritis: A systematic review. *Rheumatology* **2008**, *47*, 1747–1753. [CrossRef]
158. Wang, C.; de Pablo, P.; Chen, X.; Schmid, C.; McAlin, T. Acupuncture for pain relief in patients with rheumatoid arthritis. A systematic review. *Arthritis Rheum.* **2008**, *59*, 1249–1256. [CrossRef] [PubMed]
159. Casimiro, L.; Barnsley, L.; Brosseau, L.; Milne, S.; Welch, V.; Tugwell, P.; Wells, G.A. Acupuncture and electroacupuncture for the treatment of rheumatoid arthritis. *Cochrane Database Syst. Rev.* **2005**. [CrossRef] [PubMed]
160. Lautenschlager, J. Acupuncture in treatment of inflammatory rheumatoid diseases. *Z. Fur Rheumatol.* **1997**, *56*, 8–20. [CrossRef] [PubMed]
161. Pei, W.; Zeng, J.; Lu, L.; Lin, G.; Ruan, J. Is acupuncture an effective postherpetic neuralgia treatment: A systematic review and meta-analysis. *J. Pain Res.* **2019**, *12*, 2155–2165. [CrossRef] [PubMed]
162. Hu, H.; Chen, L.; Ma, R.; Gao, H.; Fang, J. Acupuncture for primary trigeminal neuralgia. A systematic review and PRISMA-compliant meta-analysis. *Complement. Ther. Clin. Pract.* **2019**, *34*, 254–267. [CrossRef] [PubMed]
163. Oh, P.J.; Kim, Y.L. Effectiveness of Non-Pharmacologic Interventions in Chemotherapy Induced Peripheral Neuropathy. A Systematic Review and Meta-Analysis. *J. Korean Acad. Nurs.* **2018**, *48*, 123–142. [CrossRef]
164. Wang, L.-Q.; Chen, Z.; Zhang, K.; Liang, N.; Yang, G.-Y.; Lai, L.; Liu, J.-P. Zusanli (ST36) Acupoint Injection for Diabetic Peripheral Neuropathy: A Systematic Review of Randomized Controlled Trials. *J. Altern. Complement. Med. (N. Y.)* **2018**. [CrossRef]
165. Wang, Y.; Li, W.; Peng, W.; Zhou, J.; Liu, Z. Acupuncture for postherpetic neuralgia. Systematic review and meta-analysis. *Medicine* **2018**, *97*, e11986. [CrossRef]
166. Dimitrova, A.; Murchison, C.; Oken, B. Acupuncture for the Treatment of Peripheral Neuropathy. A Systematic Review and Meta-Analysis. *J. Altern. Complement. Med. (N. Y.)* **2017**, *23*, 164–179. [CrossRef]
167. Ju, Z.Y.; Wang, K.; Cui, H.S.; Yao, Y.; Liu, S.M.; Zhou, J.; Chen, T.Y.; Xia, J. Acupuncture for neuropathic pain in adults. *Cochrane Database Syst. Rev.* **2017**. [CrossRef]
168. Franconi, G.; Manni, L.; Schröder, S.; Marchetti, P.; Robinson, N. A systematic review of experimental and clinical acupuncture in chemotherapy-induced peripheral neuropathy. *Evid.-Based Complement. Altern. Med.* **2013**, *2013*, 516916. [CrossRef] [PubMed]
169. Sim, H.; Shin, B.-C.; Lee, M.S.; Jung, A.; Lee, H.; Ernst, E. Acupuncture for Carpal Tunnel Syndrome: A Systematic Review of Randomized Controlled Trials. *J. Pain* **2011**, *12*, 307–314. [CrossRef] [PubMed]
170. Liu, H.; Li, H.; Xu, M.; Chung, K.-F.; Zhang, S.P. A systematic review on acupuncture for trigeminal neuralgia. *Altern. Ther. Health Med.* **2010**, *16*, 30–35. [PubMed]
171. Longworth, W.; McCarthy, P.W. A review of research on acupuncture for the treatment of lumbar disk protrusions and associated neurological symptomatology. *J. Altern Complement. Med.* **1997**, *3*, 55–76. [CrossRef] [PubMed]

172. Vier, C.; Almeida, M.B.d.; Neves, M.L.; Santos, A.R.S.D.; Bracht, M.A. The effectiveness of dry needling for patients with orofacial pain associated with temporomandibular dysfunction. A systematic review and meta-analysis. *Braz. J. Phys. Ther.* **2019**, *23*, 3–11. [CrossRef] [PubMed]
173. Kim, T.-H.; Kang, J.W.; Lee, T.H. Therapeutic options for aromatase inhibitor-associated arthralgia in breast cancer survivor. A systematic review of systematic reviews, evidence mapping, and network meta-analysis. *Maturitas* **2018**, *118*, 29–37. [CrossRef]
174. Pan, H.; Jin, R.; Li, M.; Liu, Z.; Xie, Q.; Wang, P. The Effectiveness of Acupuncture for Osteoporosis: A Systematic Review and Meta-Analysis. *Am. J. Chin. Med.* **2018**, *46*, 489–513. [CrossRef]
175. Chau, J.P.C.; Lo, S.H.S.; Yu, X.; Choi, K.C.; Lau, A.Y.L.; Wu, J.C.Y.; Lee, V.W.Y.; Cheung, W.H.N.; Ching, J.Y.L.; Thompson, D.R. Effects of Acupuncture on the Recovery Outcomes of Stroke Survivors with Shoulder Pain: A Systematic Review. *Front. Neurol.* **2018**, *9*, 30. [CrossRef]
176. Luo, D.; Liu, Y.; Wu, Y.; Ma, R.; Wang, L.; Gu, R.; Fu, W. Warm needle acupuncture in primary osteoporosis management. A systematic review and meta-analysis. *Acupunct. Med. J. Br. Med. Acupunct. Soc.* **2018**, *36*, 215–221. [CrossRef]
177. Hall, M.L.; Mackie, A.C.; Ribeiro, D.C. Effects of dry needling trigger point therapy in the shoulder region on patients with upper extremity pain and dysfunction. A systematic review with meta-analysis. *Physiotherapy* **2018**, *104*, 167–177. [CrossRef]
178. Chen, L.; Lin, C.-C.; Huang, T.-W.; Kuan, Y.-C.; Huang, Y.-H.; Chen, H.-C.; Kao, C.-Y.; Su, C.-M.; Tam, K.-W. Effect of acupuncture on aromatase inhibitor-induced arthralgia in patients with breast cancer. A meta-analysis of randomized controlled trials. *Breast* **2017**, *33*, 132–138. [CrossRef] [PubMed]
179. Fernandes, A.C.; Duarte Moura, D.M.; Da Silva, L.G.D.; De Almeida, E.O.; Barbosa, G.A.S. Acupuncture in Temporomandibular Disorder Myofascial Pain Treatment: A Systematic Review. *J. Oral Facial Pain Headache* **2017**, *31*, 225–232. [CrossRef] [PubMed]
180. Thiagarajah, A.G. How effective is acupuncture for reducing pain due to plantar fasciitis? *Singap. Med. J.* **2017**, *58*, 92–97. [CrossRef] [PubMed]
181. Lee, S.-H.; Lim, S.M. Acupuncture for Poststroke Shoulder Pain. A Systematic Review and Meta-Analysis. *Evid.-Based Complement. Altern. Med.* **2016**, *2016*, 3549878. [CrossRef] [PubMed]
182. Wang, K.-F.; Zhang, L.-J.; Lu, F.; Lu, Y.-H.; Yang, C.-H. Can Ashi points stimulation have specific effects on shoulder pain: A systematic review of randomized controlled trials. *Chin. J. Integr. Med.* **2016**, *22*, 467–472. [CrossRef]
183. Tang, H.; Fan, H.; Chen, J.; Yang, M.; Yi, X.; Dai, G.; Chen, J.; Tang, L.; Rong, H.; Wu, J.; et al. Acupuncture for Lateral Epicondylitis. A Systematic Review. *Evid.-Based Complement. Altern. Med.* **2015**, *2015*, 861849. [CrossRef]
184. Chang, W.-D.; Lai, P.-T.; Tsou, Y.-A. Analgesic effect of manual acupuncture and laser acupuncture for lateral epicondylalgia. A systematic review and meta-analysis. *Am. J. Chin. Med.* **2014**, *42*, 1301–1314. [CrossRef]
185. Lee, J.A.; Park, S.-W.; Hwang, P.W.; Lim, S.M.; Kook, S.; Choi, K.I.; Kang, K.S. Acupuncture for shoulder pain after stroke. A systematic review. *J. Altern. Complement. Med. (N. Y.)* **2012**, *18*, 818–823. [CrossRef]
186. Clark, R.J.; Tighe, M. The effectiveness of acupuncture for plantar heel pain: A systematic review. *Acupunct. Med. J. Br. Med. Acupunct. Soc.* **2012**, *30*, 298–306. [CrossRef]
187. Smith, C.A.; Collins, C.T.; Crowther, C.A.; Levett, K.M. Acupuncture or acupressure for pain management in labour. *Cochrane Database Syst. Rev.* **2011**, CD009232. [CrossRef]
188. Cho, S.H.; Lee, H.; Ernst, E. Acupuncture for pain relief in labour. A systematic review and meta-analysis. *BJOG Int. J. Obstet. Gynaecol.* **2010**, *117*, 907–920. [CrossRef] [PubMed]
189. La Touche, R.; Goddard, G.; De-la-Hoz, J.L.; Wang, K.; Paris-Alemany, A.; Angulo-Díaz-Parreño, S.; Mesa, J.; Hernández, M. Acupuncture in the treatment of pain in temporomandibular disorder. A systematic review and meta-analysis of randomized controlled trials. *Clin. J. Pain* **2010**, *26*, 541–550. [CrossRef] [PubMed]
190. Fink, M.; Rosted, P.; Bernateck, M.; Stiesch-Scholz, M.; Karst, M. Acupuncture in the treatment of painful dysfunction of the temporomandibular joint-a review of the literature. *Forsch. Komplement. Und Klass. Nat.* **2006**, *13*, 109–115. [CrossRef] [PubMed]
191. Green, S.; Buchbinder, R.; Hetrick, S. Acupuncture for shoulder pain. *Cochrane Database Syst. Rev.* **2005**, CD005319. [CrossRef] [PubMed]
192. Trinh, K.V.; Phillips, S.D.; Ho, E.; Damsma, K. Acupuncture for the alleviation of lateral epicondyle pain: A systematic review. *Rheumatology* **2004**, *43*, 1085–1090. [CrossRef] [PubMed]

193. Lee, H.; Ernst, E. Acupuncture for labour pain management. *Am. J. Obs. Gynecol.* **2004**, *191*, 1573–1579. [CrossRef]
194. Green, S.; Buchbinder, R.; Barnsley, L.; Hall, S.; White, M.; Smidt, N.; Assendelft, W. Acupuncture for lateral elbow pain. *Cochrane Database Syst. Rev.* **2002**, CD003527. [CrossRef]
195. Rosted, P. Practical recommendations for the use of acupuncture in the treatment of temporomandibular disorders based on the outcome of published controlled studies. *Oral Dis.* **2001**, *7*, 109–115. [CrossRef]
196. Ernst, E.; White, A.R. Acupuncture as a treatment for temporomandibular joint dysfunction-A systematic review of randomized trials. *Arch. Otolaryngol. Head Neck Surg.* **1999**, *125*, 269–272. [CrossRef]
197. Rosted, P. The use of acupuncture in dentistry: A systematic review. *Acupunct. Med.* **1998**, *16*, 43–48. [CrossRef]
198. NICE. Osteoarthritis: Care and Management. Available online: http//nice.org.uk/guidance/cg177 (accessed on 29 August 2019).
199. NICE. *Improving Supportive and Palliative Care for Adults with Cancer*; National Institute for Clinical Excellence: London, UK, 2004.
200. NICE. Endometriosis: Diagnosis and Management. Available online: http://www.nice.org.uk/guidance/NG73 (accessed on 17 October 2019).
201. NICE. Rheumatoid Arthritis in Adults. Available online: https://www.nice.org.uk/guidance/ng100 (accessed on 17 October 2019).
202. NICE. Neuropathic Pain in Adults: Pharmacological Management in Non-Specialist Settings. Available online: https://www.nice.org.uk/guidance/cg173 (accessed on 13 October 2019).
203. Turner, R.M.; Bird, S.M.; Higgins, J.P.T. The impact of study size on meta-analyses. Examination of underpowered studies in Cochrane reviews. *PLoS ONE* **2013**, *8*, e59202. [CrossRef] [PubMed]
204. Dechartres, A.; Altman, D.G.; Trinquart, L.; Boutron, I.; Ravaud, P. Association Between Analytic Strategy and Estimates of Treatment Outcomes in Meta-analyses. *JAMA* **2014**, *312*, 623–630. [CrossRef] [PubMed]
205. Roberts, I.; Ker, K. Cochran the unfinished symphony of research synthesis. *Syst. Rev.* **2016**, *5*, 115. [CrossRef] [PubMed]
206. Moore, R.A.; Moore, O.A.; Derry, S.; Peloso, P.M.; Gammaitoni, A.R.; Wang, H. Responder analysis for pain relief and numbers needed to treat in a meta-analysis of etoricoxib osteoarthritis trial. Bridging a gap between clinical trials and clinical practice. *Ann. Rheum. Dis.* **2010**, *69*, 374–379. [CrossRef] [PubMed]
207. Moore, R.A.; Derry, S.; Wiffen, P.J. Challenges in design and interpretation of chronic pain trials. *Br. J. Anaesth.* **2013**, *111*, 38–45. [CrossRef] [PubMed]
208. Campbell, J.; King, N.B. "Unsettling circularity": Clinical trial enrichment and the evidentiary politics of chronic pain. *BioSocieties* **2017**, *12*, 191–216. [CrossRef]
209. Crow, R.; Gage, H.; Hampson, S.; Hart, J.; Kimber, A.; Thomas, H. The role of expectancies in the placebo effect and their use in the delivery of health care: A systematic review. *Health Technol. Assess.* **1999**, *3*, 1–96. [CrossRef]
210. Benedetti, F. Mechanisms of Placebo and Placebo-Related Effects Across Diseases and Treatments. *Annu. Rev. Pharmacol. Toxicol.* **2008**, *48*, 33–60. [CrossRef]
211. Lund, I.; Lundeberg, T. Are minimal, superficial or sham acupuncture procedures acceptable as inert placebo controls? *Acupunct. Med.* **2006**, *24*, 13–15. [CrossRef]
212. Appleyard, I.; Lundeberg, T.; Robinson, N. Should systematic reviews assess the risk of bias from sham–placebo acupuncture control procedures? *Eur. J. Integr. Med.* **2014**, *6*, 234–243. [CrossRef]
213. Deyo, R.A.; Walsh, N.E.; Schoenfeld, L.S.; Ramamurthy, S. Can trials of physical treatments be blinded? The example of transcutaneous electrical nerve stimulation for chronic pain. *Am. J. Phys. Med. Rehabil./Assoc. Acad. Physiatr.* **1990**, *69*, 6–10. [CrossRef] [PubMed]
214. White, A.; Cummings, M.; Barlas, P.; Cardini, F.; Filshie, J.; Foster, N.E.; Lundeberg, T.; Stener-Victorin, E.; Witt, C. Defining an adequate dose of acupuncture using a neurophysiological approach-a narrative review of the literature. *Acupunct. Med.* **2008**, *26*, 111–120. [CrossRef] [PubMed]
215. MacPherson, H.; Maschino, A.C.; Lewith, G.; Foster, N.E.; Witt, C.M.; Vickers, A.J. Characteristics of acupuncture treatment associated with outcome: An individual patient meta-analysis of 17,922 patients with chronic pain in randomised controlled trials. *PLoS ONE* **2013**, *8*, e77438. [CrossRef]
216. Vas, J.; White, A. Evidence from RCTs on optimal acupuncture treatment for knee osteoarthritis—An exploratory review. *Acupunct. Med.* **2007**, *25*, 29–35. [CrossRef]

217. Schulz, K.F.; Altman, D.G.; Moher, D.; Group, T.C. CONSORT 2010 Statement. Updated guidelines for reporting parallel group randomised trials. *BMC Med.* **2010**, *8*, 18. [CrossRef]
218. MacPherson, H.; White, A.; Cummings, M.; Jobst, K.A.; Rose, K.; Niemtzow, R.C. Standards for Reporting Interventions in Controlled Trials of Acupuncture. The STRICTA Recommendations. *J. Altern. Complement. Med.* **2002**, *8*, 85–89. [CrossRef]
219. MacPherson, H.; Altman, D.G.; Hammerschlag, R.; Li, Y.; Wu, T.; White, A.; Moher, D.; on behalf of the STRICTA Revision Group. Revised STandards for Reporting Interventions in Clinical Trials of Acupuncture (STRICTA): Extending the CONSORT Statement. *PLoS Med.* **2010**, *7*, e1000261. [CrossRef]
220. Svenkerud, S.; MacPherson, H. The Impact of Stricta and Consort on Reporting of Randomised Control Trials of Acupuncture A Systematic Methodological Evaluation. *Acupunct. Med.* **2018**, *36*, 349–357. [CrossRef]
221. Ma, B.; Chen, Z.-M.; Xu, J.-K.; Wang, Y.-N.; Chen, K.-Y.; Ke, F.-Y.; Niu, J.-Q.; Li, L.; Huang, C.-B.; Zheng, J.-X.; et al. Do the CONSORT and STRICTA Checklists Improve the Reporting Quality of Acupuncture and Moxibustion Randomized Controlled Trials Published in Chinese Journals. A Systematic Review and Analysis of Trends. *PLoS ONE* **2016**, *11*, e0147244. [CrossRef]
222. Liu, Y.; Zhang, R.; Huang, J.; Zhao, X.; Liu, D.; Sun, W.; Mai, Y.; Zhang, P.; Wang, Y.; Cao, H.; et al. Reporting Quality of Systematic Reviews/Meta-Analyses of Acupuncture. *PLoS ONE* **2014**, *9*, e113172. [CrossRef]
223. Gu, J.; Wang, Q.; Wang, X.; Li, H.; Gu, M.; Ming, H.; Dong, X.; Yang, K.; Wu, H. Assessment of Registration Information on Methodological Design of Acupuncture RCT: A Review of 453 Registration Records Retrieved from WHO International Clinical Trials Registry Platform. *J. Altern. Complement. Med.* **2014**, *2014*, 614850. [CrossRef] [PubMed]
224. McQuay, H.J.; Derry, S.; Moore, R.A.; Poulain, P.; Legout, V. Enriched enrolment with randomised withdrawal (EERW): Time for a new look at clinical trial design in chronic pain. *Pain* **2008**, *135*, 217–220. [CrossRef] [PubMed]
225. Moore, R.A.; Wiffen, P.J.; Eccleston, C.; Derry, S.; Baron, R.; Bell, R.F.; Furlan, A.D.; Gilron, I.; Haroutounian, S.; Katz, N.P.; et al. Systematic review of enriched enrolment, randomised withdrawal trial designs in chronic pain. A new framework for design and reporting. *Pain* **2015**, *156*, 1382–1395. [CrossRef] [PubMed]

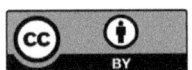

© 2019 by the authors. Licensee MDPI, Basel, Switzerland. This article is an open access article distributed under the terms and conditions of the Creative Commons Attribution (CC BY) license (http://creativecommons.org/licenses/by/4.0/).

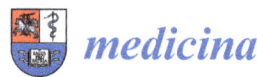

Review

Molecular Basis of Cancer Pain Management: An Updated Review

Ayappa V. Subramaniam, Ashwaq Hamid Salem Yehya and Chern Ein Oon *

Institute for Research in Molecular Medicine (INFORMM), Universiti Sains Malaysia (USM), Pulau Pinang 11800, Malaysia; ayappa725@gmail.com (A.V.S.); ashwaqlabwork@gmail.com (A.H.S.Y.)
* Correspondence: chern.oon@usm.my; Tel.: +60-4623-4879

Received: 29 June 2019; Accepted: 9 September 2019; Published: 12 September 2019

Abstract: Pain can have a significantly negative impact on the quality of life of patients. Therefore, patients may resort to analgesics to relieve the pain. The struggle to manage pain in cancer patients effectively and safely has long been an issue in medicine. Analgesics are the mainstay treatment for pain management as they act through various methods on the peripheral and central pain pathways. However, the variability in the patient genotypes may influence a drug response and adverse drug effects that follow through. This review summarizes the observed effects of analgesics on UDP-glucuronosyl (UGT) 2B7 isoenzyme, cytochrome P450 (CYP) 2D6, μ-opioid receptor μ 1 (OPRM1), efflux transporter P-glycoprotein (P-gp) and ATP-binding cassette B1 ABCB1/multiple drug resistance 1 (MDR1) polymorphisms on the mechanism of action of these drugs in managing pain in cancer. Furthermore, this review article also discusses the responses and adverse effects caused by analgesic drugs in cancer pain management, due to the inter-individual variability in their genomes.

Keywords: cancer; pain management; analgesics; adverse drug effects; polymorphism

---

1. Introduction

Pain is often experienced by cancer patients, particularly those in the advanced stage of disease where the prevalence is estimated to be more than 70% [1]. More than three decades ago, the World Health Organization (WHO) designed the 3-step "analgesic ladder" to facilitate and standardize and to advise pharmacologic cancer pain management and advising physicians worldwide on how to improve pain management in their patients (Figure 1) [1].

However, some patients with advanced cancer have inadequate control of pain with systemic analgesics. These patients may alternatively benefit from the invasive techniques such as neuraxial analgesia for vertebral pain, peripheral nerve blocks, sympathetic blocks for abdominal cancer pain and percutaneous cordotomy [2].

Non-opioids, co-analgesics (e.g., nonsteroidal anti-inflammatory drugs), and non-pharmacological measures, are frequently used to enhance analgesic control and lessen opioid requirements. In addition, they are also used to reduce adverse events related to opioid use [3]. A myriad of genes have been studied to identify biomarkers in opioid therapy. These include genes implicated in the pharmacokinetics (*CYP2D6, CYP3A4/5, ABCB1* and *UGTs,*) and pharmacodynamics (*OPRM1* and *COMT*) of opioids [3]. These genes are studied vastly because they play a key role in drug metabolism.

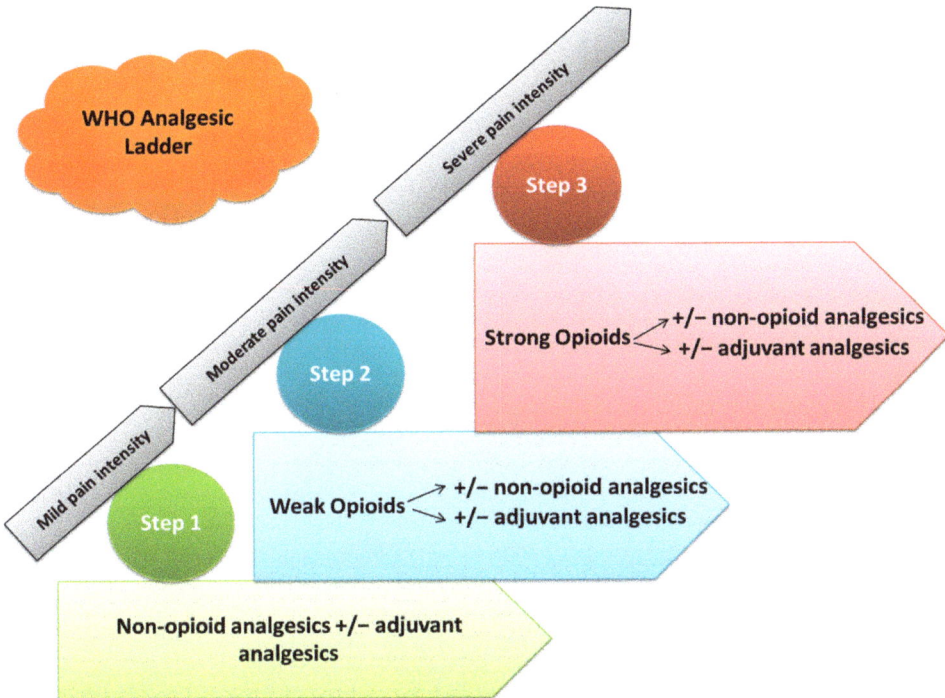

Figure 1. Overview of the analgesic ladder designed by the World Health Organization (WHO).

This review focuses on the different types of drugs that are used in cancer pain therapy and the various enzymes, which are involved in the metabolism of these drugs.

2. Cancer and Analgesics

According to the World Health Organization (WHO) in 1986, the analgesic ladder is the main reference for cancer pain management [4]. Morphine is used in the third step of the WHO analgesic ladder, which functions to treat moderate to severe pain. This step also consists of additional opioids, (e.g., fentanyl, oxycodone, buprenorphine, hydromorphone and methadone) [5]. Supportive drugs such as laxatives and antiemetics are used alongside the analgesic ladder to prevent adverse effects of opioid treatment [6], as well as non-pharmacological measures (radiotherapy, nerve blockades and neurolytic blocks) [7].

The first step the of analgesic ladder is used for treating mild pain and includes non-opioids analgesics, such as acetaminophen (paracetamol), and non-steroidal anti-inflammatory drugs (NSAIDs) with or without adjuvant analgesics [4,8–10]. The second step of the analgesic ladder consists of weak opioids, such as tramadol or codeine, which are used for mild to moderate pain. Lower doses of a step III opioid, such as morphine or oxycodone, should be administered instead of codeine or tramadol, with or without non-opioids analgesics and adjuvant analgesics [5,8–10]. The third step of the analgesic ladder treats moderate to strong pain via strong opioids, such as morphine or oxycodone, with or without non-opioids analgesics and adjuvant analgesics [5,8–10]. The correct application of the WHO pain ladder can help to successfully manage pain and provide effective analgesia for patients.

Chronic pain remains a disturbingly common consequence of cancer and its treatment. Several studies have found that more than 50% of cancer patients experience moderate to severe pain throughout their lifetime [11]. Opioid analgesia is a mainstay treatment of cancer pain. Opioids have also been associated with cancer recurrence [11,12]. Several studies have demonstrated that opioid drug abusers experience heightened sensitivity to viral and bacterial infections. Furthermore, opioids have been proven to show an effect on the function of the immune system to promote carcinogenesis. Although this is biologically plausible, clinical, in vitro and animal evidence is still inconclusive [13,14]. Recent findings have downplayed this hypothesis by stating that only particular types of tumors that possess particular receptors will be more inclined to react to opioid, either positively or negatively [11]. From these findings, it is suggested that opioids play a pivotal role in the management of moderate to severe cancer pain [11].

3. Pain Medication, Opioid Analgesics and Non-Steroidal Anti-Inflammatory Drugs (NSAID) in Cancer Pain Relief

3.1. Morphine

Morphine was first isolated from the opium poppy plant by a German pharmacist, Friedrich Sertürner, between 1803 and 1805. It is still one of the most commonly used drugs to achieve analgesia in cancer pain relief. Morphine acts on μ and κ receptors but its analgesic effect is mediated primarily by the μ receptors. This is confirmed by loss of morphine analgesia in μ receptor knockout mice [15]. The main metabolic pathway utilized by morphine is glucuronidation, which produces morphine-6-glucuronide and morphine-3-glucuronide as by-products. Morphine-6-glucuronide possesses a higher analgesic potency than its parent compound [16,17]. These metabolites are removed by the kidneys, therefore, in kidney disease patients', metabolite concentration may be high and may lead to adverse events [8,18]. A multiple regression analysis, presented maximum pain score as the crucial factor contributing to morphine usage, followed by ethnicity and A118G polymorphism [19]. Advanced cancer patients who suffered pain caused by homozygosity for the 118G allele of the μ-opioid receptor required higher morphine doses to achieve successful pain control. Although the analgesic effects are already partially decreased in heterozygous carriers, the respiratory depressive effects are decreased in homozygous carriers of the variant 118G allele [17]. It has been demonstrated that morphine does not stimulate tumor initiation, however, it does stimulate the growth of an existing breast tumor in a transgenic mouse within an experimental study [20]. Morphine is regarded as an effective analgesic for pain management amongst pediatric patients [9].

3.2. Codeine

Codeine is known as a pro-drug: An inactive metabolite that is converted to its active counterpart. Codeine is a weak opioid that is generally administered after surgery and is used alongside certain drugs to manage acute and chronic pain [21]. The analgesic properties of codeine originate from its conversion to morphine and morphine-6-glucuronide by CYP2D6 [3]. Codeine is the parent compound and has a 200× lower affinity at the opioid receptor than its morphine metabolite [22]. Poor metabolizers possess little or no CYP2D6 enzyme activity and may not achieve a sufficient level of pain control, whereas, a person with extra copies of CYP2D6 (ultra-rapid metabolizers) may convert codeine to morphine to a greater extent. However, they may be at increased risk of adverse events such as sedation or respiratory depression [3,16,18]. Codeine usage is not recommended in the presence of renal failure [8,23]. In addition, its administration in pediatric patients has shown low clinical efficacy and limited effect upon dosage escalation [9]. In August 2012, the FDA advised against prescribing codeine for children after tonsillectomy due to the risk of CYP2D6 life threatening overdose attributed to genetic variation [24].

3.3. Hydrocodone

Hydrocodone is often used in patients with advanced cancer. It is metabolized by CYP2D6 to form the active metabolite hydromorphone, which has a 10× to 33× greater affinity for μ-opioid receptors than hydrocodone [3]. A study has demonstrated an effect of CYP2D6 polymorphisms on hydrocodone metabolite production [25]. Although the effect of CYP2D6 polymorphisms on metabolite production was reported in pharmacokinetic studies, the pain relief experienced by a child who is given hydrocodone is not dependent on metabolism by CYP2D6 [22]. Adverse effects of hydrocodone are similar to other opioids [8]. Hydrocodone is a viable option for children that are known to have a poor metabolizing phenotype [22].

3.4. Hydromorphone

Hydromorphone has a similar structure to morphine and is available as parenteral and oral products [8]. Its potency and high solubility may be beneficial for patients who require a high opioid dosage and for subcutaneous administration [8,18].

3.5. Fentanyl

- Fentanyl is a highly lipophilic opioid and is used for relieving cancer pain in transdermal and transmucosal immediate-release formulations [18]. It is metabolized primarily by CYP3A4/5 to the inactive metabolite, norfentanyl [3]. A118G polymorphisms of *OPRM1* were present in various Asian cohorts' post-surgery and revealed lower fentanyl requirements in A118G-homozygous individuals [26]. The use of fentanyl for children above the age of 2 years has been approved by the FDA and it is one of the most commonly used analgesics amongst pediatric patients [9]. Comparisons made between morphine and transdermal fentanyl have shown an equal analgesic efficacy [8]. Fentanyl can be administered by continuous intravenous or subcutaneous infusion [18]. All the studies found transdermal fentanyl to be cost-effective against oral sustained release morphine with incremental cost-effectiveness ratios of £17,798, £14,487 and £1406 per quality adjusted life years in the studies by Neighbors et al. [27], Radbruch et al. [28] and Greiner et al. [29], respectively for cancer and non-cancer patients with moderate to severe chronic pain [30]. In one study of 60 adult patients with cancer receiving transdermal fentanyl, showed that polymorphisms in the gene *ABCB1* could lead to significant changes in fentanyl plasma concentrations, with the ABCB1 1236TT variant being associated with a lower need for rescue medication. To date there have been no statistically significant findings for fentanyl-related adverse effects, in the previous study or current body of literature [31,32].

3.6. Sufentanyl

Sufentanyl is often used as a replacement to fentanyl when the volume of fentanyl needed for treatment is above the range which can be administered through an injection [33–35]. Sufentanyl is more effective at a lower dose for pain control among patients [33]. It is mostly used for the treatment of patients with renal impairment [34].

3.7. Methadone

The pharmacokinetics of methadone is highly variable. Methadone is a synthetic opioid, which is commonly used as a second-line option in the presence of neuropathic pain in cancer and recognized for its use in the treatment of opioid dependency [26]. Its average half-life is approximately 24 h and can range from less than 15 hours to more than 130 hours. Results from an elegant study by Mercadante and colleagues reported that methadone achieved an analgesic effect and was more stable than morphine in a sample of 40 patients who were treated for two or three times daily according to their clinical needs [8,36]. Its increased usage has become associated with a high rate of serious adverse effects, particularly in populations with non-cancer related pain. However, methadone has a complex metabolism that involves both CYP3A4 and CYP2D6 and is a weak inhibitor of serotonin reuptake [18].

3.8. Levorphanol

Levorphanol is a potent opioid and is similar to methadone and morphine. Levorphanol has a strong affinity for µ, κ and δ opioid receptors [8]. Studies have indicated that levorphanol is an effective treatment for chronic neuropathic pain [8].

3.9. Buprenorphine

Buprenorphine has a high affinity for the µ receptor. Transdermal buprenorphine is available at a higher dosage formulation in other countries compared to the United States and is used for managing cancer pain [18]. Buprenorphine is converted to an active metabolite called norbuprenorphine by CYP3A4 and CYP2C8 metabolism, which is a weaker but full-opioid agonist [8]. Liver disease can affect the metabolism of buprenorphine [8]. Administration of buprenorphine to opioid naive patients or those receiving low-dosage opioid regimen, may induce withdrawal symptoms if physical dependence is present. Therefore, it is wise to limit treatment to cancer patients [18]. In addition, Greiner et al. [29] showed transdermal buprenorphine to be cost-effective against oral sustained release morphine with an incremental cost–effectiveness ratio of £6248 per quality adjusted to years of survival [29,30].

3.10. Oxycodone

Oxycodone is an oral opioid treatment choice for chronic cancer pain, and it is a semi-synthetic opioid prescribed for moderate to severe pain [25]. Oxycodone binds to both µ and κ receptors, but there is uncertainty surrounding the clinical implications of this dual binding [18]. Like hydrocodone, the parent compound possesses identical levels of activity at the opioid receptor as the metabolites [22]. CYP3A4 metabolizes most of the oxycodone to noroxycodone. A smaller percentage is metabolized by CYP2D6 to the active metabolite, oxymorphone, which has a 40× higher affinity and 8× higher potency for µ-opioid receptors than oxycodone [3]. The response of poor metabolizers was from 2× to 20× less than those individuals who were extensive metabolizers [26,37]. Catalyzed by CYP3A4 and CYP2D6, oxycodone is undergoing metabolism in the liver through four different metabolic pathways. When compared to morphine, the resulting metabolites, had different affinities for the µ-opioid receptor, from highest to lowest: oxymorphone > morphine > noroxymorphone > oxycodone > noroxycodone [26]. Oxycodone was more effective than other strong opioids at decreasing pain intensity scores and resulted in a lower incidence of nausea and constipation, suggesting that this drug offers better pain management among cancer patients [10]. Oxycodone was reported to be effective in patients with pancreatic cancer and this was indicated by a significant drop in pain score within 4 weeks [10,38]. The ultra-rapid metabolizer group experienced side effects such as sedation and reduced oxygen saturation more frequently compared to the poor metabolizer group [37]. Patients who are administered oxycodone often experience opioid-induced constipation (OIC) as a side effect of the treatment. In order to counter this, naloxone is co-administered to alleviate or reduce the occurrence of OIC [39]. Naloxone works in terms of binding to the µ-receptor in the gastrointestinal tract. A clinical study comprising 128 patients has revealed that there is no difference in analgesic efficacy between the control group, oxycodone only, and the oxycodone/naloxone treated group [40].

3.11. Tramadol

Tramadol is recommended for patients with moderate, severe nociceptive or neuropathic pain. It is used widely in certain countries, particularly amongst cancer patients who are opioid naive or have limited opioid exposure [18]. It consists of two enantiomers and is a synthetic analog of codeine and morphine, both of which promote analgesic activity via different mechanisms [26]. Tramadol undergoes CYP2D6 dependent O-methylation to demethyltramadol (M1) [26]. However, M1 however has a much higher affinity for the µ-receptor compared to the parent compound but a lower affinity compared to strong opioids [8,17,26]. A higher tramadol dosage will be required to achieve satisfactory pain relief in CYP2D6 PMs compared with Ems [3,41]. (−)-Tramadol inhibits norepinephrine reuptake and (+)-tramadol inhibits serotonin reuptake, thus, pain transmission in the spinal cord is greatly inhibited [26]. Poor metabolizers are characterized by deficient O-demethylation and displays two inactive alleles, resulting in their inability to convert tramadol to O-demethyltramadol and as a consequence, inadequate analgesia [17]. A case report documented that a pediatric ultra-rapid metabolizer experienced respiratory depression following tramadol administration, despite tramadol being a partial opioid [25,26,42]. It has been reported that tramadol is not commonly used to manage pain in pediatric patients and very little data exists for young patients below 16 years of age [9]. Examples of adverse effects produced by tramadol include: Constipation, dizziness, nausea, sedation, dry mouth and vomiting [8].

3.12. Tapentadol

Tapentadol is structurally similar to tramadol and is approved for use in the treatment of severe chronic pain in cancer patients [8]. Tapentadol binds with high affinity to μ, κ and δ opioid receptors. It acts on the μ-opioid receptor and inhibits noradrenaline reuptake [43]. Tapentadol provides analgesic efficacy similar to that of oxycodone when it is first administered at low doses in opioid-naïve patients [43]. However, the incidence of gastrointestinal adverse effects has been reported to be lower in the tapentadol group than in the oxycodone group [43]. Limited occurrence of gastrointestinal adverse side effects from tapentadol may serve as a great advantage in pain management in the context of multifactorial diseases, such as cancer, where other drugs can contribute to induce nausea, vomiting or constipation. However, tapentadol is a relatively new drug and there is minimal published information on its use in cancer pain management [18].

3.13. Non-Steroidal Anti-Inflammatory Drugs (NSAID)

NSAIDs are a group of non-opioid analgesics, which are commonly used for the treatment of acute pain, following surgery or chronic pain [21]. NSAIDs are used alone or alongside opioids, which treat moderate to severe pain. Many NSAIDs are metabolized by the cytochrome enzyme CYP2C9 [44]. Poor metabolizers possess lower CYP2C9 activity compared to wild-type. This results in increased area under the plasma drug concentration–time curve, decreased NSAID clearance and feasibly an increased risk of adverse effects [42]. For multiple NSAIDs, which include flurbiprofen, piroxicam, R-ibuprofen, tenoxicam and celecoxib (a COX-2 inhibitor), the CYP2C9 genotype is an important indicator of metabolic clearance. Individuals who possess the wild-type CYP2C9*1 genotype have a significantly lower systemic exposure compared with individuals that have possessed the CYP2C9*3 genotype [41,45]. Variations in CYP2C9 and CYP2C8 impair the clearance of ibuprofen from the body. This means that the medication remains in the body for much longer than it should, potentially leading to adverse effects, such as gastrointestinal bleeding [46]. Hussain and colleagues reported that NSAIDs have a strong, potential anti-cancer effect. Inhibition of PGE2 production (in addition to COX-2 inhibition) may play a vital role in cancer cell mutation and proliferation. Ultimately, inhibition of PGE2 could possibly stimulate cell mediated immune response, in so doing increasing the cytotoxic abilities of NK cells [20,47].

3.14. Paracetamol (Acetaminophen)

Paracetamol (N-(4-hydroxyphenyl)-acetamide) is one of the most widely used over-the-counter analgesics [48]. Paracetamol has been frequently co-administered with analgesics for treating cancer patients [8,10,18,26,49]. Paracetamol is regarded as the drug of choice for children with pain of a non-inflammatory nature [9]. Glucuronidation was initially recognized to be impaired in patients with Gilbert's syndrome, which is an inherited bilirubin disglucuronidation condition that increases the risk of paracetamol toxicity in affected individuals. A toxic intermediary metabolite, N-acetyl-p-benzoquinoneimine (NAPQI) is produced from cytochrome P450 2E1 and 3A4 metabolism of paracetamol [48]. NAPQI is a toxic compound. An overdose of paracetamol may cause a build-up of NAPQI, leading to paracetamol-induced acute liver failure. A systematic review carried out by

Wiffen and colleagues, have reported that there is no clear evidence that paracetamol used alone or in combination with opioid was able to provide significant pain relief to cancer patients [50].

3.15. Nefopam

Nefopam is a common postoperative non-opioid, non-steroidal analgesia. The main mechanism of analgesic action of nefopam is through the inhibition of serotonin, norepinephrine and dopamine reuptake [51–55]. A clinical study conducted by Kim and colleagues have demonstrated that patients who were administered nefopam 48 hours post renal transplant operation consumed 19% less fentanyl compared to the control group. This study suggests that nefopam as an adjunct to standard analgesia, fentanyl, reduced postoperative fentanyl consumption besides also providing better analgesia [54]. In a novel review by Girard et al. [55], they have compiled the studies where nefopam was used in combinations with opioids, paracetamol and non-steroidal anti-inflammatory drugs in both preclinical and clinical setting. The results have shown that nefopam used in combination with all these drugs has a significantly better analgesic effect in both settings [55]. Nefopam has also shown to reduce acute and chronic postoperative breast cancer surgery for a study group involving 41 patients, where the patients were administered preventive nefopam. In addition, nefopam has also been reported to reduce chronic pain [56]. Another study conducted by Hwang and colleagues have demonstrated that nefopam used in combination with oxycodone reduced the incidence of nausea among 60 patients 6 h post gynecologic surgery [57].

3.16. Metamizole (Dipyrone)

Metamizole is a widely used non-opioid analgesics for the treatment of cancer pain however it is banned in several countries due to its toxicity towards patients who have agranulocytosis [58,59]. Gaertner and colleagues reported a systematic review, which highlighted that metamizole used alone or in combination with opioid were effective in reducing cancer pain. They also reported that at higher doses, metamizole was as effective as morphine 60 mg/day [58,60]. Metamizole in combination with magnesium chloride was shown to reduce cancer pain while also preventing tolerance in a study conducted with murine model of cancer [61]. Hearn and colleagues detailed in their systematic review, from eight studies, 70% of the adult patients with acute postoperative pain who were treated with a single dose of metamizole experienced at least 50% of maximum pain relief over 4–6 h [59].

4. Adjuvant Analgesics in Cancer

Adjuvant analgesic refers to drugs that are marketed for indications other than pain but with analgesic properties in some painful conditions [49]. Drugs such as opioids, non-steroidal anti-inflammatory drugs (NSAIDS), and acetaminophen are usually co-administered with analgesics when treating cancer pain, although they can be used alone. Adjuvant analgesics are usually added to an opioid to reduce adverse effects and to enhance pain relief from opioid [49]. Over the past three decades, the use of these drugs used in clinic has increased dramatically and several are administered as first-line drugs in the treatment of chronic non-malignant pain. However, in cancer pain management, conventional practice has evolved to view opioids as first-line drugs and adjuvant analgesics are usually considered after opioid therapy has been optimized [49]. Adjuvant analgesics are specific for neuropathic pain, which was most recently defined by the International Association for the Study of Pain (IASP) as "Pain arising as a direct consequence of a lesion or disease affecting the somatosensory system" [13,62]. Of cancer pain 40%–50% was characterized by surveys to be wholly or partially neuropathic [49]. The adjuvant analgesics consist of classes of medications with different primary indications (Figure 2). According to conventional use, a group of non-specific analgesics can be differentiated from those used for specific indications, including bone and neuropathic pain.

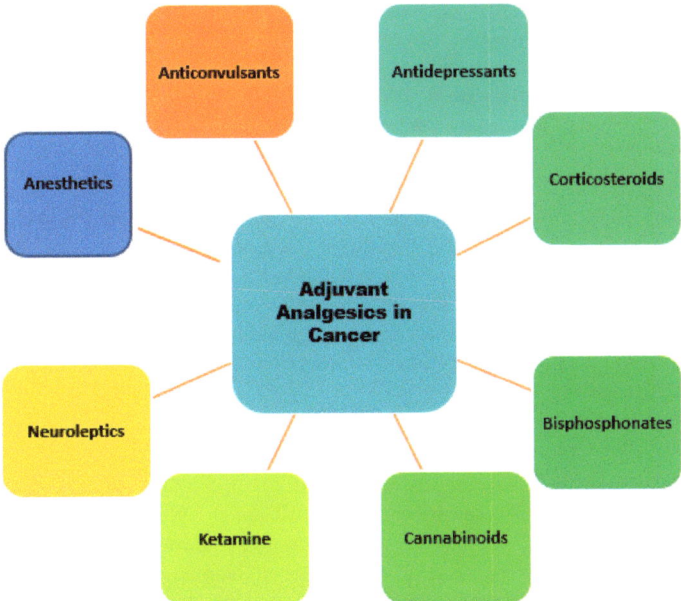

Figure 2. Schematic diagram of adjuvant analgesic drug categories for cancer pain therapy.

4.1. Antidepressants

Antidepressants are a mainstay treatment for neuropathic pain. Antidepressants are most commonly used to treat patients with a history of depression cases. Tricyclic antidepressants (TCA) and the selective serotonin reuptake inhibitors (SSRIs) are common antidepressants used in pain management among patients [8,63]. Serotonin norepinephrine reuptake inhibitors (SNRIs) is a new class of antidepressant used for the treatment of neuropathic pain and is more effective than SSRIs [63]. Antidepressant drugs used in combination with opioid has shown an opioid-sparing effect [63]. TCAs are not recommended to be used for elderly and heart disease patients due to frequent adverse side effects [8,49]. TCA could also potentially exacerbate hypotension among the elderly patients [8]. There are limited studies conducted on antidepressant effects on cancer pain now, as such, future studies should explore this area to provide better pain management among cancer patients.

4.2. Corticosteroids

Corticosteroids are usually used for cancer pain management. Studies have shown that corticosteroid treatment improves the patient's appetite and reduces nausea [49,63]. Bone pain associated metastasis are commonly treated by corticosteroids [63]. Patients who are treated by this treatment may experience sides effects such as hypertension, hyperglycemia, osteoporosis and immunosuppression [63]. High doses of corticosteroids treatment are administered for patients who experience acute pain or spinal cord compression [49,63].

4.3. Anticonvulsants (Gabapentinoids)

The most common anticonvulsant drugs used for managing cancer induced neuropathic pain are gabapentin and pregabalin [8]. Gabapentin must be dose adjusted to avoid the occurrence of adverse events [8,49]. Gabapentin has been shown to reduce cancer induced bone pain, which is caused by bone metastasis besides also, reducing postoperative bone pain [64–66]. Pregabalin is structurally similar to gabapentin but is more potent than its predecessor [63]. Both gabapentin and pregabalin were reported to provide effective pain relief post breast surgery [67–70]. Gabapentinoids are excreted through the renal route, hence patients with renal failure will require lower doses [13]. Phenytoin is another drug in this category that can be used to treat cancer pain [49]. Other anticonvulsant agents have not been studied extensively with regards to cancer pain management [8]. A novel study by Bugan et al. [71] has reported that gabapentin causes pro- and antimetastatic effect.

4.4. Anesthetics

Lidocaine may be administered through the oral, subcutaneous, parenteral and transdermal route [8]. Cancer pain was significantly reduced in a study conducted by Sharma and his colleagues [8,72]. Lidocaine provided prolonged pain relief. Lidocaine are more commonly used for non-neuropathic pains [49]. Lidocaine can be used in combination with other anticonvulsant drugs for patients who response positively to intravenous lidocaine treatment [63]. Another study has reported that the application of topical lidocaine before the surgery has significantly reduced post-surgery pain for breast cancer patients [63,73].

4.5. Ketamine

The use of ketamine in the management of cancer related neuropathic pain produced opioid-sparing effect [8,49,74]. Patients under hospice care are usually administered ketamine on a long-term basis until they pass on [49]. In a contradictory a review written by Jonkman et al. [75], they summarized from four controlled trials that there is lack of evidence that ketamine provides opioid-sparing effect for cancer pain. However, they have also argued that the efficacy of ketamine as a treatment for cancer pain management was not completely ruled out [74–78].

4.6. Neuroleptics

Patients administered with olanzapine was shown to have reduced pain scores and improved cognitive function besides also reduced anxiety [8]. Consumption of opioid after administration of neuroleptics was reported to be decreased [49].

4.7. Bisphosphonates

Bisphosphonates are used in adjunction during treatment of cancer due to the high occurrence of cancer induced bone pain. Patients under palliative care often experience bone pain. Bisphosphonates have been shown to improve pain management among patients with breast, prostate or lung cancer [8]. One bisphosphonate that has been studied widely is pamidronate, which has shown its efficacy in breast cancer patients [49]. The bone density of patients treated with pamidronate improved over time [63]. Another drug, zoledronic acid, which is more potent compared to pamidronate, also decreased cancer induced bone pain in breast, lung, myeloma and prostate cancer [49].

4.8. Cannabinoids

There are limited studies on cannabinoids use in cancer pain management as of now. Tetrahydrocannabinol (THC) and cannabidiol are the two most abundant compounds found in the cannabis plant. Some studies have suggested that the use of cannabinoids as adjunct to opioid, provided significant pain relief [64,79]. Cannabinoids efficacy in treatment of cancer pain may vary based on the population race [80]. Appetite of patients who are under cannabinoid treatment are improved [79,81]. Based on a summarized table produced by Bennett et al. [82], it was clear that the use of cannabinoids for the treatment of neuropathic and cancer related pain, decreased pain with mild adverse effects. The combination of THC and cannabidiol as a treatment has shown to provide significant pain relief among patients [81]. In a recent systematic review by Tateo [83], from eight low or moderate quality randomized clinical trials, cannabinoids were reported to effectively manage cancer pain when administered in combination with opioid. Nonetheless, further investigations must be carried out on the effectiveness of cannabinoids as adjuvant analgesics. There is no clear evidence that cannabinoids are beneficial for the treatment of cancer pain [80,83–85].

4.9. Dexmedetomidine

Dexmedetomidine is sedative drug that is usually used in the intensive care units or for patients who are under hospice or palliative care. Based on a case study reported by Hilliard and colleagues [86], the drug managed to clear the patient's pain and delirium towards the end of her life while also allowing the patient to maintain wakefulness and interact with family members. Two other case studies also revealed that administration of dexmedetomidine, provides opioid-sparing effect and essential for end-of-life care [87,88]. In an elegant study by Yuan and colleagues [89], they have proven that the combination treatment of dexmedetomidine with tramadol provided a better analgesic effect compared to the high dose treatment of tramadol alone in bone cancer rat models. Dexmedetomidine used as an adjunct along with bupivacaine for a single-shot paravertebral block was shown to improve analgesia lasting duration post breast cancer surgery. The combination also reduced opioid consumption and the nausea episodes among patients [90].

5. Enzymes Involved in Drug Metabolism

5.1. CYP2D6

One of the most common CYPs involved in drug metabolism is cytochrome P450 family 2, subfamily D, polypeptide 6 (CYP2D6). In this enzyme in which the metabolic rate can fluctuate by over 100× between the allelic variants expressed in different ethnic groups [21,91]. The genetic polymorphism of this enzyme may result in the generation of four different phenotypes. These are poor metabolizers, intermediate metabolizers, extensive metabolizers and ultra-rapid metabolizers. An individual with a genotype of two non-functioning alleles is a poor metabolizer (PM); at least one reduced functioning allele is an intermediate metabolizer (IM); at least one functional allele is an extensive metabolizer (EM) and multiple copies of a functional allele is an ultra-rapid metabolizer (UM). EM is the most common phenotype [22]. It has been shown that opioids have adverse events in patients at both extremes of function, ultra-rapid and poor. It is for this reason, that we consider both metabolizer extremes (ultra-rapid and poor) as dysfunctional and recommend that CYP2D6 substrate drugs and prodrugs be avoided in these patients [92]. In one non-lethal case, a cancer patient with pneumonia given codeine for cough suppression went into respiratory arrest. Genotyping characterized the patient as a CYP2D6 ultra-rapid metabolizer with a functional gene expansion. Death was averted when the patient was treated with naloxone and fully recovered [92,93]. Analysis on the genetic makeup of patients is crucial in determining the effectiveness and safety of the treatment to avoid adverse events or death (Table 1). The distribution of the CYP2D6 phenotypes varies by ethnicity, mainly due to differences in inherited SNPs [42]. Therefore, determining the status of CYP2D6, could provide guidance in giving out prescriptions and optimize overall cost effectiveness of health care services [24].

Table 1. Genetic variants analyzed on the effectiveness and safety of the administered treatment.

Analgesics	Study Type	Genetic Variants	Side Effect	References
Morphine	Non-randomized clinical trial	Multidrug resistance-1 gene (*MDR-1*)	Moderate or severe drowsiness and confusion or hallucinations.	[94]
		Catechol-O-methyltransferase (COMT) enzyme		
		Single nucleotide polymorphisms (SNPs) in intron 1		
	In vitro study- breast cancer cell lines	*NET1* gene expression (mediating the direct effect of morphine on breast cancer cell migration)		[95]
Codeine	Non-randomized clinical trial	*CYP2D6* gene	Sedation, addiction, dizziness and constipation	[96]
Hydrocodone	Observational study	*CYP2D6* gene	Dizziness and constipation	[97,98]
Hydromorphone	Non-randomized clinical trial	*CYP2D6* gene	Dizziness and constipation	[97,99]
Fentanyl	Non-randomized clinical trial	*CYP3A5* and *ABCB1* gene polymorphisms	Dry mouth, wheal and flare	[100]
	Observational study	Genetic variants rs12948783 (*RHBDF2*) and rs7016778 (*OPRK1*)		[101]
Methadone	Randomized double-blind study	*ABCB1*, *OPRM1* gene polymorphisms	Constipation, nausea, dizziness and delirium	[102,103]
Levorphanol	Non-randomized clinical trial	-	Nausea and vomiting	[104]
Buprenorphine	Non-randomized clinical trial	Polymorphisms in *OPRD1*	Dizziness, dry mouth, thirst and nausea	[105,106]
Oxycodone	Non-randomized clinical trial	*CYP3A5*	Nausea, vomiting, constipation, lightheadedness, dizziness or drowsiness	[107]
Tramadol	Randomized double-blind placebo controlled cross over study	*CYP2D6*	Dizziness, headache, drowsiness, nausea, vomiting, constipation, lack of energy, sweating and dry mouth	[108]
Tapentadol	Non-randomized clinical trial	No genetic variation	Nausea, vomiting, constipation, fatigue, dizziness, sleepiness, drowsiness and dry mouth	[109]
Paracetamol (Acetaminophen)	Randomized double-blind placebo controlled parallel group study	COX-3	Low fever with nausea, stomach pain and loss of appetite	[50]
Non-steroidal Anti-Inflammatory Drugs (NSAID)	Randomized, double-blind, placebo-controlled	COX-1/COX-2	Stomach pain, heartburn, stomach ulcers, a tendency to bleed, headaches, dizziness and ringing in the ears	[110,111]

5.2. CYP2C9

CYP2C9 is the most abundant P450 cytochrome in the liver. Almost 15% of clinically useful drugs, including various NSAIDs is metabolized by this enzyme in the first phase of drug metabolism [48]. Phase 1 metabolism of xenobiotic compounds is important to introduce functional groups or polar groups into the compounds. The products of phase 1 metabolism will readily couple with an endogenous conjugating molecule, which makes the metabolite less toxic and easily eliminated from the body [112]. Over 50 variants have been identified from the highly polymorphic gene that codes for CYP2C9. CYP2C9 polymorphisms may play a significant role in NSAID toxicity. Although many non-steroidal anti-inflammatory drugs (NSAIDs) are metabolized by CYP2C9, such as suprofen, naproxen, diclofenac, ibuprofen, ketoprofen, meloxicam, piroxicam, flurbiprofen, indometacin and tenoxicam. There is a difference in the effectiveness of metabolic clearance between the different NSAIDs [41]. CYP2C9 activity in poor metabolizers are lower compared to the wild type [42].

5.3. Opioid Receptors

Opioid receptors belong to a family of G-protein-coupled receptors (GPCRs), which are located in the brain and spinal cord [25,48]. There are three types of classical opioid receptors: mu (μ), kappa (κ) and delta (δ). The μ-opioid receptor (OPRM1) is the main binding site for various opioid drugs and beta-endorphins [21]. A common polymorphism of OPRM1 is a single nucleotide substitution at position 118, where an adenine is substituted for a guanine (A118G). It was reported that among Caucasians these substitutions occur with an allelic frequency of 10%–30%, with a higher prevalence amongst Asians, and a lower in African Americans [19]. The binding affinity for b-endorphin is increased with this polymorphism, which results in the change of an amino acid (asparagine for aspartate). This affects the action of opioids at the receptor [37]. Adverse effects of the drugs, such as vomiting, pupil dilation, nausea and sedation, are reduced in association with the G allele. Therefore, carriers of the G118 allele may accept higher opiate doses than non-carriers [44,91]. 118A homozygotes or heterozygotes consumed considerably less morphine than patients with 118G homozygotes [91]. Cancer patients with an 118GG polymorphism in the *OPRM1* gene need a higher morphine dose than patients with 118AA (1,2,3). Other genes, such as *CREB1*, *GIRK2* and *CACNA1E*, have similar consequences on the pain-relieving effects of opioids. Genotypes related to morphine's ability to treat pain, such as the GG genotype for *OPRM1*, may help inform appropriate dose selection. In one study, patients with the GG genotype often require higher daily doses of morphine to achieve appropriate levels of analgesia, in comparison to the wild-type A allele (225 + 143 mg/day vs. 97 + 89 mg/day in those with the A allele for *OPRM1*, $p = 0.006$) [31,32,93]. More than 100 variants of the receptor gene (*OPRM1*) have been identified [113].

5.4. Adenosine Triphosphate-Binding Cassette, Sub-Family B, Member 1 (ABCB1)

Adenosine triphosphate (ATP)-binding cassette subfamily B or multi-drug resistance gene (*MDR1*) encodes for P-glycoprotein [48]. P-glycoprotein is an efflux transporter that actively pumps substrates out of tissues to decrease concentrations of drugs on the body [113]. These proteins are present in a variety of human tissues, including the kidney, liver, gastrointestinal tract and brain [42]. Decreased renal excretion, increased bioavailability of oral medications, or in central nervous system concentrations are result of damaged the P-glycoprotein transporters. Specifically, variations in ABCB1 transporters in the brain may affect the transport of opioids into the brain through the blood–brain barrier [3].

5.5. Catechol-O-Methyltransferase (COMT)

The catechol-O-methyltransferase (COMT) enzyme is one of the enzymes that metabolizes the catecholamines, norepinephrine, epinephrine and dopamine. Therefore, the COMT enzyme acts as the main modulator of dopaminergic and adrenergic/noradrenergic neurotransmission [15]. Patients who are treated for cancer-related pain may experience opioid-related side effects if they possess a genetic variation in COMT [48]. Improved dopaminergic transmission was reported in Val158 allele, which exhibits a high COMT activity, which has been suggested to confer an advantage in the processing of aversive stimuli or in stressful conditions. In contrast, advantage in memory and attention tasks may be associated with the Met158 allele [19]. The Met158 variant is the most widely studied variant, where a G to A nucleotide substitution at codon 158 may produce an amino acid change from valine to methionine, resulting in individuals who have homozygous methionine-158 genotype [42,91]. Cancer patients with the Met/Met genotype have demonstrated a lower need for morphine compared with those with a Val/Val genotype [91]. The effect of polymorphisms in the OPRM1 and COMT genes, which transcribe opioid receptor μ 1 and catechol-O-methyltransferase respectively, are relatively well categorized in their effect on acute postoperative, cancer-related and chronic pain. When patients are homozygous for the common amino acid substitution val158met, they require a dose of morphine that is significantly higher than homozygous met/met patients [31,32,93].

5.6. Uridine Diphosphate Glucuronosyltransferases (UGTs)

The uridine diphosphate glucuronosyltransferases (UGTs) family serves a major role in the conjugation of potentially toxic drugs and endogenous compounds. UGTs catalyze the glucuronidation reaction, resulting in the addition of glucuronic acid to several lipophilic compounds [15]. Although abundant in the liver, UGTs are also found throughout different parts of the body, including the kidneys, colon, prostate, stomach and small intestines [113]. Uridine glucuronyl transferase (UGT) enzymes are subdivided into four families, and each of these into subfamilies [16]. Morphine is primarily metabolized by UDP-Glucuronosyltransferase-2B7 (UGT2B7), a phase 2 isoenzyme. It is metabolized in the liver into two metabolites: Morphine-3-glucuronide (M3G) and morphine-6-glucuronide (M6G) [42]. UGT2B7 is linked to altered levels of mRNA expression and enzymatic activity with different metabolite production [48]. The polymorphism in UGT2B7 may lead to different rates of morphine glucuronidation resulting in higher or lower levels of morphine/metabolite ratios [17,42]. Genotypic differences in UGT2B7, which is responsible for metabolizing morphine into morphine-6-glucuronide and morphine-3-glucuronide, can impact codeine's therapeutic effect. In particular, the UGT2B7*2/*2 genotype, which results in a reduced function of the enzyme, has been associated with higher toxicity. Several pharmacokinetic studies have illustrated the effects of these phenotypes on metabolite formation. In one study, a single dose of 30 mg codeine was administered to 12 UM individuals in comparison to 11 EMs and three PMs. Significant differences were detected between EM and UM groups for areas under the plasma concentration versus time curves (AUCs) for morphine with a median (range) AUC of 11 (5–17) $\mu g \cdot h \cdot L^{-1}$ in EMs and 16 (10–24) $\mu g \cdot h \cdot L^{-1}$ in UMs relative to individuals with the PM phenotype (0.5 $\mu g \cdot h \cdot L^{-1}$, $p = 0.02$) [31,32].

5.7. Melanocortin-1 Receptor Gene

Variation in the *MC1R* gene indicated the potential for highly targeted analgesia on gender and other differences. There is evidence that women, respond to κ-induced analgesia more than men [91]. Women with either one or no MC1R variants, or to men with two inactivating MC1R variants was reported to experience a weaker analgesic effect from pentazocine (k-opioid agonist) compared to women with two non-functional MC1R alleles [37,41]. Women with redhead and pale skin phenotypes have been shown to have this MC1R gene variation [41,91].

6. Conclusions and Future Perspective

Pain management regimes are established to care for post-operative and palliative patients to improve their quality of life. Patients suffering from cancer are usually subjected to chemotherapy treatment, which can be painful and cause uneasiness. Therefore, patients will resort to analgesics. The human genome is highly complex and consists of various types of polymorphisms that differ from one individual to another. A plethora of drugs are discovered and introduced into the market to counter this issue because there is not a specific drug that is suitable for every patient. Administering an incorrect drug to a patient can be life threatening. Hence, it is crucial to have the correct information on individual patient pharmacogenomics at the time of a care decision so that the data can be used to guide therapeutic decision-making. Pharmacogenomics can be employed as the future of analgesic administration to investigate the drug metabolizing enzymes or disease genes, RNA expression or protein translation of genes affecting drug response, inter-individual genetic variability in DNA sequence of drug targets and drug safety [25]. Serious adverse drug reactions (ADRs) or unsuccessful therapeutic effect in some patients may still occur from a medication with proven efficacy and safety [21]. The variation in the reaction to the drugs is often caused by the genetic composition of the individual, which could possibly be an inherited variance or an acquired variance due to mutations in their DNA. Each patient's genetic coding may be used as a basis for an individualized pain management treatment plan for analgesic metabolism and pain sensitivity allowing efficient and accurate treatments for patients [114]. Opioids like morphine, codeine and tramadol [3] are potent analgesics and serve as the foundation for severe pain management in cancer. The pursuit of personalized medicine has always been the main objective for both physicians and pharmaceutical industries. The main objective in the era of personalized medicine is to administer the correct drug at the precise dose for the "right patient" as the human genome becomes easily accessible [21,42].

7. Limitations

The limitation to this review is that the data and information collected are from low or moderate quality articles. In addition, more studies need to be carried out to fully understand the interactions of cancer drugs and painkillers that may affect therapeutic outcome. Hence, this article should only serve as a baseline and reference for future research to be carried out.

Author Contributions: A.V.S. took the lead in writing and designed the overall idea of the manuscript. A.H.S.Y. designed the figures and contributed in the subsections of the manuscript. C.E.O. was involved in the planning, drafting and designing of the whole manuscript while also providing insights on the relation among the subsections and overall idea of the manuscript.

Funding: Ayappa V. Subramaniam is supported by the Universiti Sains Malaysia Graduate Assistant Scheme and the Fundamental Research Grant Scheme (203/CIPPM/6711542). We would like to acknowledge the Union for International Cancer Control ICRETT Fellowship for facilitating the international transfer and knowledge exchange between Chern Ein Oon (USM) and Xiaomeng Wang (NTU).

Acknowledgments: We thank Mataka Banda from Keele University, UK for helping with the manuscript proofreading.

Conflicts of Interest: The authors declare no conflict of interest.

References

1. Nersesyan, H.; Slavin, K.V. Current aproach to cancer pain management: Availability and implications of different treatment options. *Ther. Clin. Risk Manag.* **2007**, *3*, 381–400. [PubMed]
2. Kurita, G.P.; Sjøgren, P.; Klepstad, P.; Mercadante, S. Interventional Techniques to Management of Cancer-Related Pain: Clinical and Critical Aspects. *Cancers* **2019**, *11*, 443. [CrossRef] [PubMed]
3. Bell, G.C.; Donovan, K.A.; McLeod, H.L. Clinical Implications of Opioid Pharmacogenomics in Patients with Cancer. *Cancer Control J. Moffitt Cancer Cent.* **2015**, *22*, 426–432. [CrossRef] [PubMed]
4. World Health Organization. *Cancer Pain Relief and Palliative Care: Report of a WHO Expert Committee [Meeting Held in Geneva from 3 to 10 July 1989]*; World Health Organization: Geneva, Switzerland, 1990; ISBN 978-92-4-120804-8.
5. Hanks, G.W.; Conno, F.; Cherny, N.; Hanna, M.; Kalso, E.; McQuay, H.J.; Mercadante, S.; Meynadier, J.; Poulain, P.; Ripamonti, C.; et al. Morphine and alternative opioids in cancer pain: The EAPC recommendations. *Br. J. Cancer* **2001**, *84*, 587–593. [CrossRef] [PubMed]
6. Leppert, W. Progress in pharmacological pain treatment with opioid analgesics. *Contemp. Oncol. Onkol.* **2009**, *13*, 66–73.
7. Eidelman, A.; White, T.; Swarm, R.A. Interventional therapies for cancer pain management: Important adjuvants to systemic analgesics. *J. Natl. Compr. Cancer Netw. JNCCN* **2007**, *5*, 753–760. [CrossRef] [PubMed]

8. Prommer, E.E. Pharmacological Management of Cancer-Related Pain. *Cancer Control J. Moffitt Cancer Cent.* **2015**, *22*, 412–425. [CrossRef]
9. Constance, J.E.; Campbell, S.C.; Somani, A.A.; Yellepeddi, V.; Owens, K.H.; Sherwin, C.M.T. Pharmacokinetics, pharmacodynamics and pharmacogenetics associated with nonsteroidal anti-inflammatory drugs and opioids in pediatric cancer patients. *Expert Opin. Drug Metab. Toxicol.* **2017**, *13*, 715–724. [CrossRef]
10. Pergolizzi, J.V.; Gharibo, C.; Ho, K.-Y. Treatment Considerations for Cancer Pain: A Global Perspective. *Pain Pract. Off. J. World Inst. Pain* **2015**, *15*, 778–792. [CrossRef]
11. Juneja, R. Opioids and cancer recurrence. *Curr. Opin. Support. Palliat. Care* **2014**, *8*, 91–101. [CrossRef]
12. Bruera, E.; Paice, J.A. Cancer pain management: Safe and effective use of opioids. *Am. Soc. Clin. Oncol. Educ. Book* **2015**, *35*, e593–e599. [CrossRef] [PubMed]
13. Kurita, G.P.; Sjøgren, P. Pain management in cancer survivorship. *Acta Oncol. Stockh. Swed.* **2015**, *54*, 629–634. [CrossRef] [PubMed]
14. Carmona-Bayonas, A.; Jiménez-Fonseca, P.; Castañón, E.; Ramchandani-Vaswani, A.; Sánchez-Bayona, R.; Custodio, A.; Calvo-Temprano, D.; Virizuela, J.A. Chronic opioid therapy in long-term cancer survivors. *Clin. Transl. Oncol. Off. Publ. Fed. Span. Oncol. Soc. Natl. Cancer Inst. Mex.* **2017**, *19*, 236–250. [CrossRef] [PubMed]
15. Anand, K.J.S.; Stevens, B.J.; McGrath, P.J. *Pain in Neonates and Infants*; Elsevier Health Sciences: Amsterdam, The Netherlands, 2007; ISBN 978-0-444-52061-6.
16. Jimenez, N.; Galinkin, J.L. Personalizing pediatric pain medicine: Using population-specific pharmacogenetics, genomics, and other -omics approaches to predict response. *Anesth. Analg.* **2015**, *121*, 183–187. [CrossRef] [PubMed]
17. Allegaert, K.; van den Anker, J.N. How to use drugs for pain management: From pharmacokinetics to pharmacogenomics. *Eur. J. Pain Suppl.* **2008**, *2*, 25–30. [CrossRef]
18. Portenoy, R.K.; Ahmed, E. Principles of opioid use in cancer pain. *J. Clin. Oncol. Off. J. Am. Soc. Clin. Oncol.* **2014**, *32*, 1662–1670. [CrossRef] [PubMed]
19. Landau, R. Pharmacogenomic Considerations in Opioid Analgesia. Available online: https://www.dovepress.com/pharmacogenomic-considerations-in-opioid-analgesia-peer-reviewed-article-PGPM (accessed on 12 November 2016).
20. Moradkhani, M.R.; Karimi, A. Role of Drug Anesthesia and Cancer. *Drug Res.* **2018**, *68*, 125–131. [CrossRef] [PubMed]
21. Ko, T.-M.; Wong, C.-S.; Wu, J.-Y.; Chen, Y.-T. Pharmacogenomics for personalized pain medicine. *Acta Anaesthesiol. Taiwan* **2016**, *54*, 24–30. [CrossRef] [PubMed]
22. Drendel, A. Pharmacogenomics of Analgesic Agents. *Clin. Pediatr. Emerg. Med.* **2007**, *8*, 262–267. [CrossRef]
23. Dean, M. Opioids in renal failure and dialysis patients. *J. Pain Symptom Manag.* **2004**, *28*, 497–504. [CrossRef] [PubMed]
24. Manworren, R.C.B.; Jeffries, L.; Pantaleao, A.; Seip, R.; Zempsky, W.T.; Ruaño, G. Pharmacogenetic Testing for Analgesic Adverse Effects: Pediatric Case Series. *Clin. J. Pain* **2016**, *32*, 109–115. [CrossRef] [PubMed]
25. Yiannakopoulou, E. Pharmacogenomics and Opioid Analgesics: Clinical Implications. *Int. J. Genomics* **2015**, *2015*, e368979. [CrossRef] [PubMed]
26. Vuilleumier, P.H.; Stamer, U.M.; Landau, R. Pharmacogenomic considerations in opioid analgesia. *Pharm. Pers. Med.* **2012**, *5*, 73–87.
27. Neighbors, D.M.; Bell, T.J.; Wilson, J.; Dodd, S.L. Economic evaluation of the fentanyl transdermal system for the treatment of chronic moderate to severe pain. *J. Pain Symptom Manag.* **2001**, *21*, 129–143. [CrossRef]
28. Radbruch, L.; Lehmann, K.; Gockel, H.-H.; Neighbors, D.; Nuyts, G. Costs of opioid therapy for chronic nonmalignant pain in Germany: an economic model comparing transdermal fentanyl (Durogesic) with controlled-release morphine. *Eur. J. Health Econ.* **2002**, *3*, 111–119. [CrossRef] [PubMed]
29. Greiner, W.; Lehmann, K.; Earnshaw, S.; Bug, C.; Sabatowski, R. Economic evaluation of Durogesic in moderate to severe, nonmalignant, chronic pain in Germany. *Eur. J. Health Econ.* **2006**, *7*, 290–296. [CrossRef]
30. National Collaborating Centre for Cancer (UK). *Opioids in Palliative Care: Safe and Effective Prescribing of Strong Opioids for Pain in Palliative Care of Adults*; National Institute for Health and Clinical Excellence: London, UK, 2012.
31. Wendt, F.R.; Sajantila, A.; Budowle, B. Predicted activity of UGT2B7, ABCB1, OPRM1, and COMT using full-gene haplotypes and their association with the CYP2D6-inferred metabolizer phenotype. *Forensic Sci. Int. Genet.* **2018**, *33*, 48–58. [CrossRef] [PubMed]

32. Kaye, A.D.; Garcia, A.J.; Hall, O.M.; Jeha, G.M.; Cramer, K.D.; Granier, A.L.; Kallurkar, A.; Cornett, E.M.; Urman, R.D. Update on the pharmacogenomics of pain management. *Pharm. Pers. Med.* **2019**, *12*, 125. [CrossRef] [PubMed]
33. Paix, A.; Coleman, A.; Lees, J.; Grigson, J.; Brooksbank, M.; Thorne, D.; Ashby, M. Subcutaneous fentanyl and sufentanil infusion substitution for morphine intolerance in cancer pain management. *Pain* **1995**, *63*, 263–269. [CrossRef]
34. White, C.; Hardy, J.; Boyd, A.; Hall, A. Subcutaneous sufentanil for palliative care patients in a hospital setting. *Palliat. Med.* **2008**, *22*, 89–90. [CrossRef]
35. Sande, T.A.; Laird, B.J.A.; Fallon, M.T. The use of opioids in cancer patients with renal impairment-a systematic review. *Support. Care Cancer Off. J. Multinatl. Assoc. Support. Care Cancer* **2017**, *25*, 661–675. [CrossRef] [PubMed]
36. Mercadante, S.; Casuccio, A.; Agnello, A.; Serretta, R.; Calderone, L.; Barresi, L. Morphine versus methadone in the pain treatment of advanced-cancer patients followed up at home. *J. Clin. Oncol. Off. J. Am. Soc. Clin. Oncol.* **1998**, *16*, 3656–3661. [CrossRef] [PubMed]
37. Fernandez Robles, C.R.; Degnan, M.; Candiotti, K.A. Pain and genetics. *Curr. Opin. Anaesthesiol.* **2012**, *25*, 444–449. [CrossRef] [PubMed]
38. Koyyalagunta, D.; Bruera, E.; Solanki, D.R.; Nouri, K.H.; Burton, A.W.; Toro, M.P.; Bruel, B.M.; Manchikanti, L. A systematic review of randomized trials on the effectiveness of opioids for cancer pain. *Pain Physician* **2012**, *15*, ES39–ES58. [PubMed]
39. Kim, E.S. Oxycodone/Naloxone Prolonged Release: A Review in Severe Chronic Pain. *Clin. Drug Investig.* **2017**, *37*, 1191–1201. [CrossRef] [PubMed]
40. Lee, K.-H.; Kim, T.W.; Kang, J.-H.; Kim, J.-S.; Ahn, J.-S.; Kim, S.-Y.; Yun, H.-J.; Eum, Y.-J.; Koh, S.A.; Kim, M.K.; et al. Efficacy and safety of controlled-release oxycodone/naloxone versus controlled-release oxycodone in Korean patients with cancer-related pain: A randomized controlled trial. *Chin. J. Cancer* **2017**, *36*, 74. [CrossRef]
41. Muralidharan, A.; Smith, M.T. Pain, analgesia and genetics. *J. Pharm. Pharmacol.* **2011**, *63*, 1387–1400. [CrossRef]
42. Ting, S.; Schug, S. The pharmacogenomics of pain management: Prospects for personalized medicine. *J. Pain Res.* **2016**, *9*, 49–56.
43. Mercadante, S. The role of tapentadol as a strong opioid in cancer pain management: A systematic and critical review. *Curr. Med. Res. Opin.* **2017**, *33*, 1965–1969. [CrossRef]
44. Palmer, S.N.; Giesecke, N.M.; Body, S.C.; Shernan, S.K.; Fox, A.A.; Collard, C.D. Pharmacogenetics of Anesthetic and Analgesic Agents. *J. Am. Soc. Anesthesiol.* **2005**, *102*, 663–671. [CrossRef]
45. Dobosz, Ł.; Kaczor, M.; Stefaniak, T.J. Pain in pancreatic cancer: Review of medical and surgical remedies. *ANZ J. Surg.* **2016**, *86*, 756–761. [CrossRef] [PubMed]
46. Analgesics Mixed with Pharmacogenomics: The Pain of It all. Available online: http://www.lateralmag.com/columns/gene-dosage/analgesics-mixed-with-pharmacogenomics-the-pain-of-it-all (accessed on 12 November 2016).
47. Hussain, M.; Javeed, A.; Ashraf, M.; Al-Zaubai, N.; Stewart, A.; Mukhtar, M.M. Non-steroidal anti-inflammatory drugs, tumour immunity and immunotherapy. *Pharmacol. Res.* **2012**, *66*, 7–18. [CrossRef] [PubMed]
48. Cregg, R.; Russo, G.; Gubbay, A.; Branford, R.; Sato, H. Pharmacogenetics of analgesic drugs. *Br. J. Pain* **2013**, *7*, 189–208. [CrossRef] [PubMed]
49. Lussier, D.; Huskey, A.G.; Portenoy, R.K. Adjuvant analgesics in cancer pain management. *Oncologist* **2004**, *9*, 571–591. [CrossRef] [PubMed]
50. Wiffen, P.J.; Derry, S.; Moore, R.A.; McNicol, E.D.; Bell, R.F.; Carr, D.B.; McIntyre, M.; Wee, B. Oral paracetamol (acetaminophen) for cancer pain. *Cochrane Database Syst. Rev.* **2017**, *7*, 1–39.
51. Fuller, R.W.; Snoddy, H.D. Evaluation of nefopam as a monoamine uptake inhibitor in vivo in mice. *Neuropharmacology* **1993**, *32*, 995–999. [CrossRef]
52. Gray, A.M.; Nevinson, M.J.; Sewell, R.D. The involvement of opioidergic and noradrenergic mechanisms in nefopam antinociception. *Eur. J. Pharmacol.* **1999**, *365*, 149–157. [CrossRef]
53. Hunskaar, S.; Fasmer, O.B.; Broch, O.J.; Hole, K. Involvement of central serotonergic pathways in nefopam-induced antinociception. *Eur. J. Pharmacol.* **1987**, *138*, 77–82. [CrossRef]

54. Kim, S.Y.; Huh, K.H.; Roh, Y.H.; Oh, Y.J.; Park, J.; Choi, Y.S. Nefopam as an adjunct to intravenous patient-controlled analgesia after renal transplantation: A randomised trial. *Acta Anaesthesiol. Scand.* **2015**, *59*, 1068–1075. [CrossRef]
55. Girard, P.; Chauvin, M.; Verleye, M. Nefopam analgesia and its role in multimodal analgesia: A review of preclinical and clinical studies. *Clin. Exp. Pharmacol. Physiol.* **2016**, *43*, 3–12. [CrossRef]
56. Na, H.-S.; Oh, A.-Y.; Koo, B.-W.; Lim, D.-J.; Ryu, J.-H.; Han, J.-W. Preventive Analgesic Efficacy of Nefopam in Acute and Chronic Pain After Breast Cancer Surgery. *Medicine (Baltimore)* **2016**, *95*, e3705. [CrossRef] [PubMed]
57. Hwang, B.-Y.; Kwon, J.-Y.; Lee, D.-W.; Kim, E.; Kim, T.-K.; Kim, H.-K. A Randomized Clinical Trial of Nefopam versus Ketorolac Combined with Oxycodone in Patient-Controlled Analgesia after Gynecologic Surgery. *Int. J. Med. Sci.* **2015**, *12*, 644–649. [CrossRef] [PubMed]
58. Gaertner, J.; Stamer, U.M.; Remi, C.; Voltz, R.; Bausewein, C.; Sabatowski, R.; Wirz, S.; Müller-Mundt, G.; Simon, S.T.; Pralong, A.; et al. Metamizole/dipyrone for the relief of cancer pain: A systematic review and evidence-based recommendations for clinical practice. *Palliat. Med.* **2017**, *31*, 26–34. [CrossRef] [PubMed]
59. Hearn, L.; Derry, S.; Moore, R.A. Single dose dipyrone (metamizole) for acute postoperative pain in adults. *Cochrane Database Syst. Rev.* **2016**, *4*, CD011421. [CrossRef] [PubMed]
60. Rodríguez, M.; Barutell, C.; Rull, M.; Gálvez, R.; Pallarés, J.; Vidal, F.; Aliaga, L.; Moreno, J.; Puerta, J.; Ortiz, P. Efficacy and tolerance of oral dipyrone versus oral morphine for cancer pain. *Eur. J. Cancer* **1994**, *30*, 584–587. [CrossRef]
61. Brito, B.E.; Vazquez, E.; Taylor, P.; Alvarado, Y.; Vanegas, H.; Millan, A.; Tortorici, V. Antinociceptive effect of systemically administered dipyrone (metamizol), magnesium chloride or both in a murine model of cancer. *Eur. J. Pain Lond. Engl.* **2017**, *21*, 541–551. [CrossRef] [PubMed]
62. Jensen, T.S.; Baron, R.; Haanpää, M.; Kalso, E.; Loeser, J.D.; Rice, A.S.C.; Treede, R.-D. A new definition of neuropathic pain. *Pain* **2011**, *152*, 2204–2205. [CrossRef] [PubMed]
63. Mitra, R.; Jones, S. Adjuvant analgesics in cancer pain: A review. *Am. J. Hosp. Palliat. Care* **2012**, *29*, 70–79. [CrossRef]
64. Chwistek, M. Recent advances in understanding and managing cancer pain. *F1000Research* **2017**, *6*, 945. [CrossRef]
65. Caraceni, A.; Zecca, E.; Martini, C.; Pigni, A.; Bracchi, P. Gabapentin for breakthrough pain due to bone metastases. *Palliat. Med.* **2008**, *22*, 392–393. [CrossRef]
66. Hamal, P.K.; Shrestha, A.B.; Shrestha, R.R. Efficacy of Preemptive Gabapentin for Lower Extremity Orthopedic surgery under Subarachnoid Block. *JNMA J. Nepal Med. Assoc.* **2015**, *53*, 210–213. [CrossRef] [PubMed]
67. Cheng, G.S.; Ilfeld, B.M. An Evidence-Based Review of the Efficacy of Perioperative Analgesic Techniques for Breast Cancer-Related Surgery. *Pain Med. Malden Mass* **2017**, *18*, 1344–1365. [CrossRef] [PubMed]
68. Freedman, B.M.; O'Hara, E. Pregabalin has opioid-sparing effects following augmentation mammaplasty. *Aesthet. Surg. J.* **2008**, *28*, 421–424. [CrossRef] [PubMed]
69. Kim, S.Y.; Song, J.W.; Park, B.; Park, S.; An, Y.J.; Shim, Y.H. Pregabalin reduces post-operative pain after mastectomy: A double-blind, randomized, placebo-controlled study. *Acta Anaesthesiol. Scand.* **2011**, *55*, 290–296. [CrossRef] [PubMed]
70. Grover, V.K.; Mathew, P.J.; Yaddanapudi, S.; Sehgal, S. A single dose of preoperative gabapentin for pain reduction and requirement of morphine after total mastectomy and axillary dissection: Randomized placebo-controlled double-blind trial. *J. Postgrad. Med.* **2009**, *55*, 257–260. [PubMed]
71. Bugan, I.; Karagoz, Z.; Altun, S.; Djamgoz, M.B.A. Gabapentin, an Analgesic Used Against Cancer-Associated Neuropathic Pain: Effects on Prostate Cancer Progression in an In Vivo Rat Model. *Basic Clin. Pharmacol. Toxicol.* **2016**, *118*, 200–207. [CrossRef] [PubMed]
72. Sharma, S.; Rajagopal, M.R.; Palat, G.; Singh, C.; Haji, A.G.; Jain, D. A phase II pilot study to evaluate use of intravenous lidocaine for opioid-refractory pain in cancer patients. *J. Pain Symptom Manag.* **2009**, *37*, 85–93. [CrossRef] [PubMed]
73. Fassoulaki, A.; Sarantopoulos, C.; Melemeni, A.; Hogan, Q. EMLA reduces acute and chronic pain after breast surgery for cancer. *Reg. Anesth. Pain Med.* **2000**, *25*, 350–355. [CrossRef] [PubMed]
74. Mercadante, S.; Arcuri, E.; Tirelli, W.; Casuccio, A. Analgesic effect of intravenous ketamine in cancer patients on morphine therapy: A randomized, controlled, double-blind, crossover, double-dose study. *J. Pain Symptom Manag.* **2000**, *20*, 246–252. [CrossRef]

75. Jonkman, K.; van de Donk, T.; Dahan, A. Ketamine for cancer pain: What is the evidence? *Curr. Opin. Support. Palliat. Care* **2017**, *11*, 88–92. [CrossRef]
76. Hardy, J.; Quinn, S.; Fazekas, B.; Plummer, J.; Eckermann, S.; Agar, M.; Spruyt, O.; Rowett, D.; Currow, D.C. Randomized, double-blind, placebo-controlled study to assess the efficacy and toxicity of subcutaneous ketamine in the management of cancer pain. *J. Clin. Oncol. Off. J. Am. Soc. Clin. Oncol.* **2012**, *30*, 3611–3617. [CrossRef]
77. Salas, S.; Frasca, M.; Planchet-Barraud, B.; Burucoa, B.; Pascal, M.; Lapiana, J.-M.; Hermet, R.; Castany, C.; Ravallec, F.; Loundou, A.; et al. Ketamine analgesic effect by continuous intravenous infusion in refractory cancer pain: Considerations about the clinical research in palliative care. *J. Palliat. Med.* **2012**, *15*, 287–293. [CrossRef]
78. Ishizuka, P.; Garcia, J.B.S.; Sakata, R.K.; Issy, A.M.; Mülich, S.L. Assessment of oral S+ ketamine associated with morphine for the treatment of oncologic pain. *Rev. Bras. Anestesiol.* **2007**, *57*, 19–31. [PubMed]
79. Birdsall, S.M.; Birdsall, T.C.; Tims, L.A. The Use of Medical Marijuana in Cancer. *Curr. Oncol. Rep.* **2016**, *18*, 40. [CrossRef]
80. Romero-Sandoval, E.A.; Kolano, A.L.; Alvarado-Vázquez, P.A. Cannabis and Cannabinoids for Chronic Pain. *Curr. Rheumatol. Rep.* **2017**, *19*, 67. [CrossRef] [PubMed]
81. Abrams, D.I.; Guzman, M. Cannabis in cancer care. *Clin. Pharmacol. Ther.* **2015**, *97*, 575–586. [CrossRef] [PubMed]
82. Bennett, M.; Paice, J.A.; Wallace, M. Pain and Opioids in Cancer Care: Benefits, Risks, and Alternatives. *Am. Soc. Clin. Oncol. Educ. Book* **2017**, *37*, 705–713. [CrossRef]
83. Tateo, S. State of the evidence: Cannabinoids and cancer pain-A systematic review. *J. Am. Assoc. Nurse Pract.* **2017**, *29*, 94–103. [CrossRef]
84. Häuser, W.; Fitzcharles, M.-A.; Radbruch, L.; Petzke, F. Cannabinoids in Pain Management and Palliative Medicine. *Dtsch. Ärztebl. Int.* **2017**, *114*, 627–634. [CrossRef] [PubMed]
85. Kramer, J.L. Medical marijuana for cancer. *CA Cancer J. Clin.* **2015**, *65*, 109–122. [CrossRef]
86. Hilliard, N.; Brown, S.; Mitchinson, S. A case report of dexmedetomidine used to treat intractable pain and delirium in a tertiary palliative care unit. *Palliat. Med.* **2015**, *29*, 278–281. [CrossRef] [PubMed]
87. Seymore, R.J.; Manis, M.M.; Coyne, P.J. Dexmedetomidine Use in a Case of Severe Cancer Pain. *J. Pain Palliat. Care Pharmacother.* **2019**, *32*, 1–8. [CrossRef] [PubMed]
88. Mupamombe, C.T.; Luczkiewicz, D.; Kerr, C. Dexmedetomidine as an Option for Opioid Refractory Pain in the Hospice Setting. *J. Palliat. Med.* **2019**, *22*, 1–4. [CrossRef]
89. Yuan, X.; Wu, J.; Wang, Q.; Xu, M. The antinociceptive effect of systemic administration of a combination of low-dose tramadol and dexmedetomidine in a rat model of bone cancer pain. *Eur. J. Anaesthesiol.* **2014**, *31*, 30–34. [CrossRef] [PubMed]
90. Mohta, M.; Kalra, B.; Sethi, A.K.; Kaur, N. Efficacy of dexmedetomidine as an adjuvant in paravertebral block in breast cancer surgery. *J. Anesth.* **2016**, *30*, 252–260. [CrossRef]
91. Webster, L.R.; Belfer, I. Pharmacogenetics and Personalized Medicine in Pain Management. *Clin. Lab. Med.* **2016**, *36*, 493–506. [CrossRef]
92. Ruano, G.; Kost, J.A. Fundamental Considerations for Genetically-Guided Pain Management with Opioids Based on CYP2D6 and OPRM1 Polymorphisms. *Pain Physician* **2018**, *21*, E611–E621.
93. Owusu Obeng, A.; Hamadeh, I.; Smith, M. Review of Opioid Pharmacogenetics and Considerations for Pain Management. *Pharmacotherapy* **2017**, *37*, 1105–1121. [CrossRef] [PubMed]
94. Ross, J.R.; Riley, J.; Taegetmeyer, A.B.; Sato, H.; Gretton, S.; du Bois, R.M.; Welsh, K.I. Genetic variation and response to morphine in cancer patients: Catechol-O-methyltransferase and multidrug resistance-1 gene polymorphisms are associated with central side effects. *Cancer* **2008**, *112*, 1390–1403. [CrossRef]
95. Ecimovic, P.; Murray, D.; Doran, P.; McDonald, J.; Lambert, D.G.; Buggy, D.J. Direct effect of morphine on breast cancer cell function in vitro: Role of the NET1 gene. *Br. J. Anaesth.* **2011**, *107*, 916–923. [CrossRef] [PubMed]
96. Kirchheiner, J.; Schmidt, H.; Tzvetkov, M.; Keulen, J.-T.H.A.; Lötsch, J.; Roots, I.; Brockmöller, J. Pharmacokinetics of codeine and its metabolite morphine in ultra-rapid metabolizers due to CYP2D6 duplication. *Pharm. J.* **2007**, *7*, 257–265. [CrossRef] [PubMed]
97. Agarwal, D.; Udoji, M.A.; Trescot, A. Genetic Testing for Opioid Pain Management: A Primer. *Pain Ther.* **2017**, *6*, 93–105. [CrossRef] [PubMed]

98. Raji, M.A.; Kuo, Y.-F.; Adhikari, D.; Baillargeon, J.; Goodwin, J.S. Decline in opioid prescribing after federal rescheduling of hydrocodone products. *Pharmacoepidemiol. Drug Saf.* **2018**, *27*, 513–519. [CrossRef] [PubMed]
99. Oldenmenger, W.H.; Lieverse, P.J.; Janssen, P.J.J.M.; Taal, W.; van der Rijt, C.C.D.; Jager, A. Efficacy of opioid rotation to continuous parenteral hydromorphone in advanced cancer patients failing on other opioids. *Support. Care Cancer* **2012**, *20*, 1639–1647. [CrossRef] [PubMed]
100. Takashina, Y.; Naito, T.; Mino, Y.; Yagi, T.; Ohnishi, K.; Kawakami, J. Impact of CYP3A5 and ABCB1 gene polymorphisms on fentanyl pharmacokinetics and clinical responses in cancer patients undergoing conversion to a transdermal system. *Drug Metab. Pharmacokinet.* **2012**, *27*, 414–421. [CrossRef] [PubMed]
101. Oosten, A.W.; Matic, M.; van Schaik, R.H.; Look, M.P.; Jongen, J.L.; Mathijssen, R.H.; van der Rijt, C.C. Opioid treatment failure in cancer patients: The role of clinical and genetic factors. *Pharmacogenomics* **2016**, *17*, 1391–1403. [CrossRef] [PubMed]
102. Bruera, E.; Palmer, J.L.; Bosnjak, S.; Rico, M.A.; Moyano, J.; Sweeney, C.; Strasser, F.; Willey, J.; Bertolino, M.; Mathias, C.; et al. Methadone versus morphine as a first-line strong opioid for cancer pain: A randomized, double-blind study. *J. Clin. Oncol. Off. J. Am. Soc. Clin. Oncol.* **2004**, *22*, 185–192. [CrossRef] [PubMed]
103. Li, Y.; Kantelip, J.-P.; Gerritsen-van Schieveen, P.; Davani, S. Interindividual variability of methadone response: Impact of genetic polymorphism. *Mol. Diagn. Ther.* **2008**, *12*, 109–124. [CrossRef] [PubMed]
104. Portenoy, R.K.; Moulin, D.E.; Rogers, A.; Inturrisi, C.E.; Foley, K.M. I.v. infusion of opioids for cancer pain: Clinical review and guidelines for use. *Cancer Treat. Rep.* **1986**, *70*, 575–581. [PubMed]
105. Clarke, T.-K.; Crist, R.C.; Ang, A.; Ambrose-Lanci, L.M.; Lohoff, F.W.; Saxon, A.J.; Ling, W.; Hillhouse, M.P.; Bruce, R.D.; Woody, G.; et al. Genetic variation in OPRD1 and the response to treatment for opioid dependence with buprenorphine in European-American females. *Pharm. J.* **2014**, *14*, 303–308. [CrossRef] [PubMed]
106. Sittl, R. Transdermal buprenorphine in cancer pain and palliative care. *Palliat. Med.* **2006**, *20* (Suppl. 1), s25–s30.
107. Naito, T.; Takashina, Y.; Yamamoto, K.; Tashiro, M.; Ohnishi, K.; Kagawa, Y.; Kawakami, J. CYP3A5*3 affects plasma disposition of noroxycodone and dose escalation in cancer patients receiving oxycodone. *J. Clin. Pharmacol.* **2011**, *51*, 1529–1538. [CrossRef]
108. Arbaiza, D.; Vidal, O. Tramadol in the Treatment of Neuropathic Cancer Pain. Available online: http://www.medscape.com/viewarticle/550883 (accessed on 4 September 2019).
109. Galiè, E.; Villani, V.; Terrenato, I.; Pace, A. Tapentadol in neuropathic pain cancer patients: A prospective open label study. *Neurol. Sci. Off. J. Ital. Neurol. Soc. Ital. Soc. Clin. Neurophysiol.* **2017**, *38*, 1747–1752. [CrossRef] [PubMed]
110. Portenoy, R.K.; Ahmed, E.; Keilson, Y.Y. Cancer pain management: Use of acetaminophen and nonsteroidal antiinflammatory drugs. *UpToDate* **2019**, *18*, 1–17.
111. Eisenberg, E.; Berkey, C.S.; Carr, D.B.; Mosteller, F.; Chalmers, T.C. Efficacy and safety of nonsteroidal antiinflammatory drugs for cancer pain: A meta-analysis. *J. Clin. Oncol. Off. J. Am. Soc. Clin. Oncol.* **1994**, *12*, 2756–2765. [CrossRef] [PubMed]
112. Stanley, L.A. Chapter 27—Drug Metabolism. In *Pharmacognosy*; Badal, S., Delgoda, R., Eds.; Academic Press: Boston, MA, USA, 2017; pp. 527–545. ISBN 978-0-12-802104-0.
113. Langman, L.J.; Dasgupta, A. *Pharmacogenomics in Clinical Therapeutics*; John Wiley & Sons: Hoboken, NJ, USA, 2012; ISBN 978-1-119-95958-8.
114. Manworren, R.C.B. Multimodal pain management and the future of a personalized medicine approach to pain. *AORN J.* **2015**, *101*, 308–314. [CrossRef] [PubMed]

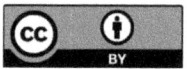

© 2019 by the authors. Licensee MDPI, Basel, Switzerland. This article is an open access article distributed under the terms and conditions of the Creative Commons Attribution (CC BY) license (http://creativecommons.org/licenses/by/4.0/).

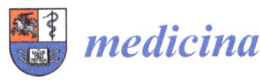

Review

Current Pharmacological Treatment of Painful Diabetic Neuropathy: A Narrative Review

Valeriu Ardeleanu [1,2,3,†], Alexandra Toma [1,4,*], Kalliopi Pafili [5,†], Nikolaos Papanas [5,†], Ion Motofei [6], Camelia Cristina Diaconu [7], Manfredi Rizzo [8,9] and Anca Pantea Stoian [10,*]

1. Department of Surgery, University "Dunarea de Jos", 800008 Galati, Romania; valeriu.ardeleanu@gmail.com
2. Department of Surgery, University "Ovidius", 900470 Constanta, Romania
3. Arestetic Clinic, 800098 Galati, Romania
4. Department of Surgery, Emergency County Clinical Hospital "Sf. Apostol Andrei", 800578 Galati, Romania
5. Second Department of Internal Medicine, Diabetes Centre-Diabetic Foot Clinic, Democritus University of Thrace, University Hospital of Alexandroupolis, 681 00 Alexandroupolis, Greece; kpafili@hotmail.com (K.P.); papanasnikos@yahoo.gr (N.P.)
6. Department of Surgery, "Carol Davila" University of Medicine and Pharmacy, 050474 Bucharest, Romania; igmotofei@gmail.com
7. Internal Medicine Department, Clinical Emergency Hospital of Bucharest, "Carol Davila" University of Medicine and Pharmacy, 050474 Bucharest, Romania; drcameliadiaconu@gmail.com
8. Biomedical Department of Internal Medicine and Medical Specialties School of Medicine, University of Palermo, 90133 Palermo, Italy; manfredi.rizzo@unipa.it
9. Division of Endocrinology, Diabetes and Metabolism, University of South Carolina School of Medicine Columbia, Columbia, SC 29209, USA
10. Diabetes, Nutrition and Metabolic Diseases Department, "Carol Davila" University of Medicine and Pharmacy, 050474 Bucharest, Romania
* Correspondence: dr.alexandratoma@gmail.com (A.T.); ancastoian@yahoo.com (A.P.S.)
† These authors have contributed equally to the present work.

Received: 29 December 2019; Accepted: 6 January 2020; Published: 9 January 2020

Abstract: *Background and Objectives*: Distal symmetrical polyneuropathy (DSPN) is one of the most common chronic complications of diabetes mellitus. Although it is usually characterized by progressive sensory loss, some patients may develop chronic pain. Assessment of DSPN is not difficult, but the biggest challenge is making the correct diagnosis and choosing the right treatment. The treatment of DSPN has three primary objectives: glycemic control, pathogenic mechanisms, and pain management. The aim of this brief narrative review is to summarize the current pharmacological treatment of painful DSPN. It also summarizes knowledge on pathogenesis-oriented therapy, which is generally overlooked in many publications and guidelines. *Materials and Methods*: The present review reports the relevant information available on DSPN treatment. The search was performed on PubMed, Cochrane, Semantic Scholar, Medline, Scopus, and Cochrane Library databases, including among others the terms "distal symmetrical polyneuropathy", "neuropathic pain treatment", "diabetic neuropathy", "diabetes complications", "glycaemic control", "antidepressants", "opioids", and "anticonvulsants". *Results*: First-line drugs include antidepressants (selective serotonin reuptake inhibitors and tricyclic antidepressants) and pregabalin. Second- and third-line drugs include opioids and topical analgesics. While potentially effective in the treatment of neuropathic pain, opioids are not considered to be the first choice because of adverse reactions and addiction concerns. *Conclusions*: DSPN is a common complication in patients with diabetes, and severely affects the quality of life of these patients. Although multiple therapies are available, the guidelines and recommendations regarding the treatment of diabetic neuropathy have failed to offer a unitary consensus, which often hinders the therapeutic options in clinical practice.

Keywords: diabetes mellitus; neuropathy; pain; pharmacological treatment

1. Introduction

Diabetic neuropathy is one of the most common chronic complications of diabetes mellitus [1]. It is defined as the presence of signs and/or symptoms of nerve dysfunction in patients with diabetes mellitus after exclusion of other causes [1,2]. The most frequent clinical manifestation is distal symmetrical polyneuropathy (DSPN), with a prevalence of 20–30% [2]. The precise pathophysiology of DSPN is multifactorial and complicated. Its main risk factors include diabetes duration, patient age, and vascular risk factors [3].

DSPN has an insidious course, characterized by chronic sensory loss with stocking and glove distribution [1]. However, it may also lead to chronic neuropathic pain [1]. DSPN treatment is complex, including both an optimal glycemic status, as well as the treatment of pain. Pain management in DSPN does not yet include specific medication to prevent or limit the reversibility of DSPN. Most often, clinical guidelines recommend symptomatic therapy, with the primary goal of pain reduction.

The present narrative review summarizes the current pharmacological treatment of painful DSPN. It includes brief references to emerging concepts and concerns such as opioid dependency and pathogenesis-oriented therapy (mainly α-lipoic acid), which are generally overlooked in many publications and guidelines.

2. Materials and Methods

We performed a review of the literature starting from 1990 by searching PubMed, Cochrane, Semantic Scholar, Medline, Scopus, and Cochrane Library databases for all observational studies, randomized clinical trials, and meta-analyses including the terms "distal symmetrical polyneuropathy", "neuropathic pain treatment", "diabetic neuropathy", "diabetes complications", "glycaemic control", "antidepressants", "opioids", and "anticonvulsants", as well as their combinations regarding DSPN. All currently available original studies, abstracts, and review articles including systematic reviews and meta-analyses were examined. Case reports and letters to the editor were excluded. Publications in English were studied in full, whereas those in other languages only in abstract form.

3. Results and Discussion

3.1. Pharmacotherapy of Diabetic Neuropathy

There are several guidelines on the optimal pharmacological treatment of painful DSPN [4–6]. There is currently a general agreement on first-line drugs and other options.

3.2. Glycemic Control

An optimal early glycemic control may delay or even prevent DSPN in type 1 diabetes mellitus and prediabetes [7–11]. In type 2 diabetes mellitus, this is less effective [12–15]. Interestingly, specific glucose-lowering strategies may have different effects. In a post-hoc analysis of the BARI 2D clinical trial (Bypass Angioplasty Revascularization Investigation in Type 2 Diabetes), subjects treated with insulin sensitizers exhibited a reduced incidence of DSPN at 4 years, as compared with those receiving insulin or sulphonylureas [16].

3.3. Antidepressants

Duloxetine is a selective norepinephrine and serotonin reuptake inhibitor. It is used with a dose of 60–120 mg daily [5,17–19]. Duloxetine appears to improve the quality of life of patients with painful DSPN [20]. Its main metabolic adverse events include modest increases of fasting plasma glucose in both short- (12 weeks) and long-term (52 weeks) treatment, a modest increase in glycated hemoglobin A1c, and small non-significant weight gain in extension studies (52 weeks) [21]. Other common side effects include dry mouth, decreased appetite, sleepiness, sweating, and gastrointestinal problems [22]. Duloxetine was approved by the US Food and Drug Administration (FDA) for painful DSPN [23].

Tricyclic antidepressants may be used as well, especially amitriptyline. Amitriptyline appears to relieve pain in comparison to placebo in patients with DSPN [24] and seems non-inferior to pregabalin [25], gabapentin [26], and duloxetine [27]. Its precise mechanism of action remains to be clarified. Nonetheless, two hypotheses have been proposed: (1) inhibition of serotonin and norepinephrine reuptake [28] and (2) antagonism of N-methyl-d-aspartate receptors, which mediate hyperalgesia and allodynia [29,30]. Amitriptyline may be considered for DSPN at a single dose of 25 to 100 mg [31], although a dosage range of 25 to 150 mg per day has been suggested [28]. Amitriptyline has FDA approval only for the treatment of depression [32,33]. The side effects include dry mouth, water retention, constipation, and vertigo. Furthermore, clinicians should assess the QTc interval, to avoid the risk of torsades de pointes, especially among subjects with additional cardiovascular risk factors [33].

Although not formally approved, venlafaxine has been used as well [5], with evidence of effectiveness for the short-term management of painful DSPN [17]. It is a potent serotonin and norepinephrine reuptake inhibitor [32]. The proposed off-label dosage ranges between 75 and 225 mg per day in patients with DSPN [31]. Common side effects include sleepiness, dizziness, and mild gastrointestinal problems [34]. Patients should be regularly assessed for QTc prolongation [35].

3.4. Anticonvulsants

The leading agent of this class is pregabalin, a calcium channel subunit α2-δ binder. It has been approved by the US Food and Drug Administration (FDA) for painful DSPN [36]. The dosage ranges from 150 to 300 mg daily [36]. Many studies have reported favorable outcomes with more than 30–50% pain improvement [5,17,18,37–39]. However, not all pregabalin-related studies had positive results [5,17,19,39,40]. Untoward effects include water retention, visual disturbances, drowsiness, ataxia, euphoria, and vertigo [41].

Gabapentin also belongs to this class of agents [42]. It has the same therapeutic target as pregabalin [39]. Gabapentin has been reported to relieve pain among DSPN subjects [26,42–45], and combination with venlafaxine seems to provide additional benefit [46]. Although not formally indicated [47], guidelines of the American Academy of Neurology suggest the use of gabapentin for the treatment of DSPN as a second-line therapy after pregabalin [31]. The recommended off-label daily dosage for DSPN subjects ranges between 900 and 3600 mg [31]. In patients with chronic kidney disease, the doses of gabapentin and pregabalin need to be adjusted: the renal clearance (CrCl $\leq$ 30 mL/min) requires dose adjustment, with a recommended dose of gabapentin of 300 mg daily and pregabalin of 75 mg daily [48]. Gabapentin has been associated with sleepiness, dizziness, suicidal behaviour, withdrawal-precipitated seizure frequency, multi-organ hypersensitivity, systemic symptoms, and drug reaction with eosinophilia [47].

Other anticonvulsants have been used as well (carbamazepine, lamotrigine, lacosamide, etc.), with variable results [5,17,48–50].

3.5. Opioids

Tapentadol is a centrally acting opioid analgesic that exerts its analgesic effects by inhibiting the μ-opioid receptor and noradrenaline uptake [51]. The FDA approved prolonged-release tapentadol for painful DSPN, based on data from two clinical trials in which patients titrated with an optimal dose of tapentadol were arbitrarily requested to continue with that dose or to change it with placebo [52,53]. However, both studies used an enriched design for patients who responded to tapentadol, and therefore the results obtained are not generalizable. Importantly, a recent systematic review and meta-analysis by the Special Interest Group on Neuropathic Pain within the International Pain Study Association found that evidence supporting the effectiveness of tapentadol in reducing neuropathic pain is inconclusive [5]. Finally, addiction is a serious concern with long-term opioid use [32].

3.6. Topical Treatment

Capsaicin is a natural alkaloid [54]. This is thought to desensitize afferent Aδ and C fibers [55]. Two forms of capsaicin are available for the treatment of painful DSPN: a low-dose cream (0.075%) [31] and a high-dose (8%) patch (Qutenza, Acorda Therapeutics, Ardsley, NY, USA) [56]. A series of studies have provided evidence of pain relief among subjects who received capsaicin cream in comparison to the vehicle [57–60], although results were inconsistent [61–63]. An older study even provided evidence of equal efficacy of capsaicin cream (0.075%) to oral amitriptyline for painful DSPN [64]. In agreement with the guidelines of the American Academy of Neurology [31], a dosage of 0.075% four times daily is recommended for the treatment of painful DSPN. A notable disadvantage is local adverse effects—mainly stinging, burning, and erythema [65].

Patches with capsaicin 8% have also been studied in painful DSPN, with conflicting results [66]. Nonetheless, some evidence points to superiority in comparison with oral pregabalin, duloxetine, and gabapentin for pain relief among DSPN patients [67]. Although not formally approved [68], a single application of this patch may provide up to 12 weeks of pain relief [69]. This should be performed under specialist supervision, with appropriate local anesthesia and monitoring for blood pressure increase, especially during the first hour following application [69].

The 5% lidocaine plaster is licensed for postherpetic neuralgia in approximately 50 countries around the world and for localized neuropathic pain in 11 Latin American countries [70]. The lidocaine molecule is a voltage-gated sodium channel inhibitor which blocks abnormally functioning neuronal sodium channels (in the dermal A-δ and C fibers) [71]. Studies have provided evidence of pain relief in DSPN patients comparable to pregabalin [72,73], amitriptyline, capsaicin, and gabapentin [73]. A maximum of three lidocaine patches 5% can be applied to intact skin once for 12 h within a 24-h period [70]. Adverse events include mild and transient application-site reactions—mainly erythema, edema, and a burning sensation [74].

Finally, topical clonidine, a presynaptic α-2 adrenergic receptor agonist with antinociceptive activity, was associated with pain relief in DSPN in a small number of studies of low-to-moderate quality [75]. Clonidine gel 0.1% may be administered in single doses of 0.65 g of gel (0.65 mg of clonidine), three times daily so that the total daily dose should not exceed 3.9 mg for both feet. The administration is associated with only mild skin-site reactions [76].

3.7. Pathogenesis-Oriented Treatment

α-Lipoic acid is a natural thiol with potent antioxidant properties, and is used as a dietary supplement. In studies evaluating this indication, it has been administered orally at doses between 600 and 1800 mg and intravenously at 600 mg per day for 3 weeks, excluding weekends [77–82]. Both formulas have been recently characterized by the FDA as safe and effective treatment options for painful DSPN [83]. The efficacy of the daily administration of a 600 mg intravenous formula for 3 weeks was investigated in a meta-analysis of four randomized, placebo-controlled trials (ALADIN I, ALADIN III, SYDNEY, NATHAN II) comprising 1258 participants with painful DSPN [82]. It was shown that α-lipoic acid improved positive neuropathic symptoms (24.1% in favor of α-lipoic acid versus placebo), but failed to alter the neuropathy impairment score significantly [82,83].

Finally, actovegin is a deproteinated, pyrogen- and antigen-free ultrafiltrate obtained from calf blood. It appears to ameliorate oxidative stress and to exhibit antiapoptotic properties [79]. In a study conducted by Ziegler et al., 567 patients were treated with actovegin (n = 281) versus placebo (n = 286). After 6 months, compared with placebo, actovegin was associated with better improvement of neuropathic symptoms, but not pain specifically (OR [95% CI] of 1.73 [1.21–2.48] for patients treated with actovegin and 1.94 [1.33–2.84] for patients placebo treated). Actovegin treatment (20 daily intravenous infusions of 2000 mg/day followed by three actovegin tablets of 600 mg each for 140 days) was associated with a clinically significant response in neuropathic symptoms and vibration perception threshold in patients with symptomatic DSPN, with a good safety profile [84]. Further studies are needed to demonstrate the efficacy of α-lipoic acid and actovegin in painful DSPN. Current pharmacological agents for painful DSPN are summarized in Table 1.

Table 1. Current pharmacological agents for painful distal symmetrical polyneuropathy (DSPN) [5,6].

Pharmacotherapy	FDA Approval for DSPN	Daily Dosage	Untoward Effects	Comments
Antidepressants				
Duloxetine	Yes [23]	60–120 mg/d [5,17–19]	Xerostomia, decreased appetite, somnolence, sweating, gastrointestinal discomfort [22]	Appears to improve the quality of life of patients with painful DSPN [20]
Amitriptyline	No [33]	25–100 mg/d [31]	Xerostomia, water retention, increased appetite, weight gain, constipation, vertigo [33]	Appears non-inferior to pregabalin [25], gabapentin, [26] and duloxetin [27] in painful DSPN; monitor QTc interval [33]
Venlafaxine	No [31]	75–225 mg/d [31]	Somnolence, dizziness, mild gastrointestinal problems [34]	Evidence of effectiveness for short-term management of painful DSPN [17]; monitor QTc interval [35]
Anticonvulsants				
Pregabalin	Yes [36]	150–300 mg/d [36]	Water retention, visual disturbances, somnolence, ataxia, euphoria, vertigo [41]	DSPN-related pain improvement of >30%–50% has been reported [5,17,18,37–39]
Gabapentin	No [47]	900–3600 mg/d [31]	Somnolence, dizziness, suicidal behaviour, withdrawal-precipitated seizure frequency, multi-organ hypersensitivity [47]	DSPN-related pain relief has been repeatedly reported [26,42–46]
Opioids				
Tapentadol extended release	Yes [52,53]	100–500 mg/d [51]	Dizziness, somnolence, headache, fatigue, gastrointestinal problems [51]	Inconclusive pain reduction [5]; addiction concern [32]
Topical treatment				
Capsaicin cream	No [32]	0.075% four times/d [31]	Skin-site reactions [63]	Equal efficacy to amitriptyline [62]
Capsaicin 8% patch	No [68]	One application every 3 months [66]	Skin-site reactions [66]	Conflicting results in DSPN [66]; application can be painful [66]; monitor for transient blood pressure increase for at least one hour following application [66]
5% lidocaine plaster	No [70]	Maximum 3 lidocaine plasters 5% can be applied to intact skin once daily for a period of 12 h [70]	Skin-site reactions [74]	Comparable efficacy to pregabalin, amitriptyline, capsaicin, and gabapentin [72,73]
Clonidine gel 0.1%	No [75]	Single doses of 0.65 g of gel, three times daily [76]	Skin-site reactions [76]	Pain relief in a small number of studies of low-to-moderate quality [75]
Pathogenesis-oriented treatment				
α-Lipoic acid	No [77]	600–1800 mg orally or 600 mg/d intravenously for 3 weeks, excluding weekends [77–81]	Nausea, vomiting, abdominal discomfort, diarrhea [77]	FDA statement: safe and effective treatment option for painful DSPN [82]

Legend: FDA: Food and Drug Administration.

4. Conclusions

DSPN is a burden both from diagnostic and treatment perspectives. It is still under-diagnosed and undertreated.

As summarized in this narrative review, first-line treatment options include pregabalin and duloxetine, with gabapentin seeming a reasonable alternative to pregabalin treatment. Second- and third-line drugs include opioids and topical analgesics. Indeed, opioids are an effective alternative in the treatment of neuropathic pain; however adverse reactions and addiction concerns limit their widespread use. More recently, research has extended beyond symptom alleviation. Pathogenesis-oriented treatments, including α-lipoic acid and actovegin, appear promising, but results need to be confirmed in more extensive trials.

Author Contributions: V.A. conceived the original draft preparation. V.A., A.T., A.P.S., K.P., and N.P. were responsible for conception and design of the review. A.T., N.P., K.P., A.P.S., C.C.D., and M.R. were responsible for the data acquisition. A.T., K.P., V.A., N.P., A.P.S., and I.M. were responsible for the collection and assembly of the articles/published data, and their inclusion and interpretation in this review. V.A., A.T., K.P., N.P., and A.P.S. contributed equally to the present work. All authors contributed to the critical revision of the manuscript for valuable intellectual content. All authors have read and agreed to the published version of the manuscript.

Funding: No funding was received.

Conflicts of Interest: A.P.S. was on advisory boards and received honoraria as a speaker for Astra Zeneca, Eli Lilly, Merck, Novo Nordisk, and Sanofi. She is currently Vice President of the Romanian National Committee of Diabetes, Nutrition and Metabolic Diseases. M.R. was on advisory boards for Astra Zeneca, Eli Lilly, Merck, Novo Nordisk, and Sanofi. He is currently the Director of Clinical Medicine and Regulatory Affairs at Novo Nordisk Europe East and South. N.P. has been an Advisory Board Member of TrigoCare International, Abbott, AstraZeneca, Elpen, MSD, Novartis, Novo Nordisk, Sanofi-Aventis, and Takeda. He has participated in sponsored studies by Eli Lilly, MSD, Novo Nordisk, Novartis, and Sanofi-Aventis. He has received honoraria as a speaker for AstraZeneca, Boehringer Ingelheim, Eli Lilly, Elpen, Galenica, MSD, Mylan, Novartis, Novo Nordisk, Pfizer, Sanofi-Aventis, Takeda, and Vianex. He has attended conferences sponsored by TrigoCare International, AstraZeneca, Boehringer Ingelheim, Eli Lilly, Novartis, Novo Nordisk, Pfizer, and Sanofi-Aventis. The other authors declare no conflict of interest.

References

1. Pop-Busui, R.; Boulton, A.J.M.; Feldman, E.L.; Bril, V.; Freeman, R.; Malik, R.A.; Sosenko, J.M.; Ziegler, D. Diabetic neuropathy: A position statement by the American Diabetes Association. *Diabetes Care* **2017**, *40*, 136–154. [CrossRef] [PubMed]
2. Ziegler, D.; Papanas, N.; Vinik, A.I.; Shaw, J.E. Epidemiology of polyneuropathy in diabetes and prediabetes. In *Handbook of Clinical Neurology*; Elsevier BV: Amsterdam, The Netherlands, 2014; Volume 126, pp. 3–22.
3. Papanas, N.; Ziegler, D. Risk factors and comorbidities in diabetic neuropathy: An update 2015. *Rev. Diabet. Stud.* **2015**, *12*, 48–62. [CrossRef] [PubMed]
4. Deng, Y.; Luo, L.; Hu, Y.; Fang, K.; Liu, J. Clinical practice guidelines for the management of neuropathic pain: A systematic review. *BMC Anesthesiol.* **2016**, *16*, 12. [CrossRef] [PubMed]
5. Finnerup, N.B.; Attal, N.; Haroutounian, S.; McNicol, E.; Baron, R.; Dworkin, R.H.; Gilron, I.; Haanpää, M.; Hansson, P.; Jensen, T.S.; et al. Pharmacotherapy for neuropathic pain in adults: A systematic review and meta-analysis. *Lancet Neurol.* **2015**, *14*, 162–173. [CrossRef]
6. Dowell, D.; Haegerich, T.M.; Chou, R. CDC guideline for prescribing opioids for chronic pain—United States. *MMWR* **2016**, *65*, 1–49. [PubMed]
7. Diabetes Control and Complications Trial (DCCT) Research Group. Effect of intensive diabetes treatment on nerve conduction in the Diabetes Control and Complications Trial. *Ann. Neurol.* **1995**, *38*, 869–880. [CrossRef] [PubMed]
8. CDC Study Group. The effect of intensive diabetes therapy on measures of autonomic nervous system function in the Diabetes Control and Complications Trial (DCCT). *Diabetologia* **1998**, *41*, 416–423. [CrossRef]
9. Albers, J.W.; Herman, W.H.; Pop-Busui, R.; Feldman, E.L.; Martin, C.L.; Cleary, P.A.; Waberski, B.H.; Lachin, J.M.; Diabetes Control and Complications Trial/Epidemiology of Diabetes Interventions and Complications Research Group. Effect of prior intensive insulin treatment during the Diabetes Control and Complications Trial (DCCT) on peripheral neuropathy in type 1 diabetes during the Epidemiology of Diabetes Interventions and Complications (EDIC) study. *Diabetes Care* **2010**, *33*, 1090–1096. [CrossRef]

10. Pop-Busui, R.; Low, P.A.; Waberski, B.H.; Martin, C.L.; Albers, J.W.; Feldman, E.L.; Sommer, C.; Cleary, P.A.; Lachin, J.M.; Herman, W.H.; et al. Effects of prior intensive insulin therapy on cardiac autonomic nervous system function in type 1 diabetes mellitus:the Diabetes Control and Complications Trial/Epidemiology of Diabetes Interventions and Complications study (DCCT/EDIC). *Circulation* **2009**, *19*, 2886–2893. [CrossRef]
11. Martin, C.L.; Albers, J.W.; Pop-Busui, R.; DCCT/EDIC Research Group. Neuropathy and related findings in the Diabetes Control and Complications Trial/Epidemiology of Diabetes Interventions and Complications study. *Diabetes Care* **2014**, *37*, 31–38. [CrossRef]
12. Ismail-Beigi, F.; Craven, T.; Banerji, M.A.; Basile, J.; Calles, J.; Cohen, R.M.; Cuddihy, R.; Cushman, W.C.; Genuth, S.; Grimm, R.H., Jr.; et al. Effect of intensive treatment of hyperglycaemia on microvascular outcomes in type 2 diabetes: An analysis of the ACCORD randomised trial. *Lancet* **2010**, *376*, 419–430. [CrossRef]
13. Callaghan, B.C.; Little, A.A.; Feldman, E.L.; Hughes, R.A.C. Enhanced glucose control for preventing and treating diabetic neuropathy. *Cochrane Database Syst. Rev.* **2012**, *6*. [CrossRef] [PubMed]
14. Ang, L.; Jaiswal, M.; Martin, C.; Pop-Busui, R. Glucose control and diabetic neuropathy: Lessons from recent large clinical trials. *Curr. Diabetes Rep.* **2014**, *14*, 528. [CrossRef] [PubMed]
15. Zoungas, S.; Arima, H.; Gerstein, H.C.; Holman, R.R.; Woodward, M.; Reaven, P.; Hayward, R.A.; Craven, T.; Coleman, R.L.; Chalmers, J. Effects of intensive glucose control on microvascular outcomes in patients with type 2 diabetes: A meta-analysis of individual participant data from randomized controlled trials. *Lancet Diabetes Endocrinol.* **2017**, *5*, 431–437. [CrossRef]
16. Pop-Busui, R.; Lu, J.; Brooks, M.M.; Albert, S.; Althouse, A.D.; Escobedo, J.; Green, J.; Palumbo, P.; Perkins, B.A.; Whitehouse, F.; et al. Impact of glycemic control strategies on the progression of diabetic peripheral neuropathy in the Bypass Angioplasty Revascularization Investigation 2 Diabetes (BARI 2D) cohort. *Diabetes Care* **2013**, *36*, 3208–3215. [CrossRef]
17. Griebeler, M.L.; Morey-Vargas, O.L.; Brito, J.P.; Tsapas, A.; Wang, Z.; Leon, B.G.C.; Phung, O.J.; Montori, V.M.; Murad, M.H. Pharmacologic interventions for painful diabetic neuropathy: An umbrella systematic review and comparative effectiveness network meta-analysis. *Ann. Intern. Med.* **2014**, *161*, 639–649. [CrossRef]
18. Tesfaye, S.; Wilhelm, S.; Lledo, A.; Schacht, A.; Tölle, T.; Bouhassira, D.; Cruccu, G.; Skljarevski, V.; Freynhagen, R. Duloxetine and pregabalin: High-dose monotherapy or their combination? The "COMBO-DN study"—A multinational, randomized, double-blind, parallel-group study in patients with diabetic peripheral neuropathic pain. *PAIN* **2013**, *154*, 2616–2625. [CrossRef]
19. Quilici, S.; Chancellor, J.; Lothgren, M.; Simon, D.; Said, G.; Le, T.K.; Garcia-Cebrian, A.; Monz, B. Meta-analysis of duloxetine vs. pregabalin and gabapentin in the treatment of diabetic peripheral neuropathic pain. *BMC Neurol.* **2009**, *9*, 6. [CrossRef] [PubMed]
20. Wernicke, J.F.; Pritchett, Y.L.; D'Souza, D.N.; Waninger, A.; Tran, P.; Iyengar, S.; Raskin, J. A randomized controlled trial of duloxetine in diabetic peripheral neuropathic pain. *Neurology* **2006**, *67*, 1411–1420. [CrossRef]
21. Hardy, T.; Sachson, R.; Shen, S.; Armbruster, M.; Boulton, A.J.M. Does treatment with duloxetine for neuropathic pain impact glycemic control? *Diabetes Care* **2007**, *30*, 21–26. [CrossRef]
22. Goldstein, D.J.; Lu, Y.; Detke, M.J.; Lee, T.C.; Iyengar, S. Duloxetine vs. Placebo in patients with painful diabetic neuropathy. *PAIN* **2005**, *116*, 109–118. [CrossRef] [PubMed]
23. Vinik, A.; Casellini, C.; Nevoret, M.L. Diabetic Neuropathies. In *Endotext [Internet]*; Feingold, K.R., Anawalt, B., Boyce, A., Eds.; Table 7, Drugs Approved by the FDA for Treatment of Neuropathic Pain Syndromes; MDText.com, Inc.: South Dartmouth, MA, USA, 2000.
24. Max, M.B. Endogenous monoamine analgesic systems: Amitriptyline in painful diabetic neuropathy. *Anesth. Prog.* **1987**, *34*, 113–127. [PubMed]
25. Bansal, D.; Bhansali, A.; Hota, D.; Chakrabarti, A.; Dutta, P. Amitriptyline vs. pregabalin in painful diabetic neuropathy: A randomized double blind clinical trial. *Diabet. Med.* **2009**, *26*, 1019–1026. [CrossRef] [PubMed]
26. Morello, C.M.; Leckband, S.G.; Stoner, C.P.; Moorhouse, D.F.; Sahagian, G.A. Randomized double-blind study comparing the efficacy of gabapentin with amitriptyline on diabetic peripheral neuropathy pain. *Arch. Intern. Med.* **1999**, *159*, 1931–1937. [CrossRef]
27. Kaur, H.; Hota, D.; Bhansali, A.; Dutta, P.; Bansal, D.; Chakrabarti, A. A comparative evaluation of amitriptyline and duloxetine in painful diabetic neuropathy: A randomized, double-blind, cross-over clinical trial. *Diabetes Care* **2011**, *34*, 818–822. [CrossRef]
28. Boulton, A.J.M. Management of diabetic peripheral neuropathy. *Clin. Diabetes* **2005**, *23*, 9–15. [CrossRef]

29. Max, M.B.; Lynch, S.A.; Muir, J.; Shoaf, S.E.; Smoller, B.; Dubner, R. Effects of desipramine, amitriptyline, and fluoxetine on pain in diabetic neuropathy. *N. Engl. J. Med.* **1992**, *326*, 1250–1256. [CrossRef]
30. Ulugol, A.; Karadag, H.C.; Tamer, M.; Firat, Z.; Aslantas, A.; Dokmeci, I. Involvement of adenosine in the anti-allodynic effect of amitriptyline in streptozotocin-induced diabetic rats. *Neurosci. Lett.* **2002**, *328*, 129–132. [CrossRef]
31. American Academy of Neurology AAN Summary of Evidence-Based Guidelines for Clinicians: Treatment of Painful Diabetic Neuropathy. 2011. Available online: https://www.aan.com/Guidelines/home/GetGuidelineContent/480 (accessed on 6 August 2019).
32. Cohen, K.; Shinkazh, N.; Frank, J.; Israel, I.; Fellner, C. Pharmacological treatment of diabetic peripheral neuropathy. *Pharm. Ther.* **2015**, *40*, 372–388.
33. Thour, A.; Marwaha, R. Amitriptyline. In *StatPearls [Internet]*; StatPearls Publishing: Treasure Island, FL, USA, 2019.
34. Gallagher, H.C.; Gallagher, R.M.; Butler, M.; Buggy, D.J.; Henman, M.C. Venlafaxine for neuropathic pain in adults. *Cochrane Database Syst. Rev.* **2015**, *8*. [CrossRef]
35. Rowbotham, M.C.; Goli, V.; Kunz, N.R.; Lei, D. Venlafaxine extended release in the treatment of painful diabetic neuropathy: A double-blind, placebo-controlled study. *PAIN* **2004**, *110*, 697–706. [CrossRef] [PubMed]
36. Cross, A.L.; Sherman, A.L. Pregabalin. In *StatPearls [Internet]*; StatPearls Publishing: Treasure Island, FL, USA, 2019.
37. Freeman, R.; Durso-Decruz, E.; Emir, B. Efficacy, safety, and tolerability of pregabalin treatment for painful diabetic peripheral neuropathy: Findings from seven randomized, controlled trials across a range of doses. *Diabetes Care* **2008**, *31*, 1448–1454. [CrossRef] [PubMed]
38. Moore, R.A.; Straube, S.; Wiffen, P.J.; Derry, S.; McQuay, H.J. Pregabalin for acute and chronic pain in adults. *Cochrane Database Syst. Rev.* **2009**, *3*. [CrossRef] [PubMed]
39. Raskin, P.; Huffman, C.; Toth, C.; Asmus, M.J.; Messig, M.; Sanchez, R.J.; Pauer, L. Pregabalin in patients with inadequately treated painful diabetic peripheral neuropathy: A randomized withdrawal trial. *Clin. J. Pain* **2014**, *30*, 379–390. [CrossRef]
40. Ziegler, D.; Duan, W.R.; An, G.; Thomas, J.W.; Nothaft, W. A randomized double-blind, placebo, and active-controlled study of T-type calcium channel blocker ABT-639 in patients with diabetic peripheral neuropathic pain. *PAIN* **2015**, *56*, 2013–2020. [CrossRef]
41. Dworkin, R.H.; Jensen, M.P.; Gammaitoni, A.R.; Olaleye, D.O.; Galer, B.S. Symptom profiles differ in patients with neuropathic versus non-neuropathic pain. *J. Pain* **2007**, *8*, 118–126. [CrossRef]
42. Wiffen, P.J.; Derry, S.; Bell, R.F.; Rice, A.S.; Tölle, T.R.; Phillips, T.; Moore, R.A. Gabapentin for chronic neuropathic pain in adults. *Cochrane Database Syst. Rev.* **2017**, *6*. [CrossRef]
43. Backonja, M.; Beydoun, A.; Edwards, K.R.; Schwartz, S.L.; Fonseca, V.; Hes, M.; LaMoreaux, L.; Garofalo, E.; Gabapentin Diabetic Neuropathy Study Group. Gabapentin for the symptomatic treatment of painful neuropathy in patients with diabetes mellitus: A randomized controlled trial. *JAMA* **1998**, *280*, 1831–1836. [CrossRef]
44. Moore, R.A.; Wiffen, P.J.; Derry, S.; Toelle, T.; Rice, A.S. Gabapentin for chronic neuropathic pain and fibromyalgia in adults. *Cochrane Database Syst. Rev.* **2014**, *4*. [CrossRef]
45. Dallocchio, C.; Buffa, C.; Mazzarello, P.; Chiroli, S. Gabapentin vs. amitriptyline in painful diabetic neuropathy: An open-label pilot study. *J. Pain Symptom Manag.* **2000**, *20*, 280–285. [CrossRef]
46. Simpson, D.A. Gabapentin and venlafaxine for the treatment of painful diabetic neuropathy. *J. Clin. Neuromuscul. Dis.* **2001**, *3*, 53–62. [CrossRef]
47. *Neurontin (Gabapentin) Prescribing Information*; Pfizer, Inc.: New York, NY, USA, 2014.
48. Ziegler, D.; Fonseca, V. From guideline to patient: A review of recent recommendations for pharmacotherapy of painful diabetic neuropathy. *J. Diabetes Complicat.* **2015**, *29*, 146–156. [CrossRef] [PubMed]
49. Waldfogel, J.M.; Nesbit, S.A.; Dy, S.M.; Sharma, R.; Zhang, A.; Wilson, L.M.; Bennett, W.L.; Yeh, H.C.; Chelladurai, Y.; Feldman, D.; et al. Pharmacotherapy for diabetic peripheral neuropathy pain and quality of life: A systematic review. *Neurology* **2017**, *88*, 1958–1967. [CrossRef] [PubMed]
50. Papanas, N.; Ziegler, D. Emerging drugs for diabetic peripheral neuropathy and neuropathic pain. *Expert Opin. Emerg. Drugs* **2016**, *21*, 393–407. [CrossRef] [PubMed]

51. Vadivelu, N.; Huang, Y.; Mirante, B.; Jacoby, M.; Braveman, F.R.; Hines, R.L.; Sinatra, R. Patient considerations in the use of tapentadol for moderate to severe pain. *Drug Healthc. Patient Saf.* **2013**, *5*, 151–159. [CrossRef] [PubMed]
52. Schwartz, S.; Etropolski, M.; Shapiro, D.Y.; Okamoto, A.; Lange, R.; Haeussler, J.; Rauschkolb, C. Safety and efficacy of tapentadol ER in patients with painful diabetic peripheral neuropathy: Results of a randomized-withdrawal, placebo-controlled trial. *Curr. Med. Res. Opin.* **2011**, *27*, 151–162. [CrossRef] [PubMed]
53. Vinik, A.I.; Shapiro, D.Y.; Rauschkolb, C.; Lange, B.; Karcher, K.; Pennett, D.; Etropolski, M.S. A randomized withdrawal, placebo-controlled study evaluating the efficacy and tolerability of tapentadol extended release in patients with chronic painful diabetic peripheral neuropathy. *Diabetes Care* **2014**, *37*, 2302–2309. [CrossRef]
54. Chong, M.S.; Hester, J. Diabetic painful neuropathy: Current and future treatment options. *Drugs* **2007**, *67*, 569–585. [CrossRef]
55. Snyder, M.J.; Gibbs, L.M.; Lindsay, T.J. Treating painful diabetic peripheral neuropathy: An update. *Am. Fam. Phys.* **2016**, *94*, 227–234.
56. Anonymous. What role for capsaicin in diabetic peripheral neuropathy? *Drug Ther. Bull.* **2016**, *54*, 90–93. [CrossRef]
57. Donofrio, P.; Walker, F.; Hunt, V.; Lewis, G.; Mireles, J.A.; Hoffman, J.; Scheffler, N.; Sheitel, P.; Campbell, S.; Wendt, J.; et al. Treatment of painful diabetic neuropathy with topical capsaicin. A multicenter, double-blind, vehicle-controlled study. *Arch. Intern. Med.* **1991**, *151*, 2225–2229.
58. Capsaicin Study Group. Effect of treatment with capsaicin on daily activities of patients with painful diabetic neuropathy. *Diabetes Care* **1992**, *15*, 159–165. [CrossRef] [PubMed]
59. Tandan, R.; Lewis, G.A.; Badger, G.B.; Fries, T.J. Topical capsaicin in painful diabetic neuropathy. Effect on sensory function. *Diabetes Care* **1992**, *15*, 15–18. [CrossRef] [PubMed]
60. Tandan, R.; Lewis, G.A.; Krusinski, P.B.; Badger, G.B.; Fries, T.J. Topical capsaicin in painful diabetic neuropathy. Controlled study with long-term follow-up. *Diabetes Care* **1992**, *15*, 8–14. [CrossRef]
61. Low, P.A.; Opfer-Gehrking, T.L.; Dyck, P.J.; Litchy, W.J.; O'Brien, P.C. Double-blind, placebo-controlled study of the application of capsaicin cream in chronic distal painful polyneuropathy. *PAIN* **1995**, *62*, 163–168. [CrossRef]
62. Chad, D.A.; Aronin, N.; Lundstrom, R.; McKeon, P.; Ross, D.; Molitch, M.; Schipper, H.M.; Stall, G.; Dyess, E.; Tarsy, D. Does capsaicin relieve the pain of diabetic neuropathy? *PAIN* **1990**, *42*, 387–388. [CrossRef]
63. Kulkantrakorn, K.; Chomjit, A.; Sithinamsuwan, P.; Tharavanij, T.; Suwankanoknark, J.; Napunnaphat, P. 0.075% capsaicin lotion for the treatment of painful diabetic neuropathy: A randomized, double-blind, crossover, placebo-controlled trial. *J. Clin. Neurosci.* **2019**, *62*, 174–179. [CrossRef]
64. Biesbroek, R.; Bril, V.; Hollander, P.; Kabadi, U.; Schwartz, S.; Singh, S.P.; Ward, W.K.; Bernstein, J.E. A double-blind comparison of topical capsaicin and oral amitriptyline in painful diabetic neuropathy. *Adv. Ther.* **1995**, *12*, 111–120.
65. Zin, C.S.; Nissen, L.M.; Smith, M.T.; O'Callaghan, J.P.; Moore, B.J. An update on the pharmacological management of post-herpetic neuralgia and painful diabetic neuropathy. *CNS Drugs* **2008**, *22*, 417–442. [CrossRef]
66. Derry, S.; Rice, A.S.; Cole, P.; Tan, T.; Moore, R.A. Topical capsaicin (high concentration) for chronic neuropathic pain in adults. *Cochrane Database Syst. Rev.* **2017**, *1*. [CrossRef]
67. Van Nooten, F.; Treur, M.; Pantiri, K.; Stoker, M.; Charokopou, M. Capsaicin 8% patch versus oral neuropathic pain medications for the treatment of painful diabetic peripheral neuropathy: A systematic literature review and network meta-analysis. *Clin. Ther.* **2017**, *39*, 787–803. [CrossRef] [PubMed]
68. Baranidharan, G.; Das, S.; Bhaskar, A. A review of the high-concentration capsaicin patch and experience in its use in the management of neuropathic pain. *Ther. Adv. Neurol. Disord.* **2013**, *6*, 287–297. [CrossRef] [PubMed]
69. Mou, J.; Paillard, F.; Turnbull, B.; Trudeau, J.; Stoker, M.; Katz, N.P. Qutenza (capsaicin) 8% patch onset and duration of response and effects of multiple treatments in neuropathic pain patients. *Clin. J. Pain* **2014**, *30*, 286–294. [CrossRef] [PubMed]
70. Mick, G.; Correa-Illanes, G. Topical pain management with the 5% lidocaine medicated plaster-a review. *Curr. Med. Res. Opin.* **2012**, *28*, 937–951. [CrossRef] [PubMed]

71. Krumova, E.K.; Zeller, M.; Westermann, A.; Maier, C. Lidocaine patch (5%) produces a selective, but incomplete block of Aδ and C fibers. *PAIN* **2012**, *153*, 273–280. [CrossRef]
72. Baron, R.; Mayoral, V.; Leijon, G.; Binder, A.; Steigerwald, I.; Serpell, M. 5% lidocaine medicated plaster versus pregabalin in post-herpetic neuralgia and diabetic polyneuropathy: An open-label, non-inferiority two-stage RCT study. *Curr. Med. Res. Opin.* **2009**, *25*, 1663–1676. [CrossRef]
73. Wolff, R.F.; Bala, M.M.; Westwood, M.; Kessels, A.G.; Kleijnen, J. 5% lidocaine medicated plaster in painful diabetic peripheral neuropathy (DPN): A systematic review. *Swiss Med. Wkly.* **2010**, *140*, 297–306.
74. Navez, M.L.; Monella, C.; Bösl, I.; Sommer, D.; Delorme, C. 5% lidocaine medicated plaster for the treatment of postherpetic neuralgia: A review of the clinical safety and tolerability. *Pain Ther.* **2015**, *4*, 1–15. [CrossRef]
75. Wrzosek, A.; Woron, J.; Dobrogowski, J.; Jakowicka-Wordliczek, J.; Wordliczek, J. Topical clonidine for neuropathic pain. *Cochrane Database Syst. Rev.* **2015**, *8*. [CrossRef]
76. Campbell, C.M.; Kipnes, M.S.; Stouch, B.C.; Brady, K.L.; Kelly, M.; Schmidt, W.K.; Petersen, K.L.; Rowbotham, M.C.; Campbell, J.N. Randomized control trial of topical clonidine for treatment of painful diabetic neuropathy. *PAIN* **2012**, *153*, 1815–1823. [CrossRef]
77. Papanas, N.; Ziegler, D. Efficacy of α-lipoic acid in diabetic neuropathy. *Expert Opin. Pharmacother.* **2014**, *15*, 2721–2731. [CrossRef] [PubMed]
78. Leppert, W.; Malec–Milewska, M.; Zajaczkowska, R.; Wordliczek, J. Transdermal and Topical Drug Administration in the Treatment of Pain. *Molecules* **2018**, *23*, 681. [CrossRef] [PubMed]
79. Bönhof, G.J.; Herder, C.; Strom, A.; Papanas, N.; Roden, M.; Ziegler, D. Emerging biomarkers, tools, and treatments for diabetic polyneuropathy. *Endocr. Rev.* **2019**, *40*, 153–192. [CrossRef] [PubMed]
80. Ziegler, D.; Low, P.A.; Litchy, W.J.; Boulton, A.J.; Vinik, A.I.; Freeman, R.; Samigullin, R.; Tritschler, H.; Munzel, U.; Maus, J.; et al. Efficacy and safety of antioxidant treatment with α-lipoic acid over 4 years in diabetic polyneuropathy: The NATHAN 1 trial. *Diabetes Care* **2011**, *34*, 2054–2060. [CrossRef]
81. Papanas, N.; Maltezos, E. A-Lipoic acid, diabetic neuropathy, and Nathan's prophecy. *Angiology* **2012**, *63*, 81–83. [CrossRef]
82. Ziegler, D.; Nowak, H.; Kempler, P.; Vargha, P.; Low, P.A. Treatment of symptomatic diabetic polyneuropathy with the antioxidant alpha-lipoic acid: A meta-analysis. *Diabet. Med.* **2014**, *21*, 114–121. [CrossRef]
83. Alpha Lipoic Acid Pharmacy Compounding Advisory Committee Meeting 12 September 2018. Available online: https://www.fda.gov/media/116311/download (accessed on 12 August 2019).
84. Ziegler, D.; Edmundson, S.; Gurieva, I.; Mankovsky, B.; Papanas, N.; Strokov, I. Predictors of response to treatment with actovegin for 6 months in patients with type 2 diabetes and symptomatic polyneuropathy. *J. Diabetes Complicat.* **2017**, *31*, 1181–1187. [CrossRef]

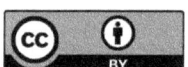

© 2020 by the authors. Licensee MDPI, Basel, Switzerland. This article is an open access article distributed under the terms and conditions of the Creative Commons Attribution (CC BY) license (http://creativecommons.org/licenses/by/4.0/).

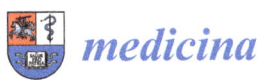

Article

A Single Site Population Study to Investigate CYP2D6 Phenotype of Patients with Persistent Non-Malignant Pain

Helen Radford [1,2], Karen H. Simpson [2], Suzanne Rogerson [2] and Mark I. Johnson [1,*]

1. Centre for Pain Research, School of Clinical and Applied Sciences, Leeds Beckett University, Leeds LS1 3HE, UK; helen.radford2@nhs.net
2. Centre for Neurosciences, Leeds Teaching Hospitals NHS Trust, Leeds LS1 3EX, UK; dr.karen.simpson@googlemail.com (K.H.S.); suzannerogerson@nhs.net (S.R.)
* Correspondence: m.johnson@leedsbeckett.ac.uk

Received: 29 March 2019; Accepted: 23 May 2019; Published: 28 May 2019

Abstract: *Background and Objectives*: Codeine requires biotransformation by the CYP2D6 enzyme, encoded by the polymorphic *CYP2D6* gene, to morphine for therapeutic efficacy. CYP2D6 phenotypes of poor, intermediate, and ultra-rapid metabolisers are at risk of codeine non-response and adverse drug reactions due to altered CYP2D6 function. The aim of this study was to determine whether genotype, inferred phenotype, and urinary and oral fluid codeine O-demethylation metabolites could predict codeine non-response following a short course of codeine. *Materials and Methods*: There were 131 Caucasians with persistent pain enrolled. Baseline assessments were recorded, prohibited medications ceased, and DNA sampling completed before commencing codeine 30 mg QDS for 5 days. Day 4 urine samples were collected 1–2 h post morning dose for codeine O-demethylation metabolites analysis. Final pain assessments were conducted on day 5. *Results*: None of the poor, intermediate, ultra-rapid metabolisers and only 24.5% of normal metabolisers responded to codeine. A simple scoring system to predict analgesic response from day 4 urinary metabolites was devised with overall prediction success of 79% (sensitivity 0.8, specificity 0.78) for morphine and 79% (sensitivity 0.76, specificity 0.83) for morphine:creatinine ratio. *Conclusions*: In conclusion, this study provides tentative evidence that day 4 urinary codeine O-demethylation metabolites could predict non-response following a short course of codeine and could be utilised in the clinical assessment of codeine response at the point of care to improve analgesic efficacy and safety in codeine therapy. We offer a scoring system to predict codeine response from urinary morphine and urinary morphine:creatinine ratio collected on the morning of day 4 of codeine 30 mg QDS, but this requires validation before it could be considered for use to assess codeine response in clinical practice.

Keywords: pain; analgesics; cytochrome P-450 *CYP2D6*; chronic pain; codeine; pharmacogenetics; pain management

---

1. Introduction

Prescriptions for codeine-based drugs increased by 10.5 percent between 2011 and 2012 in U.K. primary care settings, with an associated net increase in drug ingredient costs of £10.3 million [1]. Codeine requires biotransformation to active metabolites (morphine) via the enzyme CYP2D6. Genetic polymorphism of the *CYP2D6* gene influences the activity of the CYP2D6 enzyme resulting in inter-patient variability that may pose a risk of toxicity and sub-optimal analgesic response [2–17]. The phenotypic groups of CYP2D6 activity are poor metabolisers (PM, minimal or no CYP2D6 activity); intermediate metabolisers (IM, reduced CYP2D6 activity); normal metabolisers (NM, normal CYP2D6 activity); and ultra-rapid metabolisers (UM, greater than expected CYP2D6 activity) [18–20].

PM and IM phenotypes are at risk of sub-optimal analgesic response to codeine due to lower than expected plasma concentrations of morphine. UM phenotypes are at risk of adverse drug reactions (e.g., respiratory depression) due to higher than expected concentrations of morphine. The prevalence in Caucasian adults is ~5–10% for PMs, ~2–11% for IMs, ~77–92% for NMs and ~2–11% for UMs [21]. Prevalence of UMs in North Africans, Ethiopians, and Arabs may be as high as 40% [22,23]. There does not appear to be differences in the prevalence of CYP2D6 polymorphisms in pain patients and the general population [24].

Combining codeine with a drug that inhibits CYP2D6 can change the phenotype of an individual (i.e., phenocopying) due to competition for enzyme activity. For example, an NM may appear to be an IM or a PM due to inhibition of CYP2D6 by the confounding drug [25,26]. Knowledge about the magnitude of CYP2D6 inhibition for certain drugs aids prescribing [27–29]. Prescribing guidelines for CYP2D6 phenotypes have been published with recommendations that PM, IM, and UM phenotypes should be prescribed alternatives to codeine, tramadol, oxycodone, and nortriptyline [21,30,31]. The benefits of tailoring prescribing decisions to CYP2D6 phenotype has been demonstrated [9,14,32–36]. However, CYP2D6 screening is not part of current clinical practice. We previously reported that 19.9% of patients referred by primary care physicians to a secondary care specialist pain management clinic were at risk of drug interactions associated with co-prescription of analgesic prodrugs reliant on CYP2D6 and CYP2D6 inhibitors [37]. A method of inferring phenotype without the need for genotyping is needed at the point of care.

Accuracy of clinical CYP2D6 phenotyping has been explored using non-analgesic CYP2D6 prodrug drugs as urinary biomarkers of CYP2D6 phenotype. These drugs are not suitable to determine CYP2D6 phenotype in pain patients. Tramadol would be an unsuitable CYP2D6 phenotyping agent due to its strong opioid classification. Kirchheiner et al., [38] found that the ratio of urinary total codeine:total morphine from a 0–6 h urine sample post 30 mg codeine dose correlated to PM, NM, and UM phenotypes in healthy volunteers, although the study did not include any participants who were IM phenotypes.

The aim of our study was to determine whether genotype, inferred phenotype and urinary and oral codeine O-demethylation metabolites could predict codeine non-response in Caucasians with persistent pain following a short course of oral codeine.

2. Materials and Methods

The objectives of the study were to: (I) determine the CYP2D6 genetic profile of codeine non-response in self-reported Caucasians with persistent pain; (II) determine whether codeine non-responsiveness differs between nociceptive and neuropathic pain states; and (III) determine whether urinary and oral codeine O-demethylation metabolites predicted phenotype and codeine response.

2.1. Study Design

A single site, population study for a clinical trial of a medicinal product (CTIMP) was designed (http://www.legislation.gov.uk/uksi/2004/1031/pdfs/uksi_20041031_en.pdf). The primary endpoint was codeine non-response defined as participants who did not display a reduction in pain scores of ≥30% for 'average pain during the previous 24 h' over a course of regular codeine therapy. In addition, CYP2D6 genotype, urinary codeine O-demethylation metabolites, clinical response to codeine, and patient reported outcomes—including brief pain inventory and global impression of health—were recorded.

The study protocol was reviewed by the research team at Seacroft Hospital, Leeds Teaching Hospitals NHS Trust, Leeds U.K. and by two independent pain researchers. Study sponsorship was granted by the Research and Development department and by the Quality Assurance team at Leeds Teaching Hospitals NHS Trust. Ethical approval was granted by the Leeds East (Type 2, CTIMP flagged) Research Ethics Committee (REC: 08/H1307/132). The study was authorised by the U.K. Medicines and Healthcare Regulatory Agency, adopted by the National Institute of Health Research Clinical Research

Network portfolio (UKCRN, ID 7230), and registered on the International Standard of Randomised Controlled Trials database (ISRCTN; Trial identification number: 16874724). Amendments to study design made after the commencement of the study were approved by the Research Ethics Committee and the Medicines and Healthcare Regulatory Agency. The amendments included addition of a poster advert to aid recruitment, removal of oral fluid testing following interim analysis and change to inclusion criteria to include 'worst pain' in 24 h pain score.

2.2. Recruitment and Selection of Participants

A sample of 131 self-reported Caucasian persistent non-malignant pain patients were recruited from the Pain Clinic at Seacroft Hospital, Leeds, U.K. from October 2009 to June 2014. Potential participants were identified from the patient database held by pain service or directly from clinic by their consultant. The research nurse (S.R.) searched the database for patients with pain of moderate severity that had persisted for at least six months and who were suitable for the prescription of World Health Organisation (WHO) step 2 analgesics such as codeine. Patients with uncontrolled or escalating pain were not eligible for inclusion in the study. Each potential participant was sent a letter of invitation, a participant information pack, and a consent form. They were contacted by telephone by the research nurse (S.R.) 5–7 days later to discuss willingness and suitability to participate in the study.

2.3. Procedure

Potential participants were invited to attend the pain research clinic at the hospital on three separate occasions within a 15-day period. Visit one involved consent, screening for eligibility, enrolment and analgesic washout; visit two involved collection of samples for *CYP2D6* genotyping, analysis of urinary codeine O-demethylation metabolites and commencement of codeine treatment; and visit three involved cessation of codeine treatment and measurement of study endpoints.

2.3.1. Study Visit One

Potential participants attended the pain clinic for approximately 1 h. The visit commenced with a briefing about the study and taking signed informed consent prior to any trial procedures being conducted.

Screening for Eligibility

Participants were interviewed by the pain research nurse (S.R.) or the principal investigator (H.R.) to assess eligibility for study participation. Participants completed the modified Brief Pain Inventory short form (BPI-sf) [39] to screen for pain severity and interference. The BPI-sf has two validated elements for analysis: pain severity and pain interference. Pain severity is calculated as the mean of scores (on a 0–10 numerical rating scale) for the items 'pain at its worst in the last 24 h', 'pain at its least in the last 24 h', 'pain on the average', and 'pain right now'. Pain interference reflects how pain interferes with daily activities and is calculated as the mean of the items documenting how much pain interfered with 'general activity', 'mood', 'walking ability', 'normal work', 'relations with others', 'sleep and enjoyment of life'.

Inclusion criteria were: self-reported Caucasian; aged between 18–80 years; pain persisting greater than 3 months as diagnosed by a pain physician and recorded on the patient database; and worst pain in the last 24 h ≥ 4 points on question 3 of the BPI-sf (0 = No pain, 10 = Pain as bad as you can imagine; i.e., moderate to severe pain).

Exclusion criteria were: known sensitivity to codeine, history of experiencing intolerable side effects to opioids, persistent pain adequately controlled by weak opioids, history of recreational drug or alcohol abuse within the last two years, surgery, radiotherapy, chemotherapy, or nerve blocks less than four weeks prior to the study, pregnancy or lactation, significant anxiety or depression. Participants were excluded if they were unable to complete questionnaires in English, had participated in another clinical study within the previous four weeks, had been prescribed strong opioids that could interfere with urinalysis and who were unable to cease taking their medication for the study period. Females who were less than two years post-menopausal who were not taking adequate contraceptive precautions (i.e., an oral contraceptive, an approved hormonal implant, an intrauterine device or condoms/diaphragm and spermicide) or who had not undergone hysterectomy or surgical sterilisation (bilateral tubal ligation or bilateral oophorectomy) were excluded.

Procedures were undertaken to ensure there were no underlying medical conditions that required further investigation. A 20 mL venous blood sample was collected and analysed. Participants were excluded if they had inadequate renal function (i.e., serum creatinine as ≥130 μmol/L (females); ≥150 μmol/L (males)), liver enzymes aspartate aminotransferase or alanine aminotransferase more than twice the upper limit of normal, alkaline phosphatase more than twice the upper limit of normal, bilirubin outside of normal range, haemoglobin concentration outside normal limits, white blood cell count below the lower limit of normal or above 12×10^9/L, and abnormal plasma electrolytes. A urine sample was collected in a plain sterile container for dipstick analysis for pH, specific gravity, leukocytes, nitrates, protein, glucose, ketones, urobilinogen, bilirubin, and blood using Combur Test® (Roche Diagnostics, Risch-Rotkreuz, Switzerland) reactive strips. Participants with abnormal results were discussed with the pain consultant (K.H.S.) to ensure that the participant was safe to continue on the study, otherwise they were excluded. Females of childbearing potential were required to have a negative urine pregnancy test.

Participants also completed a self-report version of the Leeds Assessment of Neuropathic Pain Scale (S-LANSS) [40] to indicate the presence of neuropathic components of pain. A cut-point of ≥12 points on the S-LANSS was used to define the presence of neuropathic components of pain.

Analgesic Washout

At visit one, participants were asked to stop taking analgesic prodrugs requiring CYP2D6 biotransformation (codeine phosphate including combination therapies, tramadol) and CYP2D6 inhibitors identified using information from Baxter [28], Flockhart [29], and the Medicines and Healthcare Regulatory Authority [41]. Participants were allowed to continue with prescribed anti-depressants, anti-convulsants or non-steroidal anti-inflammatory drugs (NSAIDs) providing the treatment was initiated at least two weeks prior to visit one and remained at a stable dose for the study duration. Participants were allowed to continue with oral contraceptives that are a weak CYP2D6 inhibitor, and this was documented for analysis purposes.

All concomitant medication and any changes therein were recorded in the case report (data collection) form. Participants were asked not to commence any new drug therapy throughout the codeine treatment period (between visit two and visit three). Participants were dispensed 64 paracetamol tablets (500 mg) for breakthrough pain and instructed to take 1 g 4–6 hourly (maximum of 4 g in 24 h) for pain relief if required throughout the study period. Participants were asked to complete the BPI-sf and to document paracetamol consumption and any associated adverse events every day in a pain diary before retiring to bed.

2.3.2. Study Visit Two

Visit two took place 48 h after visit one and lasted approximately 3 h. On arrival eligibility to continue with the study was checked (i.e., results from blood and urine tests) and they completed the BPI-sf which was used as pre-treatment baseline measure of pain severity and interference.

CYP2D6 Genotyping

CYP2D6 genotyping was performed to determine activity scores from which phenotype was inferred. A 2 mL saliva sample was collected for *CYP2D6* genotyping after a 30-min oral fast. A Oragene•DNA Self-Collection all-in-one system (DNA Genotek, Ottawa, ON, Canada) was used for the collection, preservation, transportation, and purification of DNA from saliva. Samples were stored for no more than 6 months in the pain clinic at room temperature and protected from light (storage stability approximately 5 years: https://www.dnagenotek.com/ROW/pdf/PD-WP-005.pdf). Samples were transported ambient in batches to KBiosciences Laboratory, Hertfordshire UK for DNA extraction and processing. *CYP2D6* allele selection and base sequencing for identification was determined from allele frequencies for a Caucasian population from the literature [18,42]. A Kompetitive Allele Specific PCR genotyping system (KASP™) was used for DNA extraction and processing (competitive allele specific polymerase chain reaction) for *CYP2D6* alleles *1, *2, *3, *4, *5, *6, *9, *10, *41 and a Hybeacon assay for *CYP2D6* duplication.

The genetic data was received electronically on encrypted Excel spreadsheets from the KBiosciences Laboratory and transcribed—including deletions, duplications, and multiple SNPs/allele identification—into a study specific worksheet designed to facilitate the process of inferring phenotype from genotype (by H.R.). Alleles were allocated a CYP2D6 activity score using a scoring method by Gaedigk et al. (1999) [43]. Phenotype was inferred from the total sum of activity scores of both alleles and duplications using classifications reported by Crews et al. [44]. Worksheets were quality checked and countersigned (by K.H.S.) to ensure correct phenotype had been inferred from genotype.

Collection and Analysis of Urinary Codeine O-demethylation Metabolites

A urine sample was obtained for analysis of urinary codeine O-demethylation metabolites to confirm that no codeine had been consumed during the analgesic washout phase (i.e., at baseline). In addition, participants were instructed to collect a sample of urine in sterile a universal container 1–2 h after the morning dose of codeine on the last day of treatment to store the sample in a cool location until they returned to clinic the following day for study visit three. This sample was used to analyse urinary codeine O-demethylation metabolites when the participant was equilibrated with codeine. Samples were stored in the pain clinic at −20 °C until transported in batches to laboratories at Leeds Teaching Hospitals NHS Trust. All samples were stored frozen at −10 to −35 °C until analysis. Total urine morphine and codeine were quantified using liquid chromatography tandem mass spectroscopy (LC-MS/MS). Gradient reversed phase liquid chromatography was performed using a Shimadzu Prominence HPLC system (Shimadzu, Tokyo, Japan) fitted with a Thermo Hy-Purity C8 column (Thermo Fisher Scientific, Cheshire, UK). Drugs were detected using an ABSciex API 5000 tandem mass spectrometer (ABSciex, Warrington, UK). Quantitation was achieved using the internal standard peak area ratio method. The assay was calibrated using reference materials and deuterated internal standards purchased from LGC (Teddington, UK). All urine samples were treated with β-glucuronidase to hydrolyse glucuronide compounds prior to analysis to ensure that total morphine concentration was measured. The lower limit of morphine quantification was 50 µg/L. Lower limit of morphine detection was 10 µg/L. Results below the limit of quantification were provided with the understanding the degree of uncertainty would be high (CV >20%). Samples that contained an amount of morphine greater than the top calibration standard (500 µg/L) were diluted with deionised water and re-analysed. Urine creatinine was measured by either a Beckman LX20 automated analyser (Beckmann, High Wycombe, UK) using an alkaline picrate method or a Siemens Advia automated analyser (Siemens, Surrey, UK) using an enzymatic method. Morphine:creatinine ratios were calculated (µg morphine per mmol creatinine) to correct for differences in urine concentration.

Codeine Treatment

Codeine Phosphate tablets (30 mg, manufactured by TEVA U.K. Ltd. (Manufacturers Authorisation: PL0289/506IR), Phoenix Healthcare Distribution) were procured by the pharmacy department of Leeds Teaching Hospitals NHS Trust and stored protected from light below 25 °C. Participants received 28 tablets of 30 mg codeine phosphate (blister pack) and were instructed to take one 30 mg tablet orally every four hours to a maximum of four tablets in 24 h. This would guarantee that participants had completed three consecutive days of full dosing to ensure the participant was equilibrated with codeine when they provided their urine sample 1–2 h after the morning dose of codeine on the last day of treatment. Eight extra tablets were provided in the blister pack in case of loss or delayed clinic visit.

Participants were administered their first dose of 30 mg codeine with 200 mL of water in the clinic (dosing day 0).

Collection and Analysis of Oral Fluid O-demethylation Codeine Metabolites

Participants provided an oral fluid sample in clinic two hours after their first dose of codeine using an Intercept® collection pad (Orasure Tech Inc, Bethlehem, PA, USA). The collection pad was placed between the lower cheek and gums and gently rubbed back and forth along the gum line until the pad was moist. Once moist the collection pad was left in the mouth for 2 min and then removed and placed into a specimen vial containing 15% methanol in 4 mL ammonium acetate. Oral fluid samples were frozen and stored at −20 °C. Samples were transported in batches to laboratories at Leeds Teaching Hospitals NHS Trust for analysis of free codeine, morphine, norcodeine, and glucuronides of morphine and codeine. Analysis of oral fluid in the first 20 participants identified only one sample as positive for codeine metabolites. Following discussions with the laboratory undertaking the analysis, it was concluded this method was unsuitable to be used to infer CYP2D6 phenotype post codeine dosing. No further analysis was conducted and oral fluid sampling was removed from the study design.

At the end of study visit two, participants were issued with a pain diary to complete each day before retiring to bed. Participants were telephoned by the research nurse (S.R.) on the day before visit three so that adverse events could be assessed and to remind participants to collect their urine sample to bring to clinic.

2.3.3. Study Visit Three

During visit three, participants returned their pain diary and completed the BPI-sf and the Patient Global Impression of Change in Health. The assessors (S.R. and H.R.) completed the Clinician Global Impression of Change Scale after reviewing the participant's pain diary and any adverse events reported by the participant during the visit. The Patient Global Impression of Change questionnaire reflects the patient's belief about treatment efficacy by rating change as 'very much improved', 'much improved', 'minimally improved', 'no change', 'minimally worse', 'much worse', or 'very much worse'.

Participants were asked to return all unused study medication and empty blister packs for drug accountability and controlled destruction. Participants recommenced their regular analgesia or were prescribed codeine if their pain has been effectively controlled at the end of the study period. All study participants were followed up by telephone seven days later to ascertain any late adverse events.

2.4. Withdrawal of Participants from Study

Participants could withdraw from study at any time and without reason. It was planned that data would be collected up until the time of withdrawal and used for analysis with the consent of the participant. The investigator could to withdraw participants from the study at any time due to adverse events, violation of the study protocol, lack of efficacy, or loss to follow-up.

2.5. Pharmacovigilance and Reporting of Adverse Events

Adverse events were captured verbally through any contact with participants or in pain diaries. Serious adverse events were events resulting in death, a life-threatening situation, hospitalisation, or significant disability or incapacity. Adverse events were defined as any untoward medical occurrence observed in a participant during or following administration of codeine that did not necessarily have a causal relationship with treatment. Adverse events could include unfavourable and unintended signs and symptoms including abnormal laboratory findings that may or may not have a causal relationship with the use of codeine or paracetamol. Adverse events were recorded and assessed, and the clinical course of the adverse event was followed until resolution, stabilisation, or until it was determined that the study treatment or participation was not the cause. Adverse events were categorised according whether they were ('expected') or were not ('unexpected') listed on the codeine phosphate 30 mg "Summary of Product Characteristics" [45].

2.6. Outcome Measures

The primary endpoint in this study was codeine non-response defined as a participant who had <30% reduction in BPI-sf pain 'on the average' at the end of the course of codeine therapy. This was measured as the difference between pain 'on the average' at pre-codeine baseline (study visit two) and the mean of pain 'on the average' during codeine therapy (day 0 to day 4). Secondary endpoints used in this study were *CYP2D6* genotype, measurements of urinary codeine O-demethylation metabolites, patient reported outcomes (BPI-sf, Patient Global Impression of Change to Health) assessor determined outcomes (Clinician Global Impression of Change to Health) and frequency and severity of adverse events.

2.7. Data Management and Analysis

The protocol of statistical analyses and calculation of sample size a priori were developed with the biomedical statistical department from Napp Pharmaceuticals. The statistical protocol was peer reviewed by the biomedical statistics department from the University of Leeds as part of the Research Ethics Committee and Medicines and Healthcare Regulatory Agency approval process. The development of the database and statistical analysis of recorded data reported was undertaken by the principal investigator (H.R.). All statistical analyses were performed using IBM SPSS Statistics 21.

2.7.1. Sample Size Calculation

It was calculated that a sample size of 121 participants would give 90% power to detect a larger proportion of codeine non-responders than the null hypothesis of 10%, assuming the true proportion is 20%, using a 5% significance level for a one-sided test. Therefore, a recruitment target of 150 was set based on a drop-out rate of 20% to obtain 121 evaluable participants.

2.7.2. Statistical Analysis

The population for analysis was defined as (I) participants who attended the screening visit (enrolled population) and (II) participants who had their codeine response determined and their CYP2D6 phenotype inferred from genotype (intention-to-treat population).

2.7.3. Analysis of Primary Outcomes

The proportion of codeine non-responders (primary outcome) was calculated with 95% confidence intervals using the exact binomial distribution. A logistic regression analysis was conducted to predict codeine non-response (dependent variable, dichotomous data) from CYP2D6 activity score (independent variable, ordinal data). Analysis of variance (ANOVA) was used to compare log-transformed levels of urinary codeine O-demethylation metabolites between CYP2D6 phenotypes. Logistic regression was used to predict analgesic response using log-transformed urinary total morphine and morphine:creatinine ratio as covariates. A multivariate logistic regression model was developed to predict analgesic response using activity score and log-transformed urinary total morphine and morphine:creatinine ratio. The suitability of the model as predictor of analgesic response was assessed using receiver operating characteristic (ROC) curves.

2.7.4. Analysis of Secondary Outcomes

A descriptive analysis of data from BPI-sf, S-LANSS and Global Impression of Change was performed against codeine non-response and CYP2D6 phenotype. In this study, we used 'pain on the average', 'pain severity', and 'pain interference' in our statistical analysis of BPI-sf outcomes. Concurrent medication was analysed to determine if CYP2D6 substrates impacted on codeine response through autophenocopying. The type and number of substrates was tabulated against CYP2D6 phenotype and codeine response status and a logistic regression analysis used to determine whether CYP2D6 substrates predicted analgesic response. CYP2D6 substrate classification was determined through bioinformatics and cheminformatics databases for each drug identified [46,47]. Study medication (codeine 30 mg QDS and paracetamol 1 g PRN) was excluded from the analysis.

3. Results

3.1. Characteristics of the Sample Population at Enrolment

A total of 131 participants (age range = 23–79 years, 79 females: 52 males) were enrolled into the study (enrolled population, Figure 1). One male participant withdrew consent following visit one without giving a reason. Three females withdrew from the study due to adverse events. One female (NM phenotype, CYP2D6 activity score 2) withdrew due to moderate rash and difficulty in breathing but also experienced multiple mild adverse events such as nausea, loss of appetite, diarrhoea, restlessness, and disturbed sleep. The other females withdrew due to stomach cramps and disturbed sleep (NM phenotype, CYP2D6 activity score 2) and excessive belching and increased acid reflux (PM phenotype, CYP2D6 activity score 0). The *CYP2D6* genotype of two females could not be determined and they were unable to provide an additional DNA sample for analysis. Thus, 125 participants (age range = 23–78 years, 74 females: 51 males) had their codeine response determined and their CYP2D6 phenotype inferred from genotype (Table 1).

Table 1. Characteristics of the study from the intention to treat analysis ($n = 125$) participants at pre-codeine baseline day 0.

Variable	ITT Group		
	Male	Female	Total
Number (%)	51 (40.8%)	74 (59.2%)	125 (100%)
Age (minimum–maximum)	27–78 years	23–77 years	23–79 years
Age (Mean ± SD)	57.10 ± 12.33	55.64 ± 14.74	56.26 ± 13.71
Mean ± SD BPI-sf			
Pain severity	5.73 ± 1.61	6.25 ± 1.82	6.09 ± 1.75
Pain interference	4.99 ± 2.68	5.05 ± 2.59	5.02 ± 2.51
Pain 'on the average'	5.46 ± 1.95	5.81 ± 2.21	6.31 ± 1.76
Tally (%) S-LANSS			
≥12—Neuropathic pain	18/51 (35.30%)	35/74 (47.30%)	53/125 (42.74%)
<12—Nociceptive pain	33/51 (64.70%)	39/74 (52.71%)	71/125 (57.26%)
Medication at enrolment			
Prescribed CYP2D6 analgesic prodrug	29/51 (56.86%)	44/74 (59.46%)	73/125 (58.4%)
Tally (%) Phenotype			
PM (Activity Score = 0.0)	4/51 (7.84%)	7/74 (9.49%)	11/125 (8.8%)
IM (Activity Score = 0.5)	5/51 (9.80%)	1/74 (1.35%)	6/125 (4.8%)
NM (Activity Score = 1.0–2.0)			
• NM (Activity Score = 1.0)	12/51 (23.53%)	20/74 (27.03%)	32/125 (25.6%)
• NM (Activity Score = 1.5)	9/51 (17.65%)	9/74 (12.16%)	18/125 (14.4%)
• NM (Activity Score = 2.0)	20/51 (39.22%)	36/74 (48.65%)	56/125 (44.8%)
UM (>2.0)	1/51 (1.96%)	1/74 (1.35%)	2/125 (1.6%)

ITT, Intention to treat; SD, Standard Deviation; BPI-sf, Brief Pain Inventory short form; NRS, Numerical Rating Scale; S-LANSS, Self-report version of the Leeds Assessment of Neuropathic Pain Scale; PM, Poor metaboliser; IM, Intermediate metaboliser; NM, Normal metaboliser; UM, Ultra metaboliser.

3.2. Characteristics of Pain at Enrolment (n = 131)

Data collected for withdrawn participants were included in the analysis of the enrolled group but not the analysis of the ITT group. The mean ± SD duration of pain was 127.51 ± 133.50 months (Median: 73 months, range 9–636 months), with majority of participants diagnosed with low back pain. At enrolment 55/131 (42%) participants had a S-LANSS score ≥12 suggesting a predominantly neuropathic pain state; 76/131 (58%) participants had a S-LANSS score <12 suggesting a predominantly nociceptive pain state.

At enrolment, 125/131 (95%) participants were taking at least one analgesic and/or pain adjuvant (either prescribed or over-the-counter). There were 36/131 (27%) participants taking one analgesic or pain adjuvant, 33/131 (25%) taking two, 30/131 (23%) taking three, 21/131 (16%) taking four, 2/131 (2%) taking five, and 3/131 (2%) taking six. There were 77/131 (59%) participants taking an analgesic prodrug that was reliant on CYP2D6 activity to obtain analgesic efficacy, with co-codamol (codeine and paracetamol combined, 31/131 (24%) participants) and tramadol (26/131 (20%)) being the most commonly prescribed. Only two (1.5%) participants were prescribed more than one CYP2D6 prodrug analgesics concurrently (codeine with tramadol, and co-codamol with tramadol). There were 91/131 (70%) participants that reported they had previously failed to respond to one or more CYP2D6 analgesic prodrugs (50/131 (38%) and 46/131 (35%) respectively), with failure to respond to tramadol being the most commonly reported. There were 14/131 (11%) participants that reported failure to respond to both tramadol and co-codamol and 4/131 (3%) reporting failure to respond to tramadol, codeine, and co-codamol.

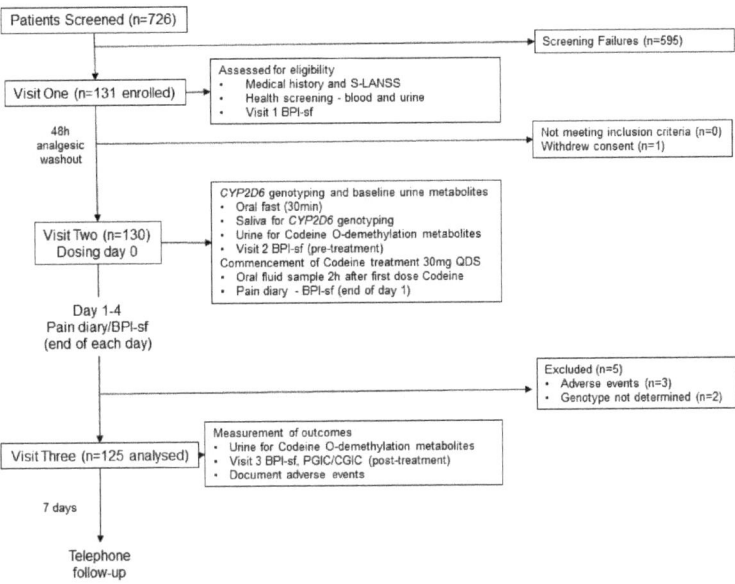

Figure 1. Flow diagram of the progress of participants through phases of the study, adapted from the Consolidated Standards of Reporting Trials (CONSORT) template [48]. PGIC, Patient Global Impression of Change to Health; CGIC, Clinician Global Impression of Change to Health.

3.3. CYP2D6 Genotyping and Inferred Phenotype at Enrolment

Two of the 131 saliva samples collected for *CYP2D6* genotyping were discarded because it was not possible to confirm the CYP2D6 activity score. In one sample, it was not possible to classify the CYP2D6 phenotype due to undetermined allele duplication indicating UM if present or NM if absent. In the other sample, it was not possible to determine the presence of the reduced functional allele *41. Phenotype was inferred from 129 of the 131 enrolled participants as follows: PM = 12/129 (9%), IM = 6/129 (5%), NM = 109/129 (85%), and UM = 2/129 (2%). The proportion of these phenotypes was within the range estimated in a general Caucasian population by Crews et al. [21]. The majority of the NM phenotype group (59/129, 46%) possessed full CYP2D6 activity (activity score of 2.0), with 32/129 (25%) having an activity score of 1.0, and 18/129 (14%) having an activity score of 1.5. The most common diplotype was CYP2D6*1/*2 (NM activity score of 2), followed by the fully functional CYP2D6*1/*1 (NM activity score of 2), CYP2D6*1/*4 (NM activity score of 1) and CYP2D6*4xN/*4 (PM activity score of 0).

A risk of suboptimal response to codeine is likely for PM, IM, or UM phenotypes. The number of participants from the enrolled sample that were taking prodrugs reliant on CYP2D6 activity were 10/12 (83%) PMs, 4/6 (67%) IMs, and 1/2 (50%) UMs. The number of participants from the enrolled sample that reported they had failed to respond to prodrug analgesic medication in the past were 9/10 (90%) PMs, 3/6 (50%) IMs, and 1/2 (50%) UMs.

3.4. Analysis of CYP2D6 Phenotype and Analgesic Response to Codeine

There were statistically significant reductions in 'pain severity', 'pain interference', and 'pain on the average', between pre-codeine baseline and the end of codeine treatment when measured as the difference between pain 'on the average' at pre-codeine baseline (study visit two) and the mean of pain 'on the average' during codeine therapy (i.e., day 0 to day 4, Table 2). However, responder analysis revealed that 99/125 (79%) participants that did not achieve a clinically meaningful reduction of pain of ≥30% from baseline and these participants were categorised as codeine non-responders (41/51 (80%) males, 58/74 (78%) females).

Table 2. Mean ± SD BPI-sf scores in the ITT population ($n = 125$).

BPI-sf	Visit 1 Pre-Analgesic Washout	Visit 2 Pre-Codeine Baseline Day 0	End of Dosing Day (Day 0)	End of Day 1	End of Day 2	End of Day 3	End of Day 4	Mean Day 0–4
Pain severity (composite)	6.31 ± 1.76	6.09 ± 1.75	5.93 ± 1.99	5.67 ± 2.27	5.54 ± 2.28	5.57 ± 2.40	5.62 ± 2.45	5.67 ± 2.17 *
Pain interference (composite)	5.02 ± 2.51	6.14 ± 2.11	5.31 ± 2.40	5.09 ± 2.58	4.90 ± 2.59	4.91 ± 2.66	4.91 ± 2.73	5.02 ± 2.51 *
Pain 'on the average'	6.09 ± 1.75	6.31 ± 1.76	6.00 ± 1.94	5.68 ± 2.28	5.55 ± 2.24	5.51 ± 2.37	5.57 ± 2.35	5.66 ± 2.11 *

The pain severity score was calculated as the mean of NRS scores for 'worst', 'least', 'average' and 'right now' pain. The pain interference score was calculated as the mean of seven items of pain interference. * $p < 0.05$ indicating statistical significance between mean day 0–4 and pre-codeine. SD, Standard Deviation; BPI-sf, Brief Pain Inventory short form; ITT, Intention to treat; NRS, Numerical Rating Scale.

There were 53/125 (42%) participants with a S-LANSS score ≥12 suggesting a predominantly neuropathic pain state; 72/125 (58%) participants had a S-LANSS score <12 suggesting a predominantly nociceptive pain state. There were 26/124 (21.0%) participants categorised as codeine responders (i.e., ≥30% reduction of pain) of which 10/26 (39%) had an S-LANSS score <12. Thus, 43/98 (44%) of participants with an S-LANSS score <12 did not respond to codeine. There were no significant differences in the frequency of response between participants categorised as having predominantly neuropathic or nociceptive pain states ($z = 0.496$, $p = 0.62$, odds ratio = 1.25 (95% CI: 0.52, 3.03)).

All PMs, IMs, and UMs were categorised as codeine non-responders (19 of 125 (15%) participants) and were negatively binomial distributed suggesting that these phenotypes would not respond to codeine in the general population (Table 3). There were 106/125 (83%) participants categorised as NMs. There were 80/106 NMs (76%) categorised as codeine non-responders. Of these, 39/56 (70%) NMs with activity scores of 2 (two fully functional alleles) were categorised as codeine non-responders, 14/18 (78%) with activity scores of 1.5 were categorised as codeine non-responders and 27/32 (84%) with activity scores of 1 were categorised as codeine non-responders.

The logistic regression analysis found that CYP2D6 activity score made a significant contribution to the prediction of codeine response (*Beta* = 0.963, Wald = 5.67 $p = 0.017$). The model Chi-square indicated that CYP2D6 activity score affected codeine response (Chi-sq = 6.78, df = 1, $p = 0.009$). The odds ratio (95% confidence interval) was 2.62 (1.186–5.790) suggesting that individuals with a high CYP2D6 activity score were 2.62 times more likely to respond to codeine than individuals with a low CYP2D6 activity score.

Table 3. Urinary codeine O-demethylation metabolites according to CYP2D6 activity score (AS) and codeine response.

Sample	PM (AS 0.0)	IM (AS 0.5)	NM (AS 1.0–2.0)	NM (AS 1.0)	NM (AS 1.5)	NM (AS 2.0)	UM (>2.0)
Total number (% non-response within phenotype)	11 (100%)	6 (100%)	96 (83.33%)	32 (84.38%)	18 (77.78%)	56 (69.64%)	2 (100%)
Codeine Responders	0	0	26	5	4	17	0
Codeine non-responders	11	6	80	27	14	39	2
Mean ± SD total morphine (μg/L)							
Codeine responders	no responders identified	no responders identified	2902.65 ± 2504.43	1754.6 ± 1661.56	2523.75 ± 1634.72	3329.47 ± 2822.71	no responders identified
Codeine non-responders #	44.18 ± 39.66	415.16 ± 317.83	2419.77 ± 2106.61	1444.65 ± 1342.90	2925.43 ± 2410.52	2846.08 ± 2226.72	5330.00 ± 3464.82
Mean ± SD morphine:creatinine ratio (μg/L)							
Codeine responders	no responders identified	no responders identified	420.04 ± 346.91	271.80 ± 228.06	347.00 ± 243.93	480.82 ± 389.56	no responders identified
Codeine non-responders #	6.91 ± 4.46	35.83 ± 7.14	311.94 ± 231.47	197.96 ± 150.23	307.00 ± 177.35	389.69 ± 263.18	646.50 ± 12.02

one sample missing from NM (AS 1.0), $n = 26$ not 27. SD, Standard Deviation; PM, Poor metaboliser; IM, Intermediate metaboliser; NM, Normal metaboliser; UM, Ultra metaboliser.

3.5. CYP2D6 Phenotype and Global Impression of Change

Analysis of the Patient Global Impression of Change to Health found that 20/26 (77%) participants who obtained an analgesic response to codeine reported improvement on the global impression of change questionnaire and 70/99 (71%) participants who did not obtain an analgesic response to codeine reported improvement on the global impression of change questionnaire. All PMs, IMs, and UMs failed to obtain an analgesic response yet 9/11 (82%) PMs reported improvement, 2/6 (33%) IMs reported improvement and 1/2 (50%) UMs reported improvement. Of the NMs who did not obtain an analgesic response 58/80 (73%) reported improvement compared with 20/26 (77%) of participants who did obtain an analgesic response. The Clinician Global Impression of Change to Health was compared with the self-reported Patient Global Impression of Change to Health for accuracy and was successfully matched in 72% of the participants.

3.6. Analysis of Adverse Events

There were no reported serious adverse events during the course of the study. The most common 'expected' adverse events were headache (46/125 (37%) participants), nausea (41/125 (33%) participants), and constipation (37/125 (30%) participants), with the majority of 'expected' adverse events reported by codeine non-responders. The most common 'unexpected' adverse events were diarrhoea (13/125 (10%) participants), stomach cramps (11/125 (9%) participants), and flu-like symptoms (11/125 participants (8%)), with a majority of 'unexpected' adverse events reported by codeine non-responders. Separate logistic regression analyses of each of these adverse events (i.e. headache, constipation, dry mouth, nausea, and drowsiness) with CYP2D6 activity score and responder status were not statistically significant.

3.7. Analysis of CYP2D6 Autophenocopying

Concurrent medication was analysed to determine if CYP2D6 substrates impacted on codeine response through autophenocopying. There were 41/125 (33%) participants not taking CYP2D6 substrates, 47 (38%) taking one CYP2D6 substrate, 23 (18%) taking two CYP2D6 substrates, 10 (8%) taking three CYP2D6 substrates, and 4 (3%) taking four CYP2D6 substrates. Logistic regression analysis found that the number of concurrent CYP2D6 substrates and log urinary transformed total morphine did not make a significant contribution to the prediction of codeine response (number CYP2D6 substrates Beta = 0.08, Wald = 0.16, p = 0.69; urinary transformed total morphine Beta = 0.000155, Wald = 2.829208, p = 0.09).

3.8. Analysis of Urinary Codeine O-demethylation Metabolites

Urine samples were collected before the first dose of codeine on study visit two (pre-codeine baseline day 0) and after the first dose of codeine on day 4. The sample of one participant was discarded due to leakage in transit from the clinic to the laboratory. Thus, 124 samples were analysed for codeine O-demethylation metabolites (Table 3). Day 4 data for each participant categorised as responder or non-responder for each CYP2D6 phenotype/activity are shown in Figures 2–5.

Data for urinary total morphine were log transformed using a base −10 logarithm to reduce skew. One urine sample from day 4 of a participant categorised as a PM was negative for urinary total morphine metabolites (<50 µg/L) and was not included in the log transformed calculation. Log transformed data was categorised according to CYP2D6 phenotype and analgesic response. There were no significant effects of responder status in the different categories of activity score for NM phenotypes (activity score = 1, $F(1,29)$ = 0.12, p = 0.73: activity score = 1.5, $F(1,16)$ = 0.59, p = 0.45: activity score = 2, $F(1,54)$ = 6.64E-10, p = 1.0). There were similar findings for morphine:creatinine ratio calculated to correct for levels of hydration. One-way ANOVA on log transformed morphine:creatinine ratio found significant effects between CYP2D6 activity scores ($F(5,117)$ = 38.43, p < 0.001). There were no significant effects of responder status in the different categories of activity score for NM phenotypes (activity score = 1, $F(1,28)$ = 0.03, p = 0.87: activity score = 1.5, $F(1,16)$ = 0.24, p = 0.63: activity score = 2, $F(1,54)$ = 0.43, p = 0.51). Logistic regression analysis found that log transformed total morphine and morphine:creatinine ratio did not make a significant contribution to the prediction of codeine response (total morphine Beta = −0.54, Wald = 0.415, p = 0.52; morphine:creatinine ratio Beta = 1.50, Wald = 2.60, p = 0.11).

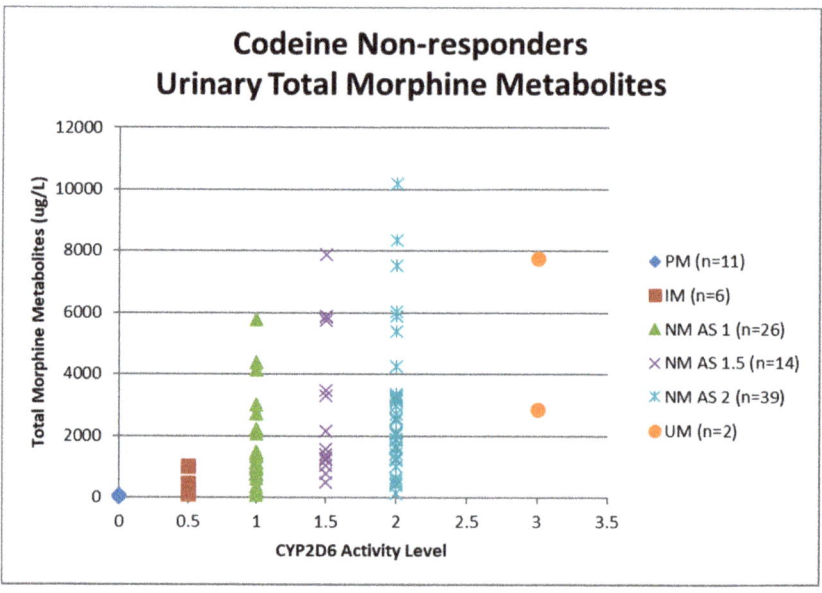

Figure 2. Individual value plot of day 4 urinary total morphine metabolites for each CYP2D6 phenotype/activity score of participants defined as codeine non-responders (<30% reduction in mean day 0–day 4 'average pain' 0–10 numerical rating scale (NRS) score when compared to baseline). AS, Activity Score; PM, Poor metaboliser; IM, Intermediate metaboliser; NM, Normal metaboliser; UM, Ultra metaboliser.

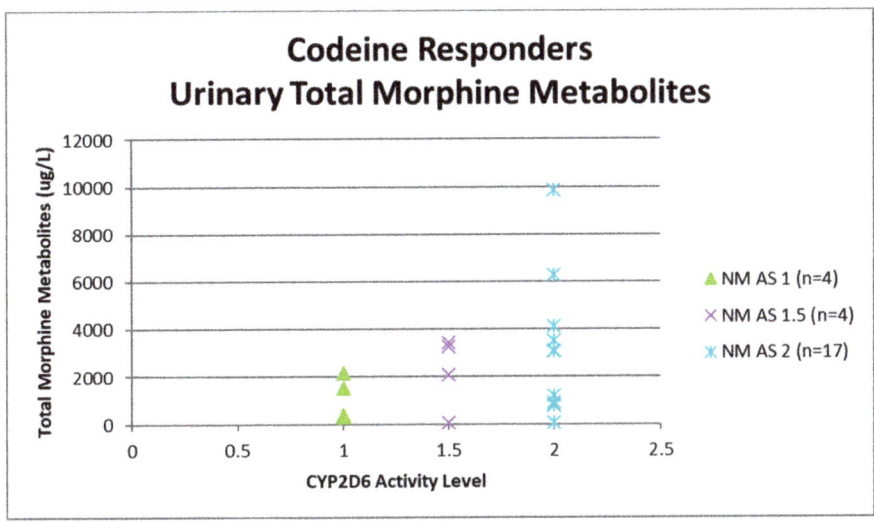

Figure 3. Individual value plot of day 4 urinary total morphine metabolites for each CYP2D6 phenotype/activity score of participants defined as codeine responders (≥30% reduction in mean day 0–day 4 'average pain' 0–10 numerical rating scale (NRS) score when compared to baseline). AS, Activity Score; NM, Normal metaboliser.

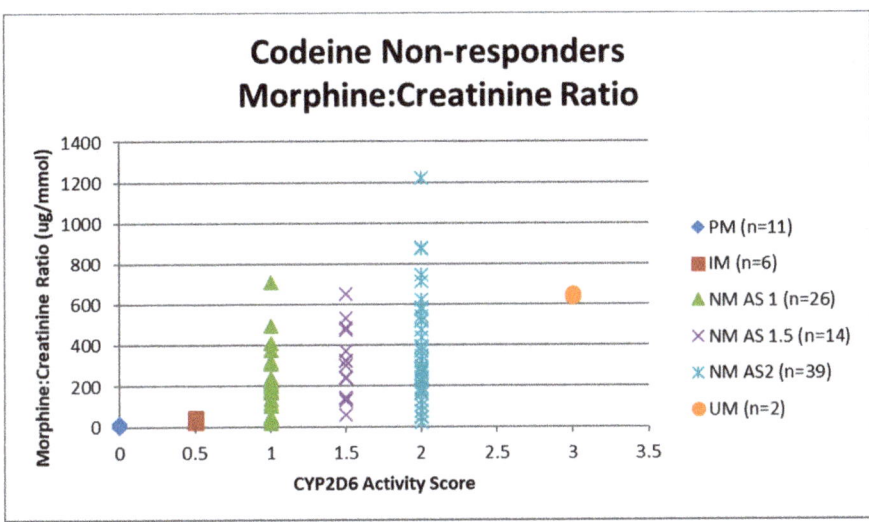

Figure 4. Individual value plot of day 4 urinary morphine:creatinine ratio for each CYP2D6 phenotype/activity score of participants defined as codeine non-responders (<30% reduction in mean day 0–day 4 'average pain' 0–10 numerical rating scale (NRS) score when compared to baseline). AS, Activity Score; PM, Poor metaboliser; IM, Intermediate metaboliser; NM, Normal metaboliser; UM, Ultra metaboliser.

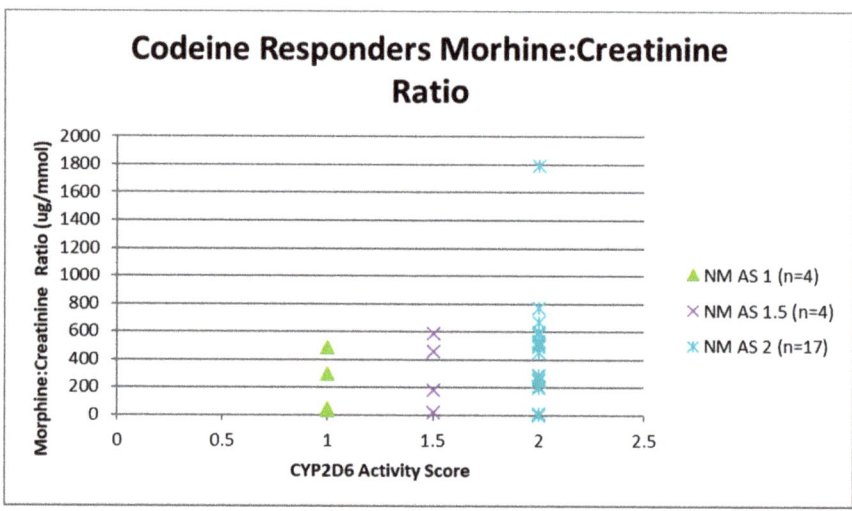

Figure 5. Individual value plot of day 4 urinary morphine:creatinine ratio for each CYP2D6 phenotype/activity score of participants defined as codeine responders (≥30% reduction in mean day 0–day 4 'average pain' 0–10 numerical rating scale (NRS) score when compared to baseline). AS, Activity Score; NM, Normal metaboliser.

3.9. Predicting Analgesic Response from Codeine Urinary Metabolites

We devised a simple scoring system in an attempt to predict analgesic response to codeine (≥30% relief) for urinary total morphine ranges and morphine:creatinine ratio for different CYP2D6 activity scores based on detected urinary metabolite (Table 4) whereby;

- 0 points = Unlikely to respond to codeine (activity score = 0 (PM) and activity score = 0.5 (IM), expected urinary total morphine <500 µg/L, expected urinary morphine:creatinine ratio = 0–100 µg/mmol);
- 1 point = Uncertain whether will respond to codeine (activity score = 1.0 (NM), expected urinary total morphine = 500–1499 µg/L, expected urinary morphine:creatinine ratio = 101–250 µg/mmol)
- 2 points = Likely to respond to codeine (activity score = 1.5 or 2.0 (NM), expected urinary total morphine = 1500–7500 µg/L, expected urinary morphine:creatinine ratio = 251–1000 µg/mmol)
- 3 points = Uncertain whether will respond to codeine and potential for adverse events (activity score >2.0 (UM), expected urinary total morphine >7500 µg/L, expected urinary morphine:creatinine ratio >1000 µg/mmol).

A multivariate logistic regression analysis was used to determine whether log-transformed mean urinary total morphine for day 4 could predict analgesic response and a ROC curve used to assess the suitability of the model. The test of the full model against a constant only model was significant at $p < 0.05$ for predicting codeine responder status using urinary total morphine for day 4 ($Beta = 2.64$, Wald = 35.46, $p < 0.001$). The model chi-square goodness of fit was significant (chi-sq. = 43.47, df = 1, $p < 0.001$). Overall prediction success was 79% with an 82% prediction success for expected codeine non-response and 75% prediction success for expected codeine response, with a sensitivity 0.8, specificity 0.78. Mean urinary morphine:creatinine ratio for day 4 the test of the full model against a constant only model was significant at $p < 0.05$ for predicting codeine responder status ($Beta = 2.77$, Wald = 34.42, $p < 0.001$). The model chi-square goodness of fit was significant (chi-sq. = 44.46, df = 1, $p < 0.001$). Overall prediction success was 79% with an 88% prediction success for expected codeine non-response and 68% prediction success for expected codeine response, with a sensitivity of 0.76, and specificity of 0.83.

Table 4. Points system for predicting codeine response from day 4 urinary total morphine metabolites (μg/L) based on detected urinary metabolite.

CYP2D6 Activity Score (AS)	CYP2D6 Phenotype	Codeine Non-Responder	Codeine Responder	Suggested Range for Predicting Codeine Response	Expected Codeine Response	Points	Rationale
		Mean total morphine (μg/L)	Mean total morphine (μg/L)	Mean total morphine (μg/L)			
0	PM	44.2	no responders identified	0–499	Probably will not respond to codeine	0	Includes PM and IM phenotypes
0.5	IM	415.2	no responders identified	0–499	Probably will not respond to codeine	0	Includes PM and IM phenotypes
1	NM	1444.7	1754.6	500–1499	May not respond to codeine	1	Includes NM AS 1 phenotype or individuals CYP2D6 phenocopying
1.5	NM	2925.4	2523	1500–7500	Should respond to codeine	2	Includes NM AS 1.5 and AS 2 phenotypes: Expected to respond to codeine
2	NM	2846.1	3329.5	1500–7500	Should respond to codeine	2	Includes NM AS 1.5 and AS 2 phenotypes: Expected to respond to codeine
3	UM	5330	no responders identified	>7500	May not respond and potential ADRs	3	Includes UM phenotypes: Potential for ADRs
		Mean morphine: creatinine ratio (μg/mmol)	Mean morphine: creatinine ratio (μg/mmol)	Mean morphine: creatinine ratio (μg/mmol)			
0	PM	6.91	no responders identified	0–100	Probably will not respond to codeine	0	Includes PM and IM phenotypes
0.5	IM	35.83	no responders identified	0–100	Probably will not respond to codeine	0	Includes PM and IM phenotypes
1	NM	197.96	271.8	101–250	May not respond to codeine	1	Includes NM AS 1 phenotype or individuals CYP2D6 phenocopying
1.5	NM	307	347	251–1000	Should respond to codeine	2	Includes NM AS 1.5 and AS 2 phenotypes: Expected to respond to codeine
2	NM	389.69	480.82	251–1000	Should respond to codeine	2	Includes NM AS 1.5 and AS 2 phenotypes: Expected to respond to codeine
3	UM	646.5	no responders identified	>1000	May not respond and potential ADRs	3	Includes UM phenotypes: Potential for ADRs

PM, Poor metaboliser; IM, Intermediate metaboliser; NM, Normal metaboliser; UM, Ultra metaboliser; AS, Activity score; ADR, Adverse drug reaction.

3.10. Predicting CYP2D6 Activity Score from Codeine Urinary Metabolites

We devised a simple scoring system in an attempt to predict CYP2D6 activity score from urinary total morphine and morphine:creatinine ratio based on detected urinary metabolite (Table 5) whereby;

- 0 points = activity score = 0 (PM), expected urinary total morphine = 0–150 µg/L, expected urinary morphine:creatinine ratio ≤20 µg/mmol);
- 0.5 points = activity score = 0.5 (IM), expected urinary total morphine 151–500 µg/L, expected urinary morphine:creatinine ratio = 21–100 µg/mmol);
- 1 point = activity score = 1.0 (NM), expected urinary total morphine = 501–2000 µg/L, expected urinary morphine:creatinine ratio = 101–300 µg/mmol)
- 1.5 points = activity score = 1.5 (NM), expected urinary total morphine = 2001–3000 µg/L, expected urinary morphine:creatinine ratio = 301–375 µg/mmol)
- 2.0 points = activity score = 2.0 (NM), expected urinary total morphine = 3001–7500 µg/L, expected urinary morphine:creatinine ratio = 376–600 µg/mmol)
- 3.0 points = activity score >2.0 (UM), expected urinary total morphine >7501 µg/L, expected urinary morphine:creatinine ratio >601 µg/mmol).

Table 5. Points system for predicting for predicting CYP2D6 activity score from day 4 urinary total morphine metabolites (µg/L) and morphine:creatinine ratio (µg/mmol) based on detected urinary metabolite.

CYP2D6 Activity Score (AS)	CYP2D6 Phenotype	Codeine Non-Responder	Codeine Responder	Suggested Range for Predicting CYP2D6 Activity Score	Points	Rationale
		Mean total morphine (µg/L)	Mean total morphine (µg/L)	Mean total morphine (µg/L)		
0	PM	44.2	no responders identified	0–150	0	<300 µg/L is a negative cut off point in codeine drug screens [49]
0.5	IM	415.2	no responders identified	151–500	0.5	Severely reduced function and comparable to PMs [50]
1	NM	1444.7	1754.6	501–2000	1	Expected to respond to codeine
1.5	NM	2925.4	2523	2001–3000	1.5	Expected to respond to codeine
2	NM	2846.1	3329.5	3001–7500	2	
3	UM	5330	no responders identified	>7501	3	Potential for ADRs
		Mean morphine: creatinine ratio (µg/L)	Mean morphine: creatinine ratio (µg/L)	Morphine: creatinine ratio (µg/L)		
0	PM	6.91	no responders identified	≤20	0	<300 µg/L is classed as a negative cut off point in codeine drug screens [49]
0.5	IM	35.83	no responders identified	21–100	0.5	Severely reduced function and comparable to PMs [50]
1	NM	197.96	271.8	101–300	1	Expected to respond to codeine
1.5	NM	307	347	301–375	1.5	
2	NM	389.69	480.82	376–600	2	
3	UM	646.5	no responders identified	>601	3	Potential for ADRs

PM, Poor metaboliser; IM, Intermediate metaboliser; NM, Normal metaboliser; UM, Ultra metaboliser; AS, Activity score; ADR, Adverse drug reaction.

A multivariate logistic regression analysis was used to determine whether log-transformed urinary total morphine could predict CYP2D6 activity score and a ROC curve used to assess the suitability of the model. Urinary total morphine and urinary Morphine:Creatinine ratio at day 4 did not make a significant contribution to the prediction of CYP2D6 activity score.

4. Discussion

This study found that 79% of participants did not achieve a clinically significant reduction of pain of ≥30% four days after commencement of codeine 30 mg QDS. The proportion of phenotypes in the sample were within the range estimated for adult Caucasians [21], with 46% of NMs having a CYP2D6 activity score of 2.0 reflecting full CYP2D6 activity. None of the PMs, IMs, and UMs, and only 24.5% of NMs responded to codeine. CYP2D6 activity score made a significant contribution to the prediction of codeine response with high CYP2D6 activity scores being 2.62 times more likely to respond than low CYP2D6 activity scores. The number of concurrent CYP2D6 substrates and urinary morphine did not make a significant contribution to the prediction of codeine response. We devised a simple scoring system to predict analgesic response (≥30% relief) from day four urinary metabolites and found that this had overall prediction success of 79% (sensitivity 0.8, specificity 0.78) for morphine and 79% (sensitivity 0.76, specificity 0.83) for morphine:creatinine ratio.

At enrolment, 59% of our sample had been prescribed analgesics dependent on CYP2D6 activity such as co-codamol and tramadol, a similar percentage to a recent service improvement project that reviewed prescribing information provided by general practitioners (GP) for new referrals to a UK National Health Service hospital pain clinic [37]. Prescribers are advised to review medication within 2–4 weeks after titration to identify patients that are unlikely to respond [51], although in our sample 70% of participants reported that they had previously failed to respond to one or more CYP2D6 analgesics despite still consuming such medication. Our study found no differences in the number of adverse events (mostly headache, dry mouth, nausea, drowsiness, and constipation) between phenotype and/or activity score. Literature on the incidence of adverse events associated with different phenotypes is sparse and contradictory [52–55].

In our responder analysis, 79% participants did not achieve a clinically meaningful reduction of pain of ≥30% to codeine 30 mg QDS, based on the cut-point for response consistent with current guidelines from Initiative on Methods, Measurement, and Pain Assessment in Clinical Trials (IMMPACT) [56,57]. Analysis of pre-post change in mean 'pain severity', 'pain interference', and 'pain on the average' of the BPI-sf found statistically significant improvements, although the use of mean data can be misleading because between-group averages may hide proportions of participants that may have responded very well, or extremely poorly to the drug [58]. This is supported by evidence from studies of pharmacological interventions that have found that pain outcomes have U-shaped distributions with some participants experiencing substantial reductions in pain and some minimal improvement [59–62]. We found that 43% (42/97) of non-responders scored ≥12 on S-LANSS in line with evidence suggesting that neuropathic pain is less likely to respond to codeine than predominantly nociceptive or mixed pain [63]. None of the PMs, IMs, or UMs responded to codeine 30mg QDS [15,17,23], although we recognise that groups samples were small with only two UMs. If the parent drug (codeine and tramadol) must be biotransformed to an active metabolite for therapeutic effect, then UM phenotypes are at risk of experiencing adverse drug reactions from high levels of the active metabolite, with IM and PM phenotypes experiencing no therapeutic effects [15,17,23]. Evidence suggests that UM phenotypes suffer lack of efficacy due to rapid metabolism whereas PM phenotypes suffer from complications from higher than desired plasma concentrations of the drug [64,65]. Ultra-rapid formation of morphine would only short-term analgesia that is not maintained for 4–6 h and would pose a risk of toxicity in UMs [23]. Therefore, codeine is not an appropriate drug for long term analgesia for persistent pain.

It is also possible that a disproportionately high number of treatment resistant participants in the sample was a consequence of polypharmacy. Participants were allowed to maintain concurrent prescribed medication during the study period providing medication was not a CYP2D6 inhibitor (excluding oral contraceptives) to prevent phenocopying through enzyme inhibition. However, five participants were taking CYP2D6 inhibitors with up to a 50% reduction in enzyme activity and all were

NMs and codeine non-responders. Three of these participants (activity score = 2) were prescribed oral contraceptives, one (activity score = 2) was prescribed diltiazem (weak inhibitor, [27]), and one (activity score = 1) was self-administrating over-the-counter diphenhydramine (Benadryl®, moderate inhibitor [29]). It is likely that CYP2D6 phenocopying occurred in these participants resulting in NMs with CYP2D6 activity scores of 2 presenting as activity scores of 1, and those with activity scores of 1 presenting with activity scores of 0.5 (i.e., as IMs). In addition, three NMs were taking strong CYP2D6 inhibitors (paroxetine or fluoxetine) of which two (activity score = 1.5 and activity score = 2) were codeine non-responders. These individuals down-titrated these CYP2D6 inhibitors so that they had ceased taking the drug three days before the baseline visit, although it is possible that this wash out period was insufficient for systemic clearance of these drugs and their metabolites.

There is debate about the combination of CYP2D6 alleles and level of CYP2D6 activity that constitutes the IM phenotype. We used an activity score of 0.5 to infer IM phenotype in-line with Clinical Pharmacogenetics Implementation Consortium guidelines (1 non-functional allele + 1 reduced function allele: activity score = 0.5). The Dutch Pharmacogenetics Working Group recommend that IM phenotype is inferred from an activity score of 0.5 or an activity score of 1 (fully functional allele + non-functional allele or homozygous partially functional alleles) because of reduced enzyme function compared with NM phenotypes with activity scores of 1.5 or 2 [30,31]. Commercially available *CYP2D6* microarrays such as the Amplichip® infer IM phenotype from activity scores of 0.5 or 1 (homozygous partially functional alleles) because of reduced enzyme function compared with NM phenotypes with activity scores of 1, 1.5, or 2 [66–69]. If we had categorised IM using an activity score of 0.5–1.0 instead of 0.5 then we would have observed codeine response in 13% participants rather than 0%. If NM was categorised using an activity score of 1.5–2.0 we would have observed a codeine response in 28% of participants rather than 24.5% of participants when categorised using activity scores 1.0–2.0. It is reasonable from these findings to suggest that a CYP2D6 activity score of 1.0 should not be categorised as an NM phenotype because codeine response was only achieved in a minority of participants. However, an activity score of 1.0 should not be categorised IM because of increased CYP2D6 enzyme activity and the possibility of responding to codeine compared with individuals with an activity score of 0.5 who will not respond to codeine. Perhaps a new phenotype classification of moderate metaboliser (MM) may be a more accurate description for an activity score of 1.0. The MM phenotype classification would represent increased enzyme activity compared with the IM phenotype and reduced enzyme activity compared with the NM phenotype.

One should be cautious when extrapolating our findings to the general pain population. The main limitations of the study were the low sample of PM, IM, and UM participants and the poor analgesic response rates in all groups. This impacts on the reliability of the predictive model. It was not possible to enrich the cohort through additional recruitment in the present study, so we recommend that the validity of our scoring system and predictive model is evaluated in a multi-centre study with larger samples. The poor response rate is likely to be due to the fact that participants had been referred to a specialist pain clinic because they were treatment resistant. Eighty individuals were excluded from participation because they had previously experienced intolerable side effects to morphine, codeine, co-codamol, or tramadol. Also, individuals may have declined to participate in the study because of intolerable side effects to codeine in the past. We suspect that these exclusions would be UMs, IMs, and PMs biasing our sample toward individuals with NM and MM phenotypes.

It was assumed that the duration of the wash-out period was sufficient to reduce potential drug interactions with CYP2D6 inhibitors. Five participants continued to take CYP2D6 inhibitors during codeine treatment and this may have reduced their responsiveness to codeine and affected urinary measurements of codeine metabolites. Medication compliance was monitored by diary entries and by counting returned medication/blister packaging at clinic visits and found to be 75–100%, with 82% of the participants categorised as fully compliant. Nevertheless, it is possible that some participants supplemented study medication with over-the-counter codeine at home that is likely to elevate concentrations of codeine metabolites. Likewise, failure to collect urine samples at the time specified by the investigators (i.e., one to two hours after the morning codeine dose) would result in lower than expected concentrations of codeine metabolites. A written reminder to the participant to collect the day 4 urine sample was printed on the day 3 pain diary.

Another confounder was the selection of *CYP2D6* alleles for the customised genotyping microarray as participants may have *CYP2D6* polymorphisms not included in the microarray or that are yet to be discovered. In these individuals, the allele *1 (no polymorphisms detected) would have been allocated indicating a fully functional allele. As scientific advancements in genotyping methodology and knowledge about *CYP2D6* polymorphisms are ongoing, it is recommended that investigators consult the Human *CYP2D6* Allele Nomenclature for an up to date overview of *CYP2D6* alleles when customising *CYP2D6* microarrays [18].

5. Conclusions

This study provides tentative evidence that day 4 urinary codeine O-demethylation metabolites could predict non-response following a short course of codeine and could be utilised in the clinical assessment of codeine response at the point of care to improve analgesic efficacy and safety in codeine therapy. We offer a scoring system to predict codeine response from urinary morphine and urinary morphine:creatinine ratio collected on the morning of day 4 of codeine 30 mg QDS but this requires validation before it could be considered for use to assess codeine response in clinical practice. Translating *CYP2D6* genotyping and/or phenotyping to clinical reality remains problematic. Whether a urine test on day 4 has clinical utility is questionable as the response at this time-point is detectable by patient self-report. Clearly, a pre-emptive urine test is desirable. Moreover, urinary concentrations of morphine may be more useful than genotype when inferring phenotype in clinical practice. There remains a need for higher standard pharmacogenomic education especially on CYP2D6 and pain management in undergraduate and post-graduate education that is relevant to clinical practice for all disciplines.

An adequately sized multi-centre study conducted in a primary care setting using samples from the general population that includes *CYP2D6* genotyping is needed to confirm our findings. Future pharmacogenomic studies using codeine in persistent pain patient populations could offer genotyping to participants who have declined to take part because of codeine intolerability. This would enable a full analysis of the frequencies of CYP2D6 phenotypes. There is also a need for a multi-centre study to validate the concentration range of codeine O-demethylation metabolites against activity scores. We recommended that participants with a non-functional allele + fully functional allele (activity score = 1) are analysed separately to those with homozygous partially functional alleles (activity score = 1) to determine whether there is a difference between the metabolic capabilities of these individuals. This would aid development of an accurate method to infer CYP2D6 phenotype in a clinical setting.

Author Contributions: Conceptualisation, H.R. and K.H.S.; Data curation, H.R. and M.I.J.; Formal analysis, H.R. and M.I.J.; Funding acquisition, H.R. and K.H.S.; Investigation, H.R. and S.R.; Methodology, H.R., K.H.S., and M.I.J.; Project administration, H.R. and K.H.S.; Resources, H.R.; Software, H.R.; Supervision, K.H.S. and M.I.J.; Validation, H.R., K.H.S., S.R., and M.I.J.; Visualisation, H.R. and M.I.J.; Writing—original draft, H.R. and M.I.J.; Writing—review & editing, H.R., K.H.S., and M.I.J.

Funding: This research was funded in part by an educational grant provided by Napp Pharmaceuticals Ltd.

Acknowledgments: The Leeds Pain Service, UK; Lynne Cooper (Clinical Trials Administrator); Steven Martin and Pauline Fitzgerald (Leeds Beckett University, UK); Department of Biomedical Statistics Napp Pharmaceuticals. We wish to express gratitude to Elizabeth Fox, St. James's University Hospital, Leeds, UK, for undertaking the laboratory analysis of samples and providing specific methodological details for the manuscript.

Conflicts of Interest: Helen Radford has received honorarium for conference symposiums from Napp Pharmaceuticals Ltd. Mark I. Johnson's institution has received research and consultancy funding for work that he has undertaken for GlaxoSmithKline. Other authors declare no conflict of interest. The funders had no role in the design of the study; in the collection, analyses, or interpretation of data; in the writing of the manuscript, or in the decision to publish the results.

References

1. Health and Social Care Information Centre. *Prescriptions Dispensed in the Community: England 2002–12*, 1st ed.; Health & Social Care Information Centre: London, UK, 2013.
2. Huttunen, K.; Raunio, H.; Rautio, J. Prodrugs—From Serendipity to Rational Design. *Pharm. Rev.* **2011**, *63*, 750–771. [CrossRef]
3. Janicki, P. Pharmacogenomics of pain management. In *Comprehensive Treatment of Chronic Pain by Medical, Interventional, and Integrative Approaches*; Deer, T., Leong, M., Buvanendran, A., Gordin, V., Kim, P., Panchal, S., Ray, A., Eds.; Springer: New York, NY, USA, 2013; pp. 23–33. [CrossRef]
4. Rosser, B.; McCracken, L.; Velleman, S.; Boichat, C.; Eccleston, C. Concerns about medication and medication adherence in patients with chronic pain recruited from general practice. *Pain* **2011**, *152*, 1201–1205. [CrossRef]
5. British Pain Society. *Opioids for Persistent Pain: Good Practice*; British Pain Society: London, UK, 2010.
6. British National Formulary. Codeine Phosphate. Available online: https://bnf.nice.org.uk/drug/codeine-phosphate.html (accessed on 27 March 2019).
7. British National Formulary. Pain Management with Opioids. Available online: https://bnf.nice.org.uk/guidance/prescribing-in-palliative-care.html (accessed on 27 March 2019).
8. Friedrichsdorf, S.; Nugent, A.P.; Strobl, Q. Codeine-associated pediatric deaths despite using recommended dosing guidelines: three case reports. *J Opioid. Manag.* **2013**, *9*, 151–155. [CrossRef]
9. Elkalioubie, A.; Allorge, D.; Robriquet, L.; Wiart, J.-F.; Garat, A.; Broly, F.; Fourrier, F. Near-fatal tramadol cardiotoxicity in a CYP2D6 ultrarapid metabolizer. *Eur. J. Clin. Pharmacol.* **2011**, *67*, 855–858. [CrossRef]
10. Madadi, P.; Amstutz, U.; Rieder, M.; Ito, S.; Fung, V.; Hwang, S.; Turgeon, J.; Michaud, V.; Koren, G.; Carleton, B. Clinical practice guideline: CYP2D6 genotyping for safe and efficacious codeine therapy. *J. Popul. Ther. Clin. Pharmacol.* **2013**, *20*, 369–396.
11. Madadi, P.; Ciszkowski, C.; Gaedigk, A.; Leeder, S.; Teitelbaum, R.; Chitayat, D.; Koren, G. Genetic transmission of cytochrome P450 2D6 (CYP2D6) ultrarapid metabolism: Iimplications for breastfeeding women taking codeine. *Curr. Drug Saf.* **2011**, *6*, 36–39. [CrossRef]
12. Ferreirós, N.; Dresen, S.; Hermanns-Clausen, M.; Auwaerter, V.; Thierauf, A.; Müller, C.; Hentschel, R.; Trittler, R.; Skopp, G.; Weinmann, W. Fatal and severe codeine intoxication in 3-year-old twins—Iinterpretation of drug and metabolite concentrations. *Int. J. Leg. Med.* **2009**, *123*, 387–394. [CrossRef]
13. Ingelman-Sundberg, M.; Sim, S.; Gomez, A.; Rodriguez-Antona, C. Influence of cytochrome P450 polymorphisms on drug therapies: Pharmacogenetic, pharmacoepigenetic and clinical aspects. *Pharmacol. Therap.* **2007**, *116*, 496–526. [CrossRef]
14. Voronov, P.; Przybylo, H.; Jagannathan, N. Apnea in a child after oral codeine: a genetic variant—An ultra-rapid metabolizer. *Paediatr. Anaesth.* **2007**, *17*, 684–687. [CrossRef]
15. Gardiner, S.; Begg, E. Pharmacogenetics, drug-metabolizing enzymes, and clinical practice. *Pharmacol. Rev.* **2006**, *58*, 521–590. [CrossRef]
16. Koren, G.; Cairns, J.; Chitayat, D.; Gaedigk, A.; Leeder, S. Pharmacogenetics of morphine poisoning in a breastfed neonate of a codeine-prescribed mother. *Lancet* **2006**, *368*. [CrossRef]
17. Weinshilboum, R. Inheritance and Drug Response. *N. Engl. J. Med.* **2003**, *348*, 529–537. [CrossRef]
18. Human Cytochrome P450 (CYP) Allele Nomenclature Database. CYP2D6 Nomenclature Database. Available online: http://www.cypalleles.ki.se/cyp2d6.htm (accessed on 27 March 2019).
19. Sim, S.; Ingelman-Sundberg, M. Update on allele nomenclature for human cytochromes P450 and the Human Cytochrome P450 Allele (CYP-allele) Nomenclature Database. *Methods Mol. Biol.* **2013**, *987*, 251–259. [CrossRef]
20. Daly, A.K.; Brockmöller, J.; Broly, F.; Eichelbaum, M.; Evans, W.E.; Gonzalez, F.J.; Huang, J.D.; Idle, J.R.; Ingelman-Sundberg, M.; Ishizaki, T.; et al. Nomenclature for human CYP2D6 alleles. *Pharmacogenetics* **1996**, *6*, 193–201. [CrossRef]
21. Crews, K.R.; Gaedigk, A.; Dunnenberger, H.M.; Leeder, J.S.; Klein, T.E.; Caudle, K.E.; Haidar, C.E.; Shen, D.D.; Callaghan, J.T.; Sadhasivam, S.; et al. Clinical Pharmacogenetics Implementation Consortium guidelines for cytochrome P450 2D6 genotype and codeine therapy: 2014 update. *Clin. Pharm.* **2014**, *95*, 376–382. [CrossRef]

22. Sistonen, J.; Sajantila, A.; Lao, O.; Corander, J.; Barbujani, G.; Fuselli, S. CYP2D6 worldwide genetic variation shows high frequency of altered activity variants and no continental structure. *Pharm. Genom.* **2007**, *17*, 93–101. [CrossRef]
23. Ingelman-Sundberg, M.; Rodriguez-Antona, C. Pharmacogenetics of drug-metabolizing enzymes: implications for a safer and more effective drug therapy. *Philos. Trans. R. Soc. Lond. B Biol. Sci.* **2005**, *360*, 1563–1570. [CrossRef]
24. Jannetto, P.; Bratanow, N. Utilization of pharmacogenomics and therapeutic drug monitoring for opioid pain management. *Pharmacogenomics* **2009**, *10*, 1157–1167. [CrossRef]
25. Owen, R.; Sangkuhl, K.; Klein, T.; Altman, R. Cytochrome P450 2D6. *Pharm. Genom.* **2009**, *19*, 559–562. [CrossRef]
26. Borges, S.; Desta, Z.; Jin, Y.; Faouzi, A.; Robarge, J.; Philip, S.; Nguyen, A.; Stearns, V.; Hayes, D.; Rae, J.; et al. Composite Functional Genetic and Comedication CYP2D6 Activity Score in Predicting Tamoxifen Drug Exposure Among Breast Cancer Patients. *J. Clin. Pharmacol.* **2010**, *50*, 450–458. [CrossRef]
27. Food & Drug Administration. CYP2D6 Inhibitors. Available online: http://www.fda.gov/Drugs/DevelopmentApprovalProcess/DevelopmentResources/DrugInteractionsLabeling/ucm093664.htm#4 (accessed on 27 March 2019).
28. Baxter, K. *Stockley's Drug Interactions: A Source Book of Interactions, Their Mechanisms, Clinical Importance, and Management*; Pharmaceutical Press: London, UK, 2008.
29. Flockhart, D. Drug Interactions: Cytochrome P450 Drug Interaction Table. Indiana University School of Medicine. Available online: http://medicine.iupui.edu/clinpharm/ddis/clinical-table (accessed on 27 March 2019).
30. Swen, J.J.; Nijenhuis, M.; de Boer, A.; Grandia, L.; Maitland-van der Zee, A.H.; Mulder, H.; Rongen, G.A.; van Schaik, R.H.; Schalekamp, T.; Touw, D.J.; et al. Pharmacogenetics: From bench to byte—An update of guidelines. *Clin. Pharmacol. Ther.* **2011**, *89*, 662–673. [CrossRef]
31. Swen, J.J.; Wilting, I.; de Goede, A.L.; Grandia, L.; Mulder, H.; Touw, D.J.; de Boer, A.; Conemans, J.M.; Egberts, T.C.; Klungel, O.H.; et al. Pharmacogenetics: from bench to byte. *Clin. Pharmacol. Ther.* **2008**, *83*, 781–787. [CrossRef]
32. Stamer, U.; Stüber, F.; Muders, T.; Musshoff, F. Respiratory Depression with Tramadol in a Patient with Renal Impairment and CYP2D6 Gene Duplication. *Anesth. Analg.* **2008**, *107*, 926–929. [CrossRef]
33. Foster, A.; Mobley, E.; Wang, Z. Complicated pain management in a CYP450 2D6 poor metabolizer. *Pain Pract.* **2007**, *7*, 352–356. [CrossRef]
34. Susce, M.; Murray-Carmichael, E.; de Leon, J. Response to hydrocodone, codeine and oxycodone in a CYP2D6 poor metabolizer. *Prog. Neuro Psychopharmacol. Biol. Psychiatry* **2006**, *30*, 1356–1358. [CrossRef]
35. Gasche, Y.; Daali, Y.; Fathi, M.; Chiappe, A.; Cottini, S.; Dayer, P.; Desmeules, J. Codeine Intoxication Associated with Ultrarapid CYP2D6 Metabolism. *N. Engl. J. Med.* **2004**, *351*, 2827–2831. [CrossRef]
36. Mason, B.J.; Blackburn, K.H. Possible serotonin syndrome associated with tramadol and sertraline coadministration. *Ann. Pharmacother.* **1997**, *31*, 175–177. [CrossRef]
37. Radford, H.; Fitzgerald, P.; Martin, S.; Johnson, M.I. A service improvement project to review prescribing information provided by general practitioners for new referrals to a UK National Health Service hospital pain clinic: Potential implications of CYP2D6 enzyme inhibition. *Br. J. Pain* **2016**, *10*, 222–231. [CrossRef]
38. Kirchheiner, J.; Schmidt, H.; Tzvetkov, M.; Keulen, J.T.; Lotsch, J.; Roots, I.; Brockmoller, J. Pharmacokinetics of codeine and its metabolite morphine in ultra-rapid metabolizers due to CYP2D6 duplication. *Pharm. J.* **2006**, *7*, 257–265. [CrossRef]
39. Mendoza, T.; Mayne, T.; Rublee, D.; Cleeland, C. Reliability and validity of a modified Brief Pain Inventory short form in patients with osteoarthritis. *Eur. J. Pain* **2006**, *10*, 353–361. [CrossRef]
40. Bennett, M.I.; Smith, B.H.; Torrance, N.; Potter, J. The S-LANSS score for identifying pain of predominantly neuropathic origin: Validation for use in clinical and postal research. *J. Pain* **2005**, *6*, 149–158. [CrossRef] [PubMed]
41. Medicines and Healthcare Regulatory Authority. UK Public Assessment Report. Tamoxifen: Reduced Effectiveness When Used with CYP2D6 Inhibitors. Available online: http://www.mhra.gov.uk/safety-public-assessment-reports/CON221598 (accessed on 27 March 2019).
42. Pharmacogenomics Knowledge Base (PharmGKB). Haplotype CYP2D6*1. Available online: https://www.pharmgkb.org/haplotype/PA165816576 (accessed on 27 March 2019).

43. Gaedigk, A.; Gotschall, R.R.; Forbes, N.S.; Simon, S.D.; Kearns, G.L.; Leeder, J.S. Optimization of cytochrome P4502D6 (CYP2D6) phenotype assignment using a genotyping algorithm based on allele frequency data. *Pharmacogenetics* **1999**, *9*, 669–682. [CrossRef] [PubMed]
44. Crews, K.R.; Gaedigk, A.; Dunnenberger, H.M.; Klein, T.E.; Shen, D.D.; Callaghan, J.T.; Kharasch, E.D.; Skaar, T.C. Clinical Pharmacogenetics Implementation Consortium (CPIC) guidelines for codeine therapy in the context of cytochrome P450 2D6 (CYP2D6) genotype. *Clin. Pharm.* **2012**, *91*, 321–326. [CrossRef] [PubMed]
45. Database, E. Codeine Phosphate 30 mg Tablets. Available online: www.medicines.org.uk/emc/medicine/23910 (accessed on 27 March 2019).
46. DrugBank. Drug and Target Database. Available online: http://www.drugbank.ca/ (accessed on 27 March 2019).
47. SuperCYP. Cytochrome P450 Database. 2012. Available online: http://bioinformatics.charite.de/supercyp/ (accessed on 27 March 2019).
48. Moher, D.; Schulz, K.F.; Altman, D.G. The CONSORT statement: Revised recommendations for improving the quality of reports of parallel-group randomised trials. *Lancet* **2001**, *357*, 1191–1194. [CrossRef]
49. Christo, P.; Manchikanti, L.; Ruan, X.; Bottros, M.; Hansen, H.; Solanki, D.; Jordan, A.; Colson, J. Urine drug testing in chronic pain. *Pain Physician* **2011**, *14*, 123–143. [PubMed]
50. Zanger, U.; Raimundo, S.; Eichelbaum, M. Cytochrome P450 2D6: overview and update on pharmacology, genetics, biochemistry. *Naunyn-Schmiedeberg's Arch. Pharmacol.* **2004**, *369*, 23–37. [CrossRef] [PubMed]
51. Smith, B.H.; Hardman, J.D.; Stein, A.; Colvin, L.; Group, S.C.P.G.D. Managing chronic pain in the non-specialist setting: A new SIGN guideline. *Br. J. Gen. Pr.* **2014**, *64*, e462–e464. [CrossRef] [PubMed]
52. Mikus, G.; Trausch, B.; Rodewald, C.; Hofmann, U.; Richter, K.; Gramatte, T.; Eichelbaum, M. Effect of codeine on gastrointestinal motility in relation to CYP2D6 phenotype[ast]. *Clin. Pharm.* **1997**, *61*, 459–466. [CrossRef]
53. Eckhardt, K.; Li, S.; Ammon, S.; Schänzle, G.; Mikus, G.; Eichelbaum, M. Same incidence of adverse drug events after codeine administration irrespective of the genetically determined differences in morphine formation. *Pain* **1998**, *76*, 27–33. [CrossRef]
54. Heintze, K.; Fuchs, W. Codeine ultra-rapid metabolizers: Age appears to be a key factor in adverse effects of codeine. *Drug Res. (Stuttg.)* **2015**, *65*, 640–644. [CrossRef]
55. Dagostino, C.; Allegri, M.; Napolioni, V.; D'Agnelli, S.; Bignami, E.; Mutti, A.; van Schaik, R.H. CYP2D6 genotype can help to predict effectiveness and safety during opioid treatment for chronic low back pain: Results from a retrospective study in an Italian cohort. *Pharmgenomics Pers. Med.* **2018**, *11*, 179–191. [CrossRef] [PubMed]
56. Dworkin, R.H.; Turk, D.C.; Wyrwich, K.W.; Beaton, D.; Cleeland, C.S.; Farrar, J.T.; Haythornthwaite, J.A.; Jensen, M.P.; Kerns, R.D.; Ader, D.N.; et al. Interpreting the clinical importance of treatment outcomes in chronic pain clinical trials: IMMPACT recommendations. *J. Pain* **2008**, *9*, 105–121. [CrossRef] [PubMed]
57. Dworkin, R.H.; Turk, D.C.; McDermott, M.P.; Peirce-Sandner, S.; Burke, L.B.; Cowan, P.; Farrar, J.T.; Hertz, S.; Raja, S.N.; Rappaport, B.A.; et al. Interpreting the clinical importance of group differences in chronic pain clinical trials: IMMPACT recommendations. *Pain* **2009**, *146*, 238–244. [CrossRef] [PubMed]
58. Moore, R.A.; Derry, S.; Wiffen, P.J. Challenges in design and interpretation of chronic pain trials. *Br. J. Anaesth.* **2013**, *111*, 38–45. [CrossRef] [PubMed]
59. Moore, R.A.; Mhuircheartaigh, R.J.; Derry, S.; McQuay, H.J. Mean analgesic consumption is inappropriate for testing analgesic efficacy in post-operative pain: Analysis and alternative suggestion. *Eur. J. Anaesthesiol.* **2011**, *28*, 427–432. [CrossRef] [PubMed]
60. Moore, R.A.; Smugar, S.S.; Wang, H.; Peloso, P.M.; Gammaitoni, A. Numbers-needed-to-treat analyses–Do timing, dropouts, and outcome matter? Pooled analysis of two randomized, placebo-controlled chronic low back pain trials. *Pain* **2010**, *151*, 592–597. [CrossRef]
61. Moore, R.A.; Moore, O.A.; Derry, S.; Peloso, P.M.; Gammaitoni, A.R.; Wang, H. Responder analysis for pain relief and numbers needed to treat in a meta-analysis of etoricoxib osteoarthritis trials: Bridging a gap between clinical trials and clinical practice. *Ann. Rheum. Dis.* **2010**, *69*, 374–379. [CrossRef]
62. Moore, R.A.; Moore, O.A.; Derry, S.; McQuay, H.J. Numbers needed to treat calculated from responder rates give a better indication of efficacy in osteoarthritis trials than mean pain scores. *Arthritis Res.* **2008**, *10*, R39. [CrossRef]

63. Chaparro, L.E.; Wiffen, P.; Moore, A.; Gilron, I. Combination pharmacotherapy for the treatment of neuropathic pain in adults. *Cochrane Database Syst. Rev.* **2012**, *7*. [CrossRef]
64. Jornil, J.; Nielsen, T.S.; Rosendal, I.; Ahlner, J.; Zackrisson, A.L.; Boel, L.W.T.; Brock, B. A poor metabolizer of both CYP2C19 and CYP2D6 identified by mechanistic pharmacokinetic simulation in a fatal drug poisoning case involving venlafaxine. *Forensic Sci. Int.* **2013**, *226*, e26–e31. [CrossRef]
65. Smith, J.C.; Curry, S. Prolonged toxicity after amitriptyline overdose in a patient deficient in CYP2D6 activity. *J. Med. Toxicol.* **2011**, *7*, 220–223. [CrossRef] [PubMed]
66. Dodgen, T.; Hochfeld, W.; Fickl, H.; Asfaha, S.; Durandt, C.; Rheeder, P.; Drogemoller, B.; Wright, G.; Warnich, L.; Labuschagne, C.; et al. Introduction of the AmpliChip CYP450 Test to a South African cohort: A platform comparative prospective cohort study. *BMC Med. Genet.* **2013**, *14*, 20. [CrossRef] [PubMed]
67. Rebsamen, M.C.; Desmeules, J.; Daali, Y.; Chiappe, A.; Diemand, A.; Rey, C.; Chabert, J.; Dayer, P.; Hochstrasser, D.; Rossier, M.F. The AmpliChip CYP450 test: Cytochrome P450 2D6 genotype assessment and phenotype prediction. *Pharm. J.* **2008**, *9*, 34–41. [CrossRef] [PubMed]
68. De Leon, J.; Susce, M.; Murray-Carmichael, E. The AmpliChip CYP450 genotyping test: Integrating a new clinical tool. *Mol. Diagn. Ther.* **2006**, *10*, 135–151. [CrossRef] [PubMed]
69. Heller, T.; Kirchheiner, J.; Armstrong, V.; Luthe, H.; Brockmuller, J.R.; Oellerich, M. Assessment of Amplichip CYP450 Based CYP2D6-Genotyping and Phenotype Prediction Compared to PCR-RFLP-genotyping and Phenotyping by Metoprolol Pharmacokinetics. *Ther. Drug Monit.* **2005**, *27*, 221. [CrossRef]

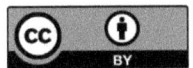 © 2019 by the authors. Licensee MDPI, Basel, Switzerland. This article is an open access article distributed under the terms and conditions of the Creative Commons Attribution (CC BY) license (http://creativecommons.org/licenses/by/4.0/).

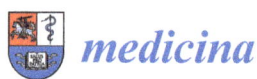

Article

Pharmacogenetic Testing in Acute and Chronic Pain: A Preliminary Study

Lorenzo Panella [1], Laura Volontè [1], Nicola Poloni [2], Antonello Caserta [1], Marta Ielmini [2], Ivano Caselli [2], Giulia Lucca [2] and Camilla Callegari [2,*]

1. Department of Rehabilitation, ASST Gaetano Pini—CTO, Via Isocrate 19, 20122 Milan, Italy; lorenzo.panella@asst-pini-cto.it (L.P.); laura.volonte@asst-pini-cto.it (L.V.); antonellovalerio.caserta@asst-pini-cto.it (A.C.)
2. Department of Medicine and Surgery, Division of Psychiatry, University of Insubria, Viale Luigi Borri 57, 21100 Varese, Italy; nicola.poloni@uninsubria.it (N.P.); marta.ielmini@hotmail.it (M.I.); ivo.ivo@aliceposta.it (I.C.); giulia1lucca@gmail.com (G.L.)
* Correspondence: camilla.callegari@uninsubria.it; Tel.: +39-0332-278727

Received: 6 March 2019; Accepted: 13 May 2019; Published: 16 May 2019

Abstract: *Background and Objectives:* Pain is one of the most common symptoms that weighs on life's quality and health expenditure. In a reality where increasingly personalized therapies are needed, the early use of genetic tests that highlights the individual response to analgesic drugs could be a valuable help in clinical practice. The aim of this preliminary study is to observe if the therapy set to 5 patients suffering of chronic or acute pain is concordant to the Pharmacogenetic test (PGT) results. *Materials and Methods:* This preliminary study compares the genetic results of pharmacological effectiveness and tolerability analyzed by the genetic test Neurofarmagen Analgesia®, with the results obtained in clinical practice of 5 patients suffering from acute and chronic pain. *Results:* Regarding the genetic results of the 5 samples analyzed, 2 reports were found to be completely comparable with the evidences of the clinical practice, while in 3 reports the profile of tolerability and effectiveness were partially discordant. *Conclusion:* In light of the data not completely overlapping with results observed in clinical practice, further studies would be appropriate in order to acquire more information on the use of Neurofarmagen in routine clinical settings.

Keywords: pain; analgesic; pharmacogenetic testing; pharmacological therapy; effectiveness; adverse effects

1. Introduction

Pain is the most common factor motivating healthcare use, as well as one of the main health care system spending factors. In particular, chronic pain is such a diffuse and disabling condition that it is considered a syndrome and not merely a symptom [1,2]. Individual sensitivity and pain perception, as well as antalgic treatment response, are influenced by numerous factors such as duration, cultural difference, weight, age, co-morbidity, concomitant therapies, psychological factors, and genetic predisposition [3–5]. Pain, especially chronic pain, includes a wide range of treatments ranging from anti-inflammatory and simple analgesics to major opioids, cannabinoids, antidepressants, antipsychotics, local anesthetics, and ketamine [6–9]. Moreover, the method of pain assessment influences acute pain diagnosis which may lead to further chronicity of underdiagnosed pain. One of the potential reasons for variability in observed clinical response to pain may be related to the method of assessment and intensity measurement for different patient populations. For example, inadequate pain evaluation may be seen in postoperative patients (assessment of pain at rest, as opposed to pain after movement) [10] and in critically ill or non-verbal patients (inadequate use of behavioral pain scales) [11].

In recent years an increased interest in the genetic and epigenetic correlates of pain was observed both for the genetic origin of pain's sensitivity threshold, and for the individual response to analgesic treatments [12,13]. A better understanding of individual sensitivity to drugs would allow a more patient-targeted approach with consequent reduction of the antalgic response time, reduction of failed treatment attempts, a remarkable reduction of healthcare costs, and therefore a more rapid improvement in quality of life [14]. Some individuals may be less responsive to therapeutic pharmacological analgesic treatments, while others may be unresponsive or exhibit adverse events. Consequently, the knowledge of individual responsiveness to antalgic drugs, besides allowing one to reach the predetermined therapeutic objective more quickly, may also reduce adverse effects [13]. The main genetic modifications implicated in different pain responses to analgesics seem to be related to drug metabolism. Genes coding for enzymes, many of which belong to the family of cytochrome P-450 with its multiple isoforms (CYP2D6, CYP2C9, CYP2C8, COMT, OPRM1) often present individual variability due to single nucleotide polymorphisms (SNPs), as confirmed by the literature [15]. The CYP2D6 gene, located on chromosome 22 and coding for a member of the cytochrome P450 enzyme superfamily (cytochrome P450, family 2, subfamily D, polypeptide 6), is responsible for the metabolism of about 25% of the drugs currently used in clinical practice. CYP2D6 is highly relevant to the metabolism of minor and major opioids [16] and for several antidepressant drugs. Several variants cause a loss of CYP2D6 function, and the homozygous subjects for these variants are called "slow metabolizers" (SM); they present, for the same dose of drug, higher plasma levels than normal [17]. The CYP2C9 gene is located on chromosome 10 that codes for a member of the cytochrome P450 enzyme superfamily (cytochrome P450, family 2, subfamily C, polypeptide 9). CYP2C9 is responsible for the metabolism of 15% of commercially available drugs. Several non-steroidal anti-inflammatory drugs (NSAIDs) are metabolized by CYP2C9 and, in some cases, the deficiency of this enzyme has been associated with an increased risk of gastrointestinal hemorrhage in patients treated with NSAIDs [18]. The CYP2C8 gene is located on chromosome 10, which codes for a member of the cytochrome P450 enzyme superfamily (cytochrome P450, family 2, subfamily C, polypeptide 8). Together with other enzymes, such as CYP2C9, CYP2C8 intervenes in the metabolism of NSAIDs, including ibuprofen and diclofenac. The gene has a variant that has been associated with a reduction in drug clearance and an increased risk of gastrointestinal hemorrhage. The COMT gene is located on chromosome 22 that encodes the catechol-O-methyltransferase enzyme, whose function is the degradation of the dopamine and norepinephrine catecholamines and the consequent modulation of the levels of these neurotransmitters in inter-synaptic space. Various polymorphisms with influence on COMT activity are known; for example, the Val158Met polymorphism has been associated with the μ opioid system response and the efficacy of morphine treatment both on acute and chronic pain [19]. The OPRM1 gene is located on chromosome 6 that encodes for μ1, the main opioid receptor target of endogenous opioid peptides (such as β-endorphin and enkephalins) and opioid analgesics (such as morphine). Several studies indicate that post-operative and oncological patients who carry at least one copy of the G allele of the gene have a lower pain threshold and experience an increase in opioid use [20]. Moreover, this polymorphism has also been associated with the susceptibility to opioid and alcohol dependence [14]. In most cases the therapeutic choices of clinicians regarding analgesic drugs are empirical, and the different individual response may represent a further step to overcome in order to obtain an adequate analgesic response. Several attempts are in fact often necessary before obtaining adequate analgesia. This leads to longer response times, greater patient distress and higher healthcare costs [21]. The rationale for this study is based on the possible clinical utility of early identification of genetic polymorphisms responsible for the different individual responses of analgesic drugs.

The aim of this preliminary study is to observe if the therapy set to 5 patients suffering of chronic or acute pain is concordant to the pharmacogenetic test (PGT) results.

2. Materials and Methods

2.1. Sample

This naturalistic study had foreseen a preliminary assessment of 5 patients affected by acute and chronic pain referring to Gaetano Pini Orthopedic Institute. Patients had to fulfill the following inclusion criteria: to be older than 18 years; to suffer from acute or chronic pain; to subscribe a generic written informed consent.

Patients were evaluated during an outpatient visit at the Gaetano Pini Institute. All patients were already taking pain medication at the time of assessment. The genetic test was performed by two investigators who did not know the clinical response at the therapy, while clinicians were not aware of the test results, carried out subsequently.

All patients provided a general written informed consent for processing personal data as part of the routine diagnostic assessment procedure and quality check processes. Assessment tools and scales were administered by clinicians at the patient's facilities, as part of clinical routine practice. As patient data was made anonymous, obscuring sensitive information used in the research to protect the recognizability of the patients, according to the Italian legislation (D.L. 196/2003, art. 110 - 24 July 2008, art. 13), the Provincial Health Ethical Review Board, consulted prior to the beginning of the study, confirmed that it did not need authorization from the Board. The study was carried out in accordance with the ethical principles of Declaration of Helsinki (with amendments) and Good Clinical Practice.

2.2. Genetic Analysis

The genetic analysis was performed by the Neurofarmagen Analgesia® kit. This test scans the genetic polymorphisms linked to the pharmacokinetics of analgesic drugs belonging to the NSAIDs, opioids, antidepressants, antiepileptic, triptans, 5HT-3 receptor antagonists, and ergotamine's derivatives. The test examines the isoforms of cytochrome CYP2B6, CYP2C8, CYP2C9, CYP2C19, CYP2D6, and CYP3A4, which are responsible for the metabolism of each of the drugs considered. The test allows us to determine the patient response both to peripheral analgesics like NSAIDs and cox-2, and to central analgesics as paracetamol, tricyclics, serotonin reuptake inhibitors (SSRI), anticonvulsants, opioids, and triptans. The genetic test's administration is carried out by taking a patient's saliva sample in an amount equal to about 1 ml. Given the same possibility to obtain the genetic information from biological material, use of saliva samples allow for greater practicality in the execution of the test, and it is less invasive. DNA was extracted from patient saliva samples with the genomic DNA Isolation kit (Norgen Biotek Corp. Thorold, ON, Canada). DNA quality was evaluated by microvolume spectrometry. The sample is collected by the patient under the doctor's guidance through the kit provided and remains stable at room temperature for a maximum of 15 days, the time required for sending it off to the laboratory to be analyzed. During the 30 min before sample collection the patient should not consume food, drink or chewing gum, must not smoke and must have completely removed the presence of any lipstick. The results are available within 10 working days from the date of arrival of the sample at Neurofarmagen laboratory (AB-BIOTICS, Barcelona, Spain) which is declared by the company as having the necessary authorization to operate as a health laboratory using biological samples. Genotyping of single nucleotide polymorphisms was performed by OpenArray® Technology on the QuantStudio™ 12K Flex Real-Time PCR System (Thermo Fisher Scientific Inc., Waltham, MA, USA) using a custom designed array. Saliva samples were marked with an electronic numerical barcode associated with the patient, and the identification code was archived at the Gaetano Pini Orthopedic Institute in Milan. The archive in question contains the correspondences necessary to associate the clinical and demographical data of each patient with the Neurofarmagen genetic record. In that way no sample was sent in association of personal data. The collected data have been used exclusively for research purposes. The test evaluates 6 different genes, putting them in relation to active 48 drugs. For each patient the report provides a table in which the molecule evaluated correspond to a color coding: (1) green—expectation of higher likelihood of the good response to treatment or a good tolerability profile than average; (2) white—index of a standard response, not different from the general population; (3) yellow—requiring more careful dose monitoring; and (4) red—for high risk of adverse effects or not expected efficacy.

2.3. Clinical Assessment

Patients were evaluated with algometric scales:

- McGill Pain Questionnaire-Short Form—MGPQ-SF [22]: this is a rating scale developed at McGill University by Melzack and Torgerson in 1971 and it is a self-report questionnaire that allows patients to give a good description of the quality and intensity of the experienced pain. It is composed of 78 words in 20 sections that are related to pain. Patients have to mark the words that best describe their pain (multiple markings are allowed). Different sections correspond to different pain's features: Sensory (sections 1–10), Affective (sections 11–15), Evaluative (section 16), and Miscellaneous (sections 17–20).
- Visual Analogue Scale—VAS [23]: the VAS scale consists of a strip of 10 cm paper which at the ends has two end points which are defined with 0 (no pain) and 10 (the worst pain that I can imagine). Patients have to mark the pain at a point on the scale as subjectively perceived at the moment of evaluation.
- Numerical Rating Scale—NRS [23]: the NRS is a 11-point scale for patient self-reporting of pain. The score is between 0 (no pain) and 10 (severe pain) and expresses the intensity of the pain perceived subjectively at the moment of evaluation.

3. Results

Clinical characteristics of the patients and treatments prescribed are shown in Table 1. The first patient (P1) was a 45-year-old woman suffering from fibromyalgia not responsive to diclofenac, paracetamol and then major opioids. The result of the test suggested for diclofenac and paracetamol a standard response without a need for dosage adjustment; the PGT highlighted a warning for the use of minor opioids (yellow response, due to an intermediate metabolism), while suggesting the possibility of a standard response to some major opioids.

The second patient (P2) was a 22-year-old woman suffering from chronic pain resulting from Ewing's femoral sarcoma resection and mega prosthesis implant replacement at the age of 16. The patient had taken several different analgesic molecules (good response to nimesulide, ineffectiveness to paracetamol, gastrointestinal intolerance to naproxen and ibuprofen, effectiveness to buprenorphine e tramadol, effectiveness to pregabalin). In this case a substantial correspondence between the report provided by the genetic analysis and effectiveness and tolerability profile observed in clinical practice was found.

The third patient (P3) was a 45-year-old woman with a diagnosis of end stage renal failure in systemic lupus erythematosus (SLE) with contraindication to the use of NSAIDs and a short-term program of renal transplantation. The patient underwent a laparoscopic abdominal operation with analgesia performed with a high dose of tramadol and without side effects, while in the post-transplant a low dose of morphine and subsequently 2 mg/day of Paracetamol for 5 days, were successfully used. Regarding tramadol, the test indicated the patient as a slow metabolizer (CYP2D6) and recommended reducing the dose by 30%, along with paying particular attention to the occurrence of adverse effects such as nausea, vomiting, constipation, respiratory depression, confusion, and urinary retention, or to choose an alternative drug (yellow response). The drug was instead used at maximal doses intravenously with complete response to pain and without collateral or treatment emergent adverse events—TEAE (emesis, as potential side effect, was not evaluated for overlapping adequate coverage with metoclopramide). With regard to the use of morphine, the test showed the presence of a variant of COMT and OPRM1 that resulted in a reduced response to opioid agonists: the patient may have needed higher dosage or more frequent administration of the drug for adequate pain control. The patient was instead subjected to post-operative therapy with morphine at minimum therapeutic doses with optimal and rapid response. With regard to paracetamol, the PGT indicated a standard response, meaning a risk of undesirable effects not higher than general population. The patient, instead, showed signs of severe hepatic toxicity as a result of maximum therapeutic antalgic dose for 5 days of treatment. The situation required clinical and instrumental hepatological monitoring; the normalization of the liver enzyme required about 60 days. In this case some discordances between the clinical setting and the PGT' suggestion emerged.

The fourth patient, (P4) was a 75-year-old woman affected by persistent osteoarthritis (OA) pain poorly responsive to common NSAIDs. The patient was clinically known as non-responsive to NSAIDs and discreetly responsive to paracetamol-codeine combination without evidence of significant adverse effects at a common therapeutic dosage. The result of the genetic test was indicative for standard response to NSAIDs and highlighted the need for specific dose monitoring and/or lower probability of positive response to codeine (yellow response). The PGT indicated the patient as an intermediate metabolizer of codeine due to the CYP2D6 gene. For the same patient, the test suggested the possibility of using major opioids (with specific reference to morphine).

The last patient (P5) was a 55-year-old man suffering from chronic pain caused by early OA. The patient presented an excellent response to the analgesic drugs used (paracetamol-codeine and NSAIDs) at the doses commonly used in clinical practice. In this case the genetic test showed a standard profile of efficacy and tolerability for the molecules used, confirming the clinical level.

Total scores of algometric scales for pain evaluation are reported for each patient in Table 2.

Table 1. Clinical characteristics of the patients and treatments prescribed.

Patient	Sex	Age	Diagnosis	Comorbidity	Therapy	Test Results
P1	F	45	Widespread pain (fibromyalgia)	Gastritis; irritable colon syndrome; depression	Aceclofenac	Not evaluated
					Diclofenac	Standard response
					Paracetamol	Standard response
P2	F	20	Chronic pain resulting from Ewing's femoral sarcoma resection and mega prosthesis implant replacement at the age of 16	Iatrogenic pulmonary restrictive syndrome caused by chemotherapy; dysthymia	Nimesulide	Not evaluated
					Paracetamol	Standard response
					Naproxen	Not evaluated
					Ibuprofen	Yellow response (increased risk of side effects)
					Buprenorphine	Standard response
					Tramadol	Yellow response (lower efficacy)
					Pregabalin	Standard response
P3	F	45	End stage renal failure with contraindication to the use of NSAIDs and a short-term program of renal transplantation	Systemic lupus erythematosus in remission	Paracetamol	Standard response
					Tramadol	Yellow response (increased risk of side effects)
P4	F	75	Persistent OA pain	Arterial hypertension; hypoacusis; recurrent and mild gastritis; irritable colon syndrome; subclinical thyroiditis	Several kinds of NSAIDs	Standard response
					Tramadol	Yellow response (lower efficacy)
					Buprenorphine	Standard response
					Codeine	Yellow response (lower efficacy)
					Paracetamol	Standard response
P5	M	55	Chronic pain caused by early OA	None	Several kinds of NSAIDs	Standard response
					Paracetamol	Standard response
					Codeine	Standard response

F: female, M: male, NSAID: non-steroidal anti-inflammatory drugs, OA: osteoarthritis.

Table 2. Total score of algometric scales McGill Pain Questionnaire-Short Form (MGPQ-SF), Numerical Rating Scale (NRS) and Visual Analogue Scale (VAS) representative of each patient.

Patient	MGPQ-SF	NRS	VAS
Patient 1 (P1)	45	8	8.07
Patient 2 (P2)	24	6	5.4
Patient 3 (P3)	7	0	0.43
Patient 4 (P4)	30	9	4.08
Patient 5 (P5)	26	5	4.7
Mean	26.4	5.6	4.69
Standard Deviation (SD)	13.61	3.5	2.74

MGPQ-SF: McGill Pain Questionnaire-Short Form, NRS: Numerical Rating Scale, VAS: Visual Analogue Scale.

4. Discussion

Pain is a syndrome that has a major impact on life's quality. It is intended as a complex phenomenon characterized by a huge subjective component and dependent on different endogenous and external factors [24,25]. An early investigation of subjective sensitivity to drug therapies could be a useful instrument in clinical practice. Over time, genetic testing has become more accessible and less expensive. However, currently available data are scarce and heterogeneous, and there are few clear evidences that genetic tests are useful tools in clinical practice [26–30].

Pain treatment is a significant challenge for clinicians and could hesitate in poor outcome, particularly among patients treated with multiple drugs, in complications and adverse drug effects [31,32], no improvement of pain, or even worsening of it, and decline in functional status. So, more accurate information could be useful in routine clinical practice. Moreover, pain therapies should be monitored regularly not only for efficacy, but also for adverse effects and addiction. In this panorama, genetic testing could be a valid tool in current practice if used in an appropriate way [30]. In pain measurement, different variables should be taken into consideration; cognitive profile of the patient, physical limitations of the patient, psychiatric comorbidity or even simulation, ethnic and cultural variations could play an important role [33–38]. In light of these elements, the use of pharmacogenetic testing could be a useful contribution to objective measurement of response in pain pharmacotherapy [30]. Our preliminary results seem to be miscellaneous. In fact, the genetic test was concordant with the clinicians' choice in two cases, but not completely overlapping in the other three cases. While in patient 2 and patient 5 the efficacy and tolerability profile provided by the test corresponded to the clinical response, in patient 1 and patient 4 the test seems to be discordant to the clinical practice. In patient 3, the PGT would have oriented the therapeutic choice quite differently from what done in clinical setting. Lastly, it is important to point out that in no case the results of genetic tests were red or green, but only standard or yellow, excluding both the higher effectiveness of the drugs and the high risk of adverse effects. Therefore, the test could be interpreted as not very sensitive but, in any case, it is evident that the sample presented is too heterogeneous and numerically limited in order to consider our descriptive analysis as indicative. Furthermore, possible pharmacodynamic and pharmacokinetic interferences related to comorbidity with other pathologies are not considered in the present study, but available in the extensive report of the pharmacogenetic test. For example, the elderly patient suffering from arthrosis assumed, at the time of recruitment, antihypertensive and antidiabetic drugs while the young patient who was recovering from a renal transplantation, took immunosuppressive anti-rejection therapies and this could be a confounding factor. The young female patient, suffering from a chronic pain syndrome consequent to the implant of femoral prosthesis, has a positive history of emotional disorder and, as confirmed by the literature, it is known that chronic pain and psychological discomfort can influence each other, also leading to a worsening of pain and of the pharmacological response [39].

Limitations of this study include the small sample size due to the pilot nature of the study and a lack of control group. The measures presented are primarily descriptive.

There is no doubt that genetic variations that involve gene coding for enzymes involved in drug metabolism, absorption, distribution, and elimination can significantly modify the therapeutic effects and tolerability profile of the drugs, and that knowing these polymorphisms would potentially allow us to customize therapy, maximize therapeutic efficacy, and minimize unwanted or adverse effects [40–46]. From the experience reached in the use of the Neurofarmagen test, it would seem that it shows a greater efficacy in predicting the side effects and need for dosage adjustment of analgesic drugs rather than therapeutic efficacy on pain symptoms. Pain is in fact greatly subjective and depends on several factors, not just genomics, so that a genetic analysis may be insufficient to evaluate this symptom in its complexity. In light of this, it seems to be desirable to intensify the studies on this subject in order to have a larger record that can be usefully utilized to help clinicians make more targeted and ultimately more effective therapeutic choices.

Author Contributions: Conceptualization, L.P.; Investigation, L.V. and A.C.; Methodology, M.I.; Supervision, C.C.; Validation, N.P.; Writing—original draft, G.L.; Writing—review & editing, I.C.

Funding: This research received no external funding.

Conflicts of Interest: The authors declare no conflict of interest.

References

1. Cordell, W.H.; Keene, K.K.; Giles, B.K.; Jones, J.B.; Jones, J.H.; Brizendine, E.J. The high prevalence of pain in emergency medical care. *Am. J. Emerg. Med.* **2002**, *20*, 165–169.
2. Phillips, C.J. The Cost and Burden of Chronic Pain. *Rev. Pain* **2009**, *3*, 2–5.
3. Callegari, C.; Bortolaso, P.; Vender, S. A single case report of recurrent surgery for chronic back pain and its implications concerning a diagnosis of Münchausen syndrome. *Funct. Neurol.* **2006**, *21*, 103–108.
4. Hermans, L.; Van Oosterwijck, J.; Goubert, D.; Goudman, L.; Crombez, G.; Calders, P.; Meeus, M. Inventory of Personal Factors Influencing Conditioned Pain Modulation in Healthy People: A Systematic Literature Review. *Pain Pract.* **2016**, *16*, 758–769.
5. Fillingim, R.B. Individual Differences in Pain: Understanding the Mosaic that Makes Pain Personal. *Pain* **2017**, *158* (Suppl. 1), S11–S18.
6. Rosenblum, A.; Marsch, L.A.; Joseph, H.; Portenoy, R.K. Opioids and the treatment of chronic pain: Controversies, current status, and future directions. *Exp. Clin. Psychopharmacol.* **2008**, *16*, 405–416.
7. Khouzam, H.R. Psychopharmacology of chronic pain: A focus on antidepressants and atypical antipsychotics. *Postgrad. Med.* **2016**, *128*, 323–330.
8. Albert, U.; Carmassi, C.; Cosci, F.; De Cori, D.; Di Nicola, M.; Ferrari, S.; Poloni, N.; Tarricone, I.; Fiorillo, A. Role and clinical implications of atypical antipsychotics in anxiety disorders, obsessive-compulsive disorder, trauma-related, and somatic symptom disorders: A systematized review. *Int. Clin. Psychopharmacol.* **2016**, *31*, 249–258.
9. Cohen, S.P.; Bhatia, A.; Buvanendran, A.; Schwenk, E.S.; Wasan, A.D.; Hurley, R.W.; Viscusi, E.R.; Narouze, S.; Davis, F.N.; Ritchie, E.C.; et al. Consensus Guidelines on the Use of Intravenous Ketamine Infusions for Chronic Pain From the American Society of Regional Anesthesia and Pain Medicine, the American Academy of Pain Medicine, and the American Society of Anesthesiologists. *Reg. Anesth. Pain Med.* **2018**, *43*, 521–546.
10. Gilron, I.; Vandenkerkhof, E.; Katz, J.; Kehlet, H.; Carley, M. Evaluating the Association Between Acute and Chronic Pain After Surgery: Impact of Pain Measurement Methods. *Clin. J. Pain* **2017**, *33*, 588–594.
11. Kotfis, K.; Zegan-Barańska, M.; Szydłowski, Ł.; Żukowski, M.; Ely, E.W. Methods of pain assessment in adult intensive care unit patients—Polish version of the CPOT (Critical Care Pain Observation Tool) and BPS (Behavioral Pain Scale). *Anaesthesiol. Intensive Ther.* **2017**, *49*, 66–72.
12. Fillingim, R.B.; Wallace, M.R.; Herbstman, D.M.; Ribeiro-Dasilva, M. Genetic contributions to pain: A review of findings in humans. *Oral Dis.* **2008**, *14*, 673–682.
13. James, S. Human pain and genetics: Some basics. *Br. J. Pain* **2013**, *7*, 171–178.
14. Young, E.E.; Lariviere, W.R.; Belfer, I. Genetic basis of pain variability: Recent advances. *J. Med. Genet.* **2012**, *49*, 1–9.
15. Cregg, R.; Russo, G.; Gubbay, A.; Branford, R.; Sato, H. Pharmacogenetics of analgesic drugs. *Br. J. Pain* **2013**, *7*, 189–208.

16. St Sauver, J.L.; Olson, J.E.; Roger, V.L.; Nicholson, W.T.; Black, J.L.; Takahashi, P.Y.; Caraballo, P.J.; Bell, E.J.; Jacobson, D.J.; Larson, N.B.; et al. CYP2D6 phenotypes are associated with adverse outcomes related to opioid medications. *Pharmgenom. Pers. Med.* **2017**, *10*, 217–227.
17. Samer, C.F.; Daali, Y.; Wagner, M.; Hopfgartner, G.; Eap, C.B.; Rebsamen, M.C.; Rossier, M.F.; Hochstrasser, D.; Dayer, P.; Desmeules, J.A. Genetic polymorphisms and drug interactions modulating CYP2D6 and CYP3A activities have a major effect on oxycodone analgesic efficacy and safety. *Br. J. Pharmacol.* **2010**, *160*, 919–930.
18. Figueiras, A.; Estany-Gestal, A.; Aguirre, C.; Ruiz, B.; Vidal, X.; Carvajal, A.; Salado, I.; Salgado-Barreira, A.; Rodella, L.; Moretti, U.; et al. CYP2C9 variants as a risk modifier of NSAID-related gastrointestinal bleeding: A case-control study. *Pharmacogenet. Genom.* **2016**, *26*, 66–73.
19. Chamorro, A.J.; Marcos, M.; Mirón-Canelo, J.A.; Pastor, I.; González-Sarmiento, R.; Laso, F.J. Association of μ-opioid receptor (OPRM1) gene polymorphism with response to naltrexone in alcohol dependence: A systematic review and meta-analysis. *Addict. Biol.* **2012**, *17*, 505–512.
20. Nielsen, L.M.; Christrup, L.L.; Sato, H.; Drewes, A.M.; Olesen, A.E. Genetic Influences of OPRM1, OPRD1 and COMT on Morphine Analgesia in a Multi-Modal, Multi-Tissue Human Experimental Pain Model. *Basic Clin. Pharmacol. Toxicol.* **2017**, *121*, 6–12.
21. Amanzio, M.; Pollo, A.; Maggi, G.; Benedetti, F. Response variability to analgesics: A role for non-specific activation of endogenous opioids. *Pain* **2001**, *90*, 205–215.
22. Melzack, R. The short-form McGill Pain Questionnaire. *Pain* **1987**, *30*, 191–197.
23. Hawker, G.A.; Mian, S.; Kendzerska, T.; French, M. Measuresof adult pain: Visual Analog Scale for Pain (VAS Pain), Numeric Rating Scale for Pain (NRS Pain), McGill Pain Questionnaire (MPQ), Short-Form McGill Pain Questionnaire (SF-MPQ), Chronic Pain Grade Scale (CPGS), Short Form-36 Bodily Pain Scale (SF-36 BPS), and Measure of Intermittent and Constant Osteoarthritis Pain (ICOAP). *Arthritis Care Res. (Hoboken)* **2011**, *63* (Suppl. 11), S240–S252.
24. Callegari, C.; Salvaggio, F.; Gerlini, A.; Vender, S. Physical and psychic elements in chronic pain. *Recenti Prog. Med.* **2007**, *98*, 239–242.
25. Crofford, L.J. Chronic Pain: Where the Body Meets the Brain. *Trans. Am. Clin. Climatol. Assoc.* **2015**, *126*, 167–183.
26. Arellano, A.L.; Martin-Subero, M.; Monerris, M.; Llerena, A.; Farré, M.; Montané, E. Multiple adverse drug reactions and genetic polymorphism testing. A case report with negative result. *Medicine (Baltimore)* **2017**, *96*, e8505.
27. Trescot, A.M.; Faynboym, S. A review of the role of genetic testing in pain medicine. *Pain Physician* **2014**, *17*, 425–445.
28. Ielmini, M.; Poloni, N.; Caselli, I.; Diurni, M.; Grecchi, A.; Callegari, C. The role of pharmacogenetic testing in the treatment of bipolar disorder: Preliminary results. *Minerva Psichiatrica* **2018**, *59*, 10–15.
29. Ielmini, M.; Poloni, N.; Caselli, I.; Espadaler, J.; Tuson, M.; Grecchi, A.; Callegari, C. The utility of pharmacogenetic testing to support the treatment of bipolar disorder. *Pharmgenom. Pers. Med.* **2018**, *11*, 35–42.
30. Agarwal, D.; Udoji, M.A.; Trescot, A. Genetic Testing for Opioid Pain Management: A Primer. *Pain Ther.* **2017**, *6*, 93–105.
31. Morales-Espinoza, E.M.; Kostov, B.; Salami, D.C.; Perez, Z.H.; Rosalen, A.P.; Molina, J.O.; Gonzalez-de Paz, L.; Momblona, J.M.; Àreu, J.B.; Brito-Zerón, P.; et al. Complexity, comorbidity, and health care costs associated with chronic widespread pain in primary care. *Pain* **2016**, *157*, 818–826.
32. Callegari, C.; Ielmini, M.; Bianchi, L.; Lucano, M.; Bertù, L.; Vender, S. Antiepileptic drug use in a nursing home setting: A retrospective study in older adults. *Funct. Neurol.* **2016**, *31*, 87–93.
33. Bates, M.S.; Edwards, W.T.; Anderson, K.O. Ethnocultural influences on variation in chronic pain perception. *Pain* **1993**, *52*, 101–112.
34. Diatchenko, L.; Slade, G.D.; Nackley, A.G.; Bhalang, K.; Sigurdsson, A.; Belfer, I.; Goldman, D.; Xu, K.; Shabalina, S.A.; Shagin, D.; et al. Genetic basis for individual variations in pain perception and the development of a chronic pain condition. *Hum. Mol. Genet.* **2005**, *14*, 135–143.
35. Blyth, F.M.; Rochat, S.; Cumming, R.G.; Creasey, H.; Handelsman, D.J.; Le Couteur, D.G.; Naganathan, V.; Sambrook, P.N.; Seibel, M.J.; Waite, L.M. Pain, frailty and comorbidity on older men: The CHAMP study. *Pain* **2008**, *140*, 224–230.
36. Marazziti, D.; Mungai, F.; Vivarelli, L.; Presta, S.; Dell'Osso, B. Pain and psychiatry: A critical analysis and pharmacological review. *Clin. Pract. Epidemiol. Ment. Health* **2006**, *6*, 31.

37. Poloni, N.; Diurni, M.; Buzzi, A.; Cazzamalli, S.; Aletti, F.; Baranzini, F.; Vender, S. Recovery style, symptoms and psychosocial functioning in psychotic patients: A preliminary study. *Riv. Psichiatr.* **2013**, *48*, 386–392.
38. Caselli, I.; Poloni, N.; Ielmini, M.; Diurni, M.; Callegari, C. Epidemiology and evolution of the diagnostic classification of factitious disorders in DSM-5. *Psychol. Res. Behav. Manag.* **2017**, *10*, 387–394.
39. Sheng, J.; Liu, S.; Wang, Y.; Cui, R.; Zhang, X. The Link between Depression and Chronic Pain: Neural Mechanisms in the Brain. *Neural Plast.* **2017**, *2017*, 9724371.
40. Diurni, M.; Baranzini, F.; Costantini, C.; Poloni, N.; Vender, S.; Callegari, C. Metabolic side effects of second generation antipsychotics in drug-naïve patients: A preliminary study. *Riv. Psichiatr.* **2009**, *44*, 176–178.
41. Hiratsuka, M.; Mizugaki, M. Genetic polymorphisms in drug-metabolizing enzymes and drug targets. *Mol. Genet. Metab.* **2001**, *73*, 298–305.
42. Stingl, J.; Viviani, R. Polymorphism in CYP2D6 and CYP2C19, members of the cytochrome P450 mixed-functionoxidase system, in the metabolism of psychotropic drugs. *J. Intern. Med.* **2015**, *277*, 167–177.
43. Jannetto, P.J.; Bratanow, N.C. Pain management in the 21st century: Utilization of pharmacogenomics and therapeutic drug monitoring. *Expert Opin. Drug Metab. Toxicol.* **2011**, *7*, 745–752.
44. Bolla, E.; Bortolaso, P.; Ferrari, M.; Poloni, N.; Callegari, C.; Marino, F.; Lecchini, S.; Vender, S.; Cosentino, M. Are CYP1A2*1F and *1C associated with clozapine tolerability?: A preliminary investigation. *Psychiatry Res.* **2011**, *189*, 483.
45. Ferrari, M.; Bolla, E.; Bortolaso, P.; Callegari, C.; Poloni, N.; Lecchini, S.; Vender, S.; Marino, F.; Cosentino, M. Association between CYP1A2 polymorphisms and clozapine-induced adverse reactions in patients with schizophrenia. *Psychiatry Res.* **2012**, *200*, 1014–1017.
46. Kozyra, M.; Ingelman-Sundberg, M.; Lauschke, V.M. Rare genetic variants in cellular transporters, metabolic enzymes, and nuclear receptors can be important determinants of interindividua differences in drug response. *Genet. Med.* **2017**, *19*, 20–29.

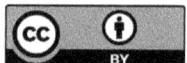

© 2019 by the authors. Licensee MDPI, Basel, Switzerland. This article is an open access article distributed under the terms and conditions of the Creative Commons Attribution (CC BY) license (http://creativecommons.org/licenses/by/4.0/).

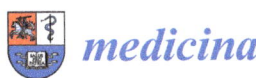

Article

Comparison of the Analgesic Effect of Ropivacaine with Fentanyl and Ropivacaine Alone in Continuous Epidural Infusion for Acute Herpes Zoster Management: A Retrospective Study

Hee Yong Kang [1], Chung Hun Lee [2,*], Sang Sik Choi [2], Mi Kyoung Lee [2], Yeon Joo Lee [2] and Jong Sun Park [2]

[1] Department of Anesthesiology and Pain Medicine, Kyung Hee University Hospital, Kyungheedae Road 23, Dongdaemun-Gu, Seoul 02447, Korea; ujuabba@gmail.com
[2] Department of Anesthesiology and Pain Medicine, Korea University Medical Center, Guro Hospital, Gurodong Road 148, Guro-Gu, Seoul 08308, Korea; clonidine@empal.com (S.S.C.); mknim@hotmail.com (M.K.L.); pipipipig@naver.com (Y.J.L.); pkjgsn@naver.com (J.S.P.)
* Correspondence: bodlch@naver.com

Received: 6 November 2019; Accepted: 6 January 2020; Published: 8 January 2020

Abstract: *Background and Objectives*: Currently, few studies have reported the effects of opioids during continuous epidural infusion (CEI) to control pain owing to herpes zoster (HZ). This study aimed to retrospectively compare the effectiveness of epidural opioids in the treatment of acute HZ pain. *Materials and Methods*: We reviewed medical records of 105 patients who were divided into two groups: R group (CEI with ropivacaine) and RF group (CEI with ropivacaine and fentanyl). Clinical efficacy was evaluated using the numeric rating scale (NRS) score for 6 months after the procedures. We compared the percentage of patients with complete remission in each group. We investigated the complication rates during CEI. *Results*: No significant differences in the NRS scores were observed between the two groups in the 6-month period. The adjusted odds ratio (OR) for patients included in the complete remission was 0.6 times lower in the RF group than in the R group (95% confidence interval: 0.22–1.71, $p = 0.35$). The OR for complications during CEI was higher in the RF group than in the R group. However, the difference was not statistically significant. *Conclusions*: No difference was observed in the management of HZ pain and the prevention of postherpetic neuralgia between the two groups. The incidence of complications tended to be higher in the RF group than in the R group.

Keywords: continuous epidural infusion; fentanyl; herpes zoster; ropivacaine; postherpetic neuralgia; neuropathic pain; intervention

1. Introduction

Neuropathic pain may be due to multiple pathologic conditions such as herpes zoster (HZ), diabetes, cancer, and radiculopathy and affects the quality of life of elderly patients [1]. In particular, pain owing to HZ, caused by the reactivation of the varicella-zoster virus (VZV), is known to be more prevalent in elderly patients with reduced T-cell immunity [2]. Pain associated with HZ is defined as acute herpetic neuralgia until 30 days after the skin rash, subacute herpetic neuralgia until 3 months after the acute phase, and postherpetic neuralgia (PHN) afterward [3]. PHN can persist for more than 12 months, and PHN can last for 6 months in 8.5% of patients and for 12 months in 6% of patients, despite early treatment with antiviral drugs [4,5]. Continuous or intermittent zoster-associated pain can also affect the quality of life and the ability to work. Therefore, effective treatments for zoster-associated pain (ZAP) are necessary to prevent negative sequelae.

Medications such as antiepileptics, tricyclic antidepressants, lidocaine patches, and analgesics may be effective in relieving pain [6,7]. However, interventional therapy is recommended for uncontrolled pain or in the case of a high likelihood of transition to PHN, even with sufficient medication [6,7]. Epidural analgesia, paravertebral block, and pulsed radiofrequency have been performed as interventional therapies to reduce pain [6–8]. Recently, it has been reported that continuous epidural infusion (CEI) using a catheter is effective for ZAP [9–11]. Most studies have shown that epidural administration of local anesthetics is effective in controlling ZAP [9–11]. However, few studies have compared the effectiveness of epidural opioids (particularly fentanyl) in controlling pain owing to HZ.

Thus, this retrospective study aimed to determine whether the addition of opioids to local anesthetics during CEI in patients with acute HZ showed synergistic effects with previously known local anesthetics and opioids.

2. Materials and Methods

2.1. Study Design

This study was performed after the approval by the Institutional Review Board of Korea University Medical Center, Guro Hospital, Seoul, Republic of Korea (2018GR0057, 8 February 2018). The study also complied with the STROBE checklist (supplementary material S1 checklist). The medical records of patients who underwent CEI for acute HZ from April 2014 to July 2018 were collected. Patients were divided into two groups: R group, in which patients were administered CEI containing ropivacaine without fentanyl, and RF group, in which patients were administered CEI containing ropivacaine with fentanyl. Inclusion criteria were patients older than 50 years with a numeric rating scale (NRS; 0 = no pain and 10 = worst possible pain) score of ≥4; patients who received only the standard drug therapy, including antiviral agents, until the administration of CEI; and patients who underwent follow-up for a period of 6 months after CEI. Exclusion criteria were patients with insufficient medical records, patients who did not maintain the catheter for more than 10 days after CEI, patients who did not receive standard medications such as antiviral agents until the procedure, and patients who discontinued the prescribed standard medication (gabapentin or pregabalin, and analgesics such as oxycodone) owing to the side effects of the drugs. Patients who underwent other procedures for pain control within 6 months after the procedure were excluded from this study but were included in the analysis of complications during the catheter maintenance period. Complication rates during the catheter maintenance period were separately analyzed.

2.2. Procedure

After placing the patient in the prone position, an aseptic dressing was applied to the procedure site. A Tuohy epidural needle (18-gauge) was inserted into the interlaminar space at the third or fourth level below the target level under fluoroscopic guidance. The loss of resistance technique was used to verify if the needle was located in the epidural space. After confirming the needle position, a 20-gauge epidural catheter (EpiStim™, length: 800 mm, Sewoon Medical Co., Ltd, Seoul, Korea) was placed at the target level through the Tuohy needle (Figure 1) with radiographic confirmation. This type of epidural catheter has a built-in conductive guidewire (Nitinol, length = 1100 mm) with 800 mm inside the catheter and 300 mm exposed for connection to an electric nerve stimulator. The cathode of the electric nerve stimulator (Life-Tech EZstim, Stafford, TX, USA) was connected to the exposed guidewire, and the anode was attached to an electrode on the patient's calf. A zero to 5 mA electric current was then delivered through the guidewire. Verbal communication with the patient confirmed that the electric stimulation had reached the HZ-affected area. The catheter was placed in the appropriate epidural space, and once electric stimulation was initiated, verbal communication with the patient confirmed the sensation. After patient confirmation, further communication established that the electric stimulus was following the HZ dermatome. If the electric stimulation was in a region other than the HZ dermatome, the epidural catheter was adjusted under fluoroscopy, and the electric stimulation was repeated to confirm its presence in the HZ-affected area. Once the stimulus was established in the correct area, the guidewire was removed. After removing the guidewire, the position of the epidural catheter tip was confirmed using a contrast agent and fluoroscopy; 0.19% ropivacaine and 1 mg dexamethasone (total 8 mL) were then administered via an epidural catheter in the R group, and 0.19% ropivacaine and 1 mg dexamethasone with 50 µg fentanyl (total 8 mL) were administered in the RF group. After initial drug injection, patients in the R group were administered CEI (total 275 mL) containing 30–45 mL of 0.75% ropivacaine (37.1 ± 4.1) and normal saline without fentanyl. Patients in the RF group were administered CEI (total 275 mL) containing 30–40 mL of 0.75% ropivacaine (36.1 ± 3.7) and normal saline with 200 µg fentanyl. In both groups, CEI was administered at a rate of 4 mL/h via a portable balloon infusion device (AutoFuser pump, ACE Medical Co., Ltd., Seoul, Korea). Concentrations of ropivacaine in the portable balloon infusion device were adjusted according to the degree of pain relief or side effects. In both groups, the epidural catheter was fixed by subcutaneous tunneling to decrease the risk of infection and catheter migration. The inserted catheter was maintained in its position for a minimum of 10 days and was removed after 2 weeks. Whether patients were undergoing catheterization as inpatients or outpatients, a physician changed the dressings daily and monitored the procedure site. Additionally, antiepileptics (pregabalin or gabapentin) and analgesics were administered to patients in both groups. Antiepileptics were prescribed by adjusting the drug dose according to age and renal function and were tapered according to symptoms. Oral oxycodone was administered as an analgesic, starting with the minimum reported effective dose for PHN [12].

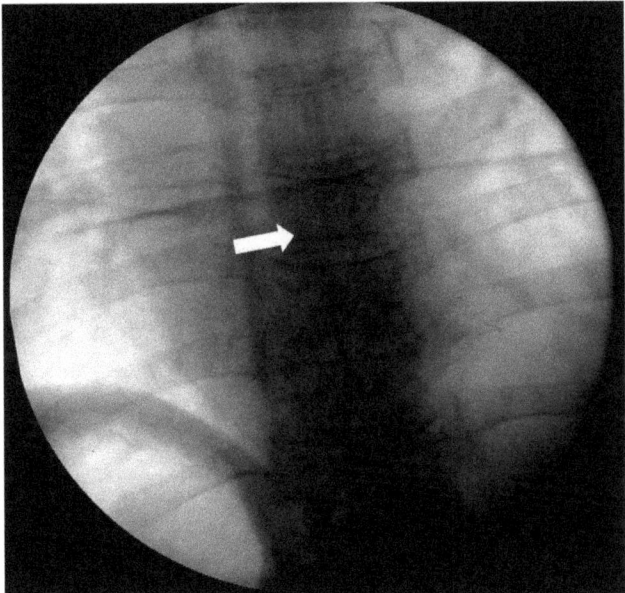

Figure 1. Fluoroscopic images of the continuous epidural block. The catheter used for the procedure had a built-in conductive guidewire that allowed the detection of the catheter tip using radiography, along with electrical stimulation. The arrow indicates the tip of the guidewire in the EpiStim™ catheter.

2.3. Data Collection

Data regarding age, sex, spinal level of catheterization, days from the onset of rash to CEI, past medical history (hypertension (HTN), diabetes mellitus (DM), liver disease, kidney disease, and asthma), and amount of 0.75% ropivacaine in the infusion device were collected. The patients' pain was assessed using an 11-point verbal NRS (0, no pain and 10, unbearable pain). We collected the

NRS score data at different times: immediately before the procedure (baseline NRS score); 1 h after the procedure; 14 days after the procedure; and 1, 3, and 6 months after the procedure from patients' medical records. Complete remission was defined as an NRS score ≤2, with no further medication prescribed at 6 months after the procedure. The number of patients included in this category during the 6-month follow-up period was recorded. We recorded whether other interventional procedures were performed owing to inadequate pain control during the 6-month follow-up period after CEI. We also collected records of complications (nausea, vomiting, dysuria, hypotension, and itching) during the epidural catheter maintenance period.

2.4. Outcome Measures

To compare analgesic effect as the primary endpoint, we compared NRS scores of the two groups at baseline; 1 h; 14 days; and 1, 3, and 6 months after the procedure, after correcting for various variables. As the secondary endpoint, we compared the percentage of patients with complete remission in each group, the proportion of patients requiring additional nerve block owing to inadequate pain control after the procedure, and the incidence of complications owing to CEI between the two groups.

2.5. Statistical Analysis

Demographic data were analyzed using the Kolmogorov–Smirnov test to assess the normality of the distribution. Normally distributed sets of demographic data were compared between the groups using an independent *t*-test, and non-normally distributed datasets were compared using the Mann–Whitney U test. After correcting for various confounding variables (age, sex, spinal level of catheterization, days from the onset of rash to CEI, past medical history (HTN, DM, liver disease, kidney disease, and asthma), average amount of 0.75% ropivacaine in the infusion device, and baseline NRS score), we analyzed the differences in NRS scores between the groups using analysis of covariance. Multivariable logistic regression analysis was used to compare the percentages of complete remission within 6 months after the procedure and to compare the percentages of patients who underwent other interventional treatments between the two groups. Univariable logistic regression analysis was performed to compare the complication rates owing to CEI. Data are presented as mean ± standard deviation or median (interquartile range). The collected data were analyzed using Statistical Package for the Social Sciences (SPSS) software (version 17.0; SPSS 157 Inc., Chicago, IL, USA). All statistical tests were two-sided, and the threshold for statistical significance was set at $p < 0.05$.

3. Results

We reviewed the medical records of 137 patients. Five patients missed the follow-up or had inadequate medical records in the 6 months after the procedure. Twelve patients underwent other interventional procedures within 6 months of CEI. In six patients, the catheter could not be maintained for more than 10 days owing to side effects associated with CEI. Two patients did not receive antiviral drugs at the beginning of the HZ episode. During the 6-month follow-up period, one patient had other pain-causing diseases. The medical records of these patients were excluded from the final analysis. Moreover, six patients discontinued using antiepileptics or analgesics owing to drug-associated side effects after the procedure. To prevent drug-induced bias, these patients were also excluded from the final analysis. After the exclusions, the medical records of the remaining 105 patients were analyzed. Sixty-two patients were assigned to the R group and 43 were assigned to the RF group (Figure 2).

No significant differences were observed in the demographic and clinical characteristics of the patients between the two groups (Table 1, supplementary file S2).

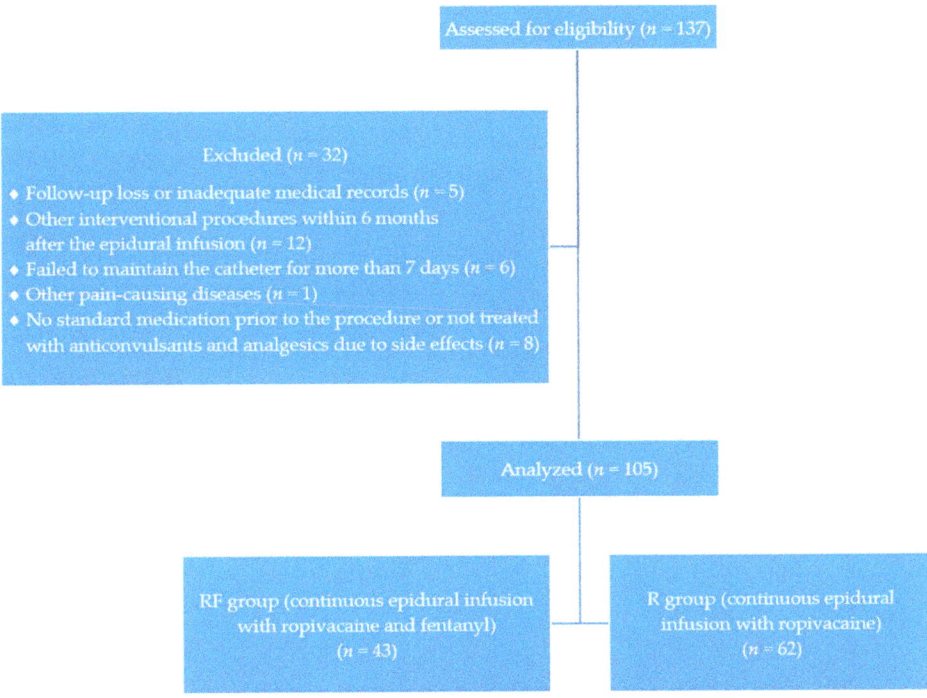

Figure 2. Flow diagram showing patient inclusion.

Table 1. Baseline demographic and clinical characteristics of the patients.

Demographic and Clinical Characteristics	Acute HZ (≤30 Days) R Group (n = 62)	Acute HZ (≤30 Days) RF Group (n = 43)	p Value
Age (years)	66.2 ± 9.3	65.3 ± 7.9	0.61
Sex (male/female)	20/42	13/30	0.84
Site of HZ infection	C: 14 (22.6%)	C: 7 (16.3%)	0.87
	T: 36 (58.1%)	T: 25 (58.1%)	
	L: 12 (19.4%)	L: 11 (25.6%)	
HTN	23 (37%)	20 (47%)	0.42
DM	18 (29%)	14 (33%)	0.83
Asthma	2 (3%)	1 (2%)	1.0
Hepatic disease	3 (5%)	1 (2%)	0.64
Kidney disease	3 (5%)	2 (5%)	1.0
Baseline NRS score	8 (6–8)	7 (6.5–8)	0.87
Avg. amount of 0.75% ropivacaine in infusion device (mL)	37.1 ± 4.1	36.1 ± 3.7	0.25

HZ: herpes zoster, Avg: average, HTN: hypertension, DM: diabetes mellitus, NRS: numeric rating scale of 0–10, C: cervical, T: thoracic, L: lumbar, R group: local anesthetic without epidural opioid, RF group: local anesthetic with epidural opioid. Data are presented as mean ± standard deviation, median (interquartile range), or number (%).

No significant difference was observed between the two groups with respect to post-procedure NRS scores after correcting for confounding variables (Table 2). There was no significant difference in the reduction ratio of NRS scores according to fentanyl use with time after CEI (Figure 3).

Table 2. Comparison of numeric rating scale scores between the groups after correction for confounding variables.

NRS Score	Acute HZ (≤30 Days) R Group (n = 62)	Acute HZ (≤30 Days) RF Group (n = 43)	p Value
Baseline NRS score	7.1 ± 1.5	7.3 ± 1.0	0.31
NRS score * 1 h after epidural procedure	2.9 ± 1.8	3.1 ± 1.3	0.26
NRS score * 14 days after epidural procedure	1.7 ± 0.8	1.9 ± 0.8	0.16
NRS score * 1 month after epidural procedure	1.9 ± 1.1	2.1 ± 0.7	0.18
NRS score * 3 months after epidural procedure	1.5 ± 1.1	1.8 ± 0.8	0.11
NRS score * 6 months after epidural procedure	1.2 ± 1.0	1.4 ± 0.9	0.18

* The NRS scores (0 = no pain and 10 = worst possible pain) are represented as means ± standard deviation, R group: local anesthetic without epidural opioid, RF group: local anesthetic with epidural opioid. Data were analyzed for the difference in the pain scores between the groups using analysis of covariance. Adjustments were made for age, sex, time from the onset of rash to epidural infusion, average amount of 0.75% ropivacaine in the infusion device, location of herpes zoster, hypertension, diabetes mellitus, asthma, hepatic disease, and kidney disease.

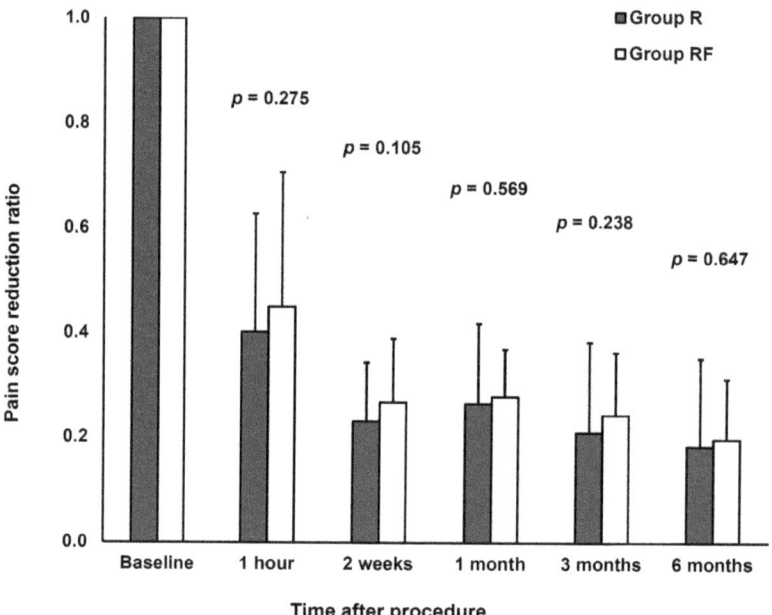

Figure 3. Comparison of the numeric rating scale score reduction ratio according to fentanyl use with time after continuous epidural infusion.

The proportion of patients showing complete remission was lower in the RF group than in the R group. However, the difference was not statistically significant (adjusted odds ratio (OR): 0.62, 95% confidence interval (CI): 0.22–1.71, p = 0.35; Table 3). The proportion of patients who underwent other interventional procedures owing to insufficient pain control within 6 months after CEI was 3.21 times higher in the RF group than in the R group (adjusted OR: 3.21, 95% CI: 0.56–18.24, p = 0.19; Table 4).

Table 3. Comparison of complete remission during the 6-month follow-up period between the groups after epidural infusion.

Complete Remission	R Group	RF Group	Adjusted OR (95% CI) Reference: R Group	p Value
Acute HZ (≤30 days)	46/62 (74%)	30/43 (70%)	0.62 (0.22–1.71)	0.35

OR: odds ratio, CI: confidence interval, R group: local anesthetic without epidural opioid, RF group: local anesthetic with epidural opioid. Complete remission is defined as a numerical rating scale score of <2 with no further medication. Data are presented as number (%). Data were analyzed using multivariable logistic regression analysis. Adjustments were made for age, sex, location of herpes zoster, days from the onset of rash to epidural infusion, average amount of 0.75% ropivacaine in the infusion device, history of hypertension, diabetes mellitus, asthma, hepatic disease, and kidney disease, and baseline pain score.

Table 4. Comparison of other interventions performed owing to insufficient pain control during the 6-month follow-up period after epidural infusion.

Performed Other Interventions	R Group	RF Group	Adjusted OR (95% CI) Reference: R Group	p Value
Acute HZ (≤30 days)	6/68 (9%)	6/49 (12%)	3.21 (0.56–18.24)	0.19

R group: local anesthetic without epidural opioid, RF group: local anesthetic with epidural opioid. Data are presented as number (%). Data included patients who underwent other procedures within the 6-month follow-up period and those who did not maintain the epidural catheter for more than 7 days owing to the side effects. Data were analyzed using multivariable logistic regression analysis. Adjustments were made for age, sex, location of herpes zoster, days from the onset of rash to epidural infusion, average amount of 0.75% ropivacaine in infusion device, history of hypertension, diabetes mellitus, asthma, hepatic disease, and kidney disease, and baseline pain score.

Complication rates (nausea, vomiting, dysuria, hypotension, and itching) during CEI were higher in the RF group than in the R group (Table 5). However, these differences were not statistically significant.

Table 5. Comparison of complication rates during continuous epidural infusion between the groups.

Side Effects	R Group	RF Group	Unadjusted OR (95% CI) Reference: R Group	p Value
Nausea	1/68 (1%)	5/53 (9%)	6.98 (0.79–61.67)	0.08
Vomiting	1/68 (1%)	3/53 (6%)	4.02 (0.41–39.80)	0.23
Dysuria	2/68 (3%)	3/53 (6%)	1.98 (0.32–12.30)	0.46
Itching sensation	0/68 (0%)	3/53 (6%)	9.50 (0.48–187.95)	0.14
Hypotension	0/68 (0%)	3/53 (6%)	9.50 (0.48–187.95)	0.14

R group: local anesthetic without epidural opioid, RF group: local anesthetic with epidural opioid. Data are presented as number (%). Data included patients who underwent other procedures within the 6-month follow-up period and those who did not maintain the epidural catheter for more than 7 days owing to the side effects. Data were analyzed using univariable logistic regression analysis.

4. Discussion

This study determined whether there was a difference in pain reduction and complication rates between local anesthetics alone and local anesthetics with opioids in CEI for patients with acute HZ. No significant difference was observed in pain reduction between the two groups during the 6-month follow-up period. Furthermore, there was no significant difference in the complete remission rate and the proportion of patients who underwent other invasive procedures owing to inadequate pain control within 6 months after CEI. The rates of complications such as nausea (unadjusted OR: 6.98), vomiting (unadjusted OR: 4.02), itching (unadjusted OR: 9.50), and hypotension (unadjusted OR: 9.50) during CEI were consistently higher in the RF group than in the R group. However, the difference was not statistically significant.

Reactivated VZV in the sensory ganglia of the spinal cord manifests as HZ and subsequently spreads out to the affected dermatome, thereby producing an inflammatory response and inducing nerve damage. A serious initial nerve damage or inability to restore normal function after the loss of nerve function can lead to PHN [13]. Therefore, active treatment before the nerve damage occurs can help prevent PHN and control pain. A recent meta-analysis reported that CEI in the acute phase of HZ is effective in controlling pain and preventing PHN [14]. The rationale behind using CEI to manage acute HZ pain and prevent PHN is that the interruption of afferent pain stimuli to the central nervous system and the improved blood flow to nerve tissue will minimize neural damage and reduce pain to the patient by blocking sympathetic nerves [15,16].

The analgesic effect of epidural opioids added to local anesthetics has been proven in several studies [17–21]. Neuraxial local anesthetics and opioids function synergistically to provide analgesia during labor [17,18]. For postoperative pain control, the addition of fentanyl to 0.1% solution of ropivacaine enhances analgesic efficacy [19]. The coadministration of fentanyl (100 µg) and 1% ropivacaine accelerated the onset of sensory and motor blocks during epidural ropivacaine [20] or lidocaine [21] anesthesia, without significant side effects related to fentanyl. The analgesic effect of epidural opioids seems to be related to the location of receptor sites in the spinal cord. These receptor sites have been identified in many areas of the brain and central nervous system, with very high densities in the substantia gelatinosa of the spinal cord [22]. Previous studies on epidural labor analgesia [17,18] and postoperative epidural analgesia [19] have also reported that opioid administration in combination with local anesthesia in the epidural space has a better effect on pain control than the administration of local anesthetics alone. However, the pain control measures in these studies were primarily performed for nociceptive pain.

Some studies have suggested that the effects of opioid-mediated analgesia in neuropathic pain may be reduced by an increase in neuropeptide cholecystokinin, an endogenous inhibitor of opioid-mediated analgesia [23]. Moreover, in neuropathic pain, the functional pool of opioid receptors is likely to be reduced at the spinal level [24].

These factors suggest that the addition of opioids during CEI for ZAP, which is a type of neuropathic pain, may not be more effective than the local anesthetic alone. Watt et al. concluded that after epidural morphine administration in 11 PHN patients, the morphine was more likely to cause side effects than pain relief [25]. In our study, no difference was observed in pain reduction between epidural infusion using local anesthetic alone and epidural infusion using local anesthetic and fentanyl to control ZAP.

Epidural opioid administration can cause several systemic side effects [26,27]. In the present study, the incidence of side effects such as nausea, vomiting, dysuria, and itching tended to be higher in the RF group than in the R group. Previous studies have reported no difference in the rate of complications with epidural opioid administration [17–21]. However, in these studies, only young participants were included in the trial. The average age of HZ patients included in the present study was 65.8 years. In other words, the higher incidence of complications in the opioid group in the present study may be because of the older age of patients.

Previous studies have reported that a single epidural block may be effective in managing ZAP; however, it has limited efficacy in preventing PHN [28,29]. Hence, patients who could not maintain the CEI catheter for more than 10 days were excluded from the analysis in the present study.

All patients included in the present study underwent CEI and received simultaneous antiepileptic and analgesic medications. To avoid bias owing to drug treatments, patients who discontinued the drugs owing to side effects were excluded from the analysis.

The complete remission rate in the present study was 74% in the R group and 70% in the RF group. Reportedly, the greater severity of acute ZAP is associated with a greater likelihood of its progression to PHN [30,31]. In our hospital, interventional treatments such as CEI were performed only for patients with HZ who had an NRS score ≥4 even after oral medication. All patients included in this study had NRS scores ≥4 (mean 7.2 ± 1.3, 7.3 ± 1.0). The higher NRS scores could be one of the reasons for the lower rates of complete remission. Additionally, the definition we adopted for complete remission (NRS score ≤2, no further medication prescribed) could possibly be another reason for the lower remission rates, as other studies have defined complete remission as a pain-free state with an NRS score <3 or have not mentioned the withdrawal of medication [11,28].

Although CEI shows excellent pain control effect in HZ patients, it is invasive; thus, there is a possibility of side effects (epidural hematoma, epidural abscess, etc.). However, none of the patients in this study reported epidural infection, possibly because of daily dressing by well-trained physicians and well-educated patients and caregivers. A previous study [6] reported a low risk of epidural hematoma associated with epidural blocks, and in this study, epidural hematoma was not reported in patients. However, it should be implemented considering risks and benefits.

This study had some limitations in the interpretation of the results. Since this was a retrospective study, unmeasured confounding variables may have influenced the results. However, to control potential confounding variables, we performed an analysis of covariance with the baseline demographics and underlying diseases of patients as covariates. We excluded patients who were treated with other interventional procedures within 6 months after CEI. This approach may have caused a selection bias in this study. However, inclusion of these patients might have resulted in uncertainty regarding whether the improvement in the patients' symptoms was because of CEI or other interventions. We excluded patients who received other interventions when calculating the complete remission rates and 6-month pain scores and separately analyzed the ratios. To overcome the selection bias, we selected only patients who underwent CEI with the same type of catheter (EpiStim™ epidural catheter) and those for whom CEI was performed by the same anesthesiologist. The study showed no significant difference between the two groups in terms of the degree of pain reduction or the complication rates owing to the limited number of patients. However, the incidence of complications was consistently higher in the RF group than in the R group. A larger sample size may result in statistically significant results, especially with respect to the complication rates. In the present study, patients were not randomly assigned to the groups because we analyzed medical records during normal practice. The patients' medical records were written without blinding. Therefore, the present study may have an inherent risk of bias.

5. Conclusions

No difference was observed in the management of ZAP and the prevention of PHN between the group with added opioid and the one without opioid in the local anesthetic during CEI. The difference in the incidence of complications was not significant; however, it was consistently higher in the group with opioid added to CEI. A well-planned prospective study with a greater number of patients to compare strategies for preventing ZAP and PHN is needed to validate the results of this study.

Supplementary Materials: The following are available online at http://www.mdpi.com/1010-660X/56/1/22/s1, S1: S1 file, and S2: STROBE checklist.

Author Contributions: Conceptualization, C.H.L. and S.S.C.; data curation, H.Y.K. and C.H.L.; formal analysis, H.Y.K. and C.H.L.; investigation, C.H.L., Y.J.L. and J.S.P.; methodology, C.H.L., Y.J.L. and J.S.P.; project administration, C.H.L.; resources, M.K.L.; software, H.Y.K.; supervision, S.S.C. and M.K.L.; validation, C.H.L. and M.K.L.; visualization, C.H.L.; writing—original draft, H.Y.K. and C.H.L.; writing—review and editing, H.Y.K., C.H.L. and M.K.L. All authors have read and agreed to the published version of the manuscript.

Funding: This research received no external funding.

Acknowledgments: Statistical analysis was conducted after consulting Soon Young Hwang (Korea University Medical Center, Guro Hospital), a statistical expert. The authors would like to thank all the participants in the study. We would like to thank Editage (www.editage.co.kr) for English language editing.

Conflicts of Interest: The authors declare no conflict of interest.

References

1. Pickering, G.; Leplege, A. Herpes zoster pain, postherpetic neuralgia, and quality of life in the elderly. *Pain Pract.* **2011**, *11*, 397–402. [CrossRef] [PubMed]
2. Arvin, A. Aging, immunity and the Varicella-zoster virus. *N. Engl. J. Med.* **2005**, *352*, 2266–2267. [CrossRef] [PubMed]

3. Bowsher, D. Factors influencing the features of postherpetic neuralgia and outcome when treated with tricyclics. *Eur. J. Pain* **2003**, *7*, 1–7. [CrossRef]
4. Bouhassira, D.; Chassany, O.; Gaillat, J.; Hanslik, T.; Launay, O.; Mann, C.; Rabaud, C.; Rogeaux, O.; Strady, C. Patient perspective on herpes zoster and its complications: An observational prospective study in patients aged over 50 years in general practice. *Pain* **2012**, *153*, 342–349. [CrossRef] [PubMed]
5. Cunningham, A.L.; Dworkin, R.H. The management of post-herpetic neuralgia. *BMJ* **2000**, *321*, 778–779. [CrossRef] [PubMed]
6. van Wijck, A.J.; Wallace, M.; Mekhail, N.; van Kleef, M. Evidence-based interventional pain medicine according to clinical diagnoses. 17. Herpes zoster and post-herpetic neuralgia. *Pain Pract.* **2011**, *11*, 88–97. [CrossRef]
7. Jeon, Y.H. Herpes zoster and postherpetic neuralgia: Practical consideration for prevention and treatment. *Korean J. Pain.* **2015**, *28*, 177–184. [CrossRef]
8. Werner, R.N.; Nikkels, A.F.; Marinović, B.; Schäfer, M.; Czarnecka-Operacz, M.; Agius, A.M.; Bata-Csörgő, Z.; Breuer, J.; Girolomoni, G.; Gross, G.E.; et al. European consensus-based (S2k) Guideline on the Management of Herpes Zoster—guided by the European Dermatology Forum (EDF) in cooperation with the European Academy of Dermatology and Venereology (EADV), Part 2: Treatment. *J. Eur. Acad. Dermatol. Venereol.* **2017**, *31*, 20–29. [CrossRef]
9. Seo, Y.G.; Kim, S.H.; Choi, S.S.; Lee, M.K.; Lee, C.H.; Kim, J.E. Effectiveness of continuous epidural analgesia on acute herpes zoster and postherpetic neuralgia: A retrospective study. *Medicine (Baltimore)* **2018**, *97*, e9837. [CrossRef]
10. Li, S.J.; Feng, D. Effect of 2% lidocaine continuous epidural infusion for thoracic or lumbar Herpes-zoster-related pain. *Medicine (Baltimore)* **2018**, *97*, e11864. [CrossRef]
11. Pasqualucci, A.; Pasqualucci, V.; Galla, F.; De Angelis, V.; Marzocchi, V.; Colussi, R.; Paoletti, F.; Girardis, M.; Lugano, M.; Del Sindaco, F. Prevention of post-herpetic neuralgia: Acyclovir and prednisolone versus epidural local anesthetic and methylprednisolone. *Acta Anaesthesiol. Scand.* **2000**, *44*, 910–918. [CrossRef] [PubMed]
12. Watson, C.P.; Babul, N. Efficacy of oxycodone in neuropathic pain: A randomized trial in postherpetic neuralgia. *Neurology* **1998**, *50*, 1837–1841. [CrossRef]
13. Winnie, A.P.; Hartwell, P.W. Relationship between time of treatment of acute herpes zoster with sympathetic blockade and prevention of postherpetic neuralgia: Clinical support for a new theory of the mechanism by which sympathetic blockade provides therapeutic benefit. *Reg. Anesth.* **1993**, *18*, 277–282.
14. Kim, H.J.; Ahn, H.S.; Lee, J.Y.; Choi, S.S.; Cheong, Y.S.; Kwon, K.; Yoon, S.H.; Leem, J.G. Effects of applying nerve blocks to prevent postherpetic neuralgia in patients with acute herpes zoster: A systematic review and meta-analysis. *Korean J. Pain* **2017**, *30*, 3–17. [CrossRef] [PubMed]
15. Doran, C.; Yi, X. The anti-inflammatory effect of local anesthetics. *Pain Clin.* **2007**, *19*, 207–213. [CrossRef]
16. Opstelten, W.; van Wijck, A.J.; Stolker, R.J. Interventions to prevent postherpetic neuralgia: Cutaneous and percutaneous techniques. *Pain* **2004**, *107*, 202–206. [CrossRef] [PubMed]
17. Lee, A.I.; McCarthy, R.J.; Toledo, P.; Jones, M.J.; White, N.; Wong, C.A. Epidural labor analgesia-fentanyl dose and breastfeeding success: A randomized clinical trial. *Anesthesiology* **2017**, *127*, 614–624. [CrossRef]
18. Kee, W.D.N.; Khaw, K.S.; Ng, F.F.; Ng, K.K.; So, R.; Lee, A. Synergistic interaction between fentanyl and bupivacaine given intrathecally for labor analgesia. *Anesthesiology* **2014**, *120*, 1126–1136.
19. Khanna, A.; Saxena, R.; Dutta, A.; Ganguly, N.; Sood, J. Comparison of ropivacaine with and without fentanyl vs bupivacaine with fentanyl for postoperative epidural analgesia in bilateral total knee replacement surgery. *J. Clin. Anesth.* **2017**, *37*, 7–13. [CrossRef]
20. Cherng, C.H.; Yang, C.P.; Wong, C.S. Epidural fentanyl speeds the onset of sensory and motor blocks during epidural ropivacaine anesthesia. *Anesth. Analg.* **2005**, *101*, 1834–1837. [CrossRef]
21. Cherng, C.H.; Wong, C.S.; Ho, S.T. Epidural fentanyl speeds the onset of sensory block during epidural lidocaine anesthesia. *Reg. Anesth. Pain Med.* **2001**, *26*, 523–526. [CrossRef]
22. Pert, C.B.; Kuhar, M.J.; Snyder, S.H. Opiate receptor: Autoradiographic localization in rat brain. *Proc. Natl. Acad. Sci. USA* **1976**, *73*, 3729–3733. [CrossRef] [PubMed]
23. Ossipov, M.; Malan, T.; Lai, J.; Porreca, F. Opioid pharmacology of acute and chronic pain. In *The Pharmacology of Pain*, 1st ed.; Dickenson, A., Besson, J.M., Eds.; Springer: Berlin/Heidelberg, Germany, 1997; pp. 305–333.
24. Dickenson, A. Spinal cord pharmacology of pain. *Br. J. Anaesth.* **1995**, *75*, 193–200. [CrossRef]

25. Watt, J.W.; Wiles, J.R.; Bowsher, D.R. Epidural morphine for postherpetic neuralgia. *Anaesthesia* **1996**, *51*, 647–651. [CrossRef] [PubMed]
26. Chaney, M.A. Side effects of intrathecal and epidural opioids. *Can. J. Anaesth.* **1995**, *42*, 891–903. [CrossRef] [PubMed]
27. Alansary, A.M.; Elbeialy, M.A.K. Dexmedetomidine versus fentanyl added to bupivacaine for epidural analgesia in combination with general anesthesia for elective lumbar disc operations: A prospective, randomized double-blinded study. *Saudi J. Anaesth.* **2019**, *13*, 119–125.
28. van Wijck, A.J.; Opstelten, W.; Moons, K.G.; van Essen, G.A.; Stolker, R.J.; Kalkman, C.J.; Verheij, T.J. The PINE study of epidural steroids and local anaesthetics to prevent postherpetic neuralgia: A randomised controlled trial. *Lancet* **2006**, *367*, 219–224. [CrossRef]
29. Kikuchi, A.; Kotani, N.; Sato, T.; Takamura, K.; Sakai, I.; Matsuki, A. Comparative therapeutic evaluation of intrathecal versus epidural methylprednisolone for long-term analgesia in patients with intractable postherpetic neuralgia. *Reg. Anesth. Pain Med.* **1999**, *24*, 287–293.
30. Kawai, K.; Rampakakis, E.; Tsai, T.F.; Cheong, H.J.; Dhitavat, J.; Covarrubias, A.O.; Yang, L.; Cashat-Cruz, M.; Monsanto, H.; Johnson, K.; et al. Predictors of postherpetic neuralgia in patients with herpes zoster: A pooled analysis of prospective cohort studies from North and Latin America and Asia. *Int. J. Infect. Dis.* **2015**, *34*, 126–131. [CrossRef]
31. Forbes, H.J.; Thomas, S.L.; Smeeth, L.; Clayton, T.; Farmer, R.; Bhaskaran, K.; Langan, S.M. A systematic review and meta-analysis of risk factors for postherpetic neuralgia. *Pain* **2016**, *157*, 30–54. [CrossRef]

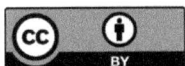

© 2020 by the authors. Licensee MDPI, Basel, Switzerland. This article is an open access article distributed under the terms and conditions of the Creative Commons Attribution (CC BY) license (http://creativecommons.org/licenses/by/4.0/).

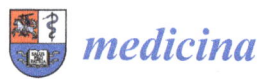

Article

Factors Predicting Favorable Short-Term Response to Transforaminal Epidural Steroid Injections for Lumbosacral Radiculopathy

Dong Yoon Park [1], Seok Kang [2] and Joo Hyun Park [3],*

[1] Department of Rehabilitation Medicine, Graduate School, The Catholic University of Korea, Seoul 06591, Korea; dyfree@naver.com
[2] Department of Physical Medicine and Rehabilitation, Korea University Guro Hospital, Seoul 08308, Korea; caprock@paran.com
[3] Department of Rehabilitation Medicine, Seoul St. Mary's Hospital, College of Medicine, The Catholic University of Korea, Seoul 06591, Korea
* Correspondence: drpjh@catholic.ac.kr; Tel.: +82-2-2258-6280; Fax: +82-2-2258-2825

Received: 23 January 2019; Accepted: 15 May 2019; Published: 18 May 2019

Abstract: *Background and Objectives:* The purpose of this retrospective study was to identify predictors of short-term outcomes associated with a lumbosacral transforaminal epidural steroid injection (TFESI). *Materials and Methods:* The medical records of 218 patients, who were diagnosed with lumbosacral radiculopathy and treated with a TFESI, were reviewed in this retrospective study. A mixture of corticosteroid, lidocaine, and hyaluronidase was injected during TFESI. Patients with >50% pain relief on the numerical rating scale compared with the initial visit constituted the good responder group. Demographic, clinical, MRI, and electrodiagnostic data were collected to assess the predictive factors for short-term outcomes of the TFESI. *Results:* A multivariate logistic regression analysis demonstrated that a shorter duration of symptoms and a positive sharp wave (PSW)/fibrillation (Fib) observed in electrodiagnostic study (EDx) increased the odds of significant improvement 2–4 weeks after the TFESI. *Conclusions:* Shorter duration of symptoms and PSW/Fib on EDx were predictors of favorable short-term response to TFESI.

Keywords: radiculopathy; epidural injection; predictor; corticosteroid; electromyography; hyalurodinase

1. Introduction

Low back pain and radiating pain are common health conditions, with a lifetime prevalence of about 40–60% [1–3]. However, no gold standard imaging or laboratory test is available for the diagnosis of lumbosacral radiculopathy. Clinicians arrive at the diagnosis based on a combination of history, physical examination, imaging, and neurophysiological studies. Decisions regarding optimal treatment are also not easy, especially given the various therapeutic approaches available: medications, physiotherapy, exercise, injections, and surgery.

There is controversy regarding the effect of a lumbosacral epidural steroid injection. Some studies have demonstrated the efficacy of epidural steroid injections for the treatment of radiating pain in patients with lumbosacral disk herniation [4–7]. Other studies have shown that the effectiveness of this procedure is limited [8,9]. Nevertheless, lumbosacral epidural injections have been widely used to treat radicular pain in clinical practice. In addition, this procedure has also been used to treat patients who have undergone previous low back surgery [10].

Three different techniques, including transforaminal, interlaminar, and caudal approaches, have been widely used in clinical practice. The transforaminal epidural steroid injection (TFESI) seems to be better than an interlaminar or a caudal approach for radicular pain [7,11].

Despite the widespread availability of epidural steroid injections, little is known about the factors predicting their success. Studies investigating the predictors of lumbar epidural steroid injections have shown conflicting results [9,12–28]. If the diagnostic information can be used to predict treatment response, it can facilitate the treatment plan. The aim of this study was to determine the factors that represent predictors of short-term outcomes of a lumbosacral TFESI.

2. Materials and Methods

2.1. Patients

The patients who had undergone lumbosacral TFESI procedures in the Department of Rehabilitation, Korea University Guro Hospital, from March 2014 to October 2017, were included in this study. The electronic medical records of symptomatic patients who were diagnosed with lumbosacral disk herniation, that presented with radiating pain, and were treated with a TFESI, were reviewed. This study was approved by the institutional review board of the relevant institution (Korea university Guro hospital, Approval code: 2017GR0017, date of approval: 16 November 2017). The inclusion criteria were: (i) patients aged over 20 years old; (ii) patients who complained of radiating pain; (iii) definitive diagnosis of lumbosacral disk herniation, which was confirmed by MRI; and (iv) TFESI treatment.

The exclusion criteria were: (i) inadequate data including history, physical examination, and MRI findings; (ii) failure to visit our clinic again 2–4 weeks after the TFESI; (iii) symptoms after traffic accident or workplace injury; (iv) prior lumbosacral epidural steroid injections in the past 3 months; (v) severe motor weakness of the lower extremity (less than a fair grade on a manual muscle test of any the following: hip flexion, knee extension, ankle dorsiflexion, great toe extension, and ankle plantar flexion); (vi) acute bladder or bowel symptoms; (vii) diagnosis of other diseases, such as diabetic polyneuropathy, in addition to lumbosacral radiculopathy, diagnosed either clinically or via electrodiagnostic study (EDx); or (viii) abnormal blood test results. Blood tests were routinely done for all the patients before the epidural injection. Blood tests included a complete blood count, blood chemistry, C-reactive protein, prothrombin time, and activated partial thromboplastin time. Patients with either severe motor weakness (less than a fair grade) or acute bladder and bowel symptoms were referred to a spine surgeon. Based on these criteria, 218 patients were included in this study. Oral analgesia was prescribed to all patients. None of the included patients were involved in other treatment, such as physical therapy.

2.2. TFESI

All of the procedures were conducted by two specialists experienced in spinal intervention under fluoroscopic guidance on an outpatient basis. Blood tests, including complete blood count, blood chemistry, erythrocyte sedimentation rate, C-reactive protein, prothrombin time, and activated partial thromboplastin time, were carried out on all the patients before the procedure to determine infection or bleeding risk. Patients taking anti-platelet agents or anticoagulants were asked to discontinue them for a week before the procedure. Informed consent was obtained from each patient. All the procedures were carried out via an extraepineural approach. With the patient lying in a prone position, the C-arm was rotated obliquely to obtain an X-ray image of pedicle and neural foramen. An 89 mm, 23-gauge spinal needle was advanced into the safe triangle. The safe triangle was defined by the pedicle superiorly, the lateral border of the vertebral body laterally, and the outer margin of spinal nerve medially. The contrast agent was spread into the epidural space and externally along the spinal nerve root. A mixture of 20 mg (0.5 cc) of triamcinolone acetonide suspension, 2 cc of 0.5% lidocaine, and 750 IU of hyaluronidase was slowly injected at each level. This mixture has been used to treat acute and chronic low back pain and radicular symptoms via various mechanisms. Corticosteroids exhibit anti-inflammatory effects, as well as interfere with nociceptive C-fiber conduction [29]. Local anesthetics impair peripheral neurotransmission of pain impulses, normalize the hyperalgesic state of the nervous system, and prevent and reduce neuronal plasticity in the central nervous system by reducing the peripheral nociceptive input [30]. Hyaluronidase is a lysing enzyme that disrupts the epidural scar tissue and adhesions. The use of hyaluronidase reduces fibrosis and facilitates the spread of injections [31]. This enzyme is reported to be effective in treating chronic low back pain or radiating pain [32].

All the patients were asked to visit the outpatient clinic 2 weeks after the TFESI to evaluate the short-term therapeutic effect. However, a few patients failed to visit on the scheduled date because of the patient's personal circumstances. Therefore, we collected the short-term outcome based on the first visit between 2 and 4 weeks after the TFESI.

2.3. Review of Clinical Data and Outcomes

A retrospective review of medical records was performed. The following data were reviewed: (i) demographics, (ii) clinical characteristics, (iii) MRI, and (iv) EDx measurements. Demographic data included age and sex. Clinical data included past medical history, symptoms, and physical examination. Past medical history, including the presence of diabetes, hypertension, and previous lumbosacral spine surgery, was reviewed. Any sprain or trauma associated with the low back was assessed just before the onset of symptoms. Duration of symptoms was classified as acute (≤4 weeks), subacute (4–24 weeks), and chronic (≥24 weeks). The nature of pain was evaluated as follows: presence of low back pain, buttock pain, or neurogenic claudication. The straight leg raise test (SLR) and motor and sensory examination were performed. The SLR was considered positive if the radiating symptoms were triggered by lifting the leg less than 60 degrees. The motor exam was considered abnormal if there was weakness associated with any of the following muscle groups on manual muscle testing: hip flexors, knee extensors, ankle dorsiflexors, great toe extensors, and ankle plantar flexors. The sensory exam was considered abnormal if allodynia, hypoesthesia, anesthesia, or paresthesia was detected along the nerve root dermatome.

All the patients underwent lumbar MRI, and all the MRI data were reviewed by a single radiologist specializing in musculoskeletal imaging at our hospital. MRI data included the level of herniated nucleus pulposus (HNP), the presence of nerve root compression or contact, foraminal stenosis, and moderate-to-severe central canal stenosis.

EDx, including a nerve conduction study and needle electromyography, was performed by qualified electromyographers. We used a needle electromyography (EMG) electrode to examine paravertebral and limb muscles, including at least six muscles: gluteus maximus, tensor fascia lata, vastus medialis, tibialis anterior, peroneus longus, and medial gastrocnemius. We reviewed the presence of radiculopathy based on the EDx report. The presence of a positive sharp wave (PSW) or fibrillation (Fib) in the lower limb, and motor unit action potential (MUAP) change, were also reviewed. A MUAP change refers to polyphasia, long duration, and/or large MUAPs in the lower limb muscles.

The short-term response of TFESI was determined by the degree of pain relief at the outpatient clinic 2 to 4 weeks after TFESI. Pain intensity at the initial and follow-up visits was assessed using the numerical rating scale (NRS) (0–10 points, 11 numeric scale). Good responders were defined as the group with a reduction greater than 50% on NRS at the follow-up visit compared with the initial visit. The others were defined as poor responders.

2.4. Statistical Analysis

Descriptive statistics were used to report the demographic and clinical data. Categorical variables were described using absolute and relative frequencies. Continuous variables were described using the mean and standard deviation, and discrete variables were described using the median and corresponding ranges. We conducted the independent *t*-test, the Mann–Whitney test, and the chi-squared test to demonstrate the statistical difference of clinical data between the good and poor response groups. The independent *t*-test and Mann–Whitney test were used for continuous variables. The chi-squared test was used for categorical variables.

Univariate logistic regression analysis was first performed for the analysis of the primary outcome. The odds ratios (ORs) and 95% confidence intervals (CIs) were determined to show the reliability of the estimates. Multiple logistic regression analysis was used to identify individual predictors of substantial response suggested by the univariate analysis. All p values <0.05 in the univariate analysis were included in the multivariate analysis. Data were analyzed using SPSS software version 20.0 (SPSS Inc., Chicago, IL, USA), and a p value <0.05 was considered significant in all analyses.

3. Results

Demographic, clinical, and MRI data were collected from all the patients. However, EDx was performed in 150 of the 218 patients. The number of patients presenting with a favorable response 2–4 weeks after TFESI was 133 (61.0%), and the number of poor responders was 85 (39.0%). Demographics, past medical history, spinal surgery history, duration and presentation of symptoms, physical examination, the number of TFESI levels, and MRI and EDx findings were compared between the favorable and poor response groups (Table 1). A statistically significant difference was observed between the two groups regarding history of lumbar surgery, duration of symptoms, neurogenic claudication, the SLR test, PSW/Fib on EDx, and central canal stenosis on MRI.

Table 1. Summary of Results.

Variables		Values		p-Value
		Poor Responders ($n = 85$)	Good Responders ($n = 133$)	
Pain at initial visit (NRS)		7.51 ± 1.297	7.91 ± 1.048	0.003
Demographic				
Sex	Male	38 (44.7%)	58 (43.6%)	0.874
	Female	47 (55.3%)	75 (56.4%)	
Age		60.31 ± 16.35	56.31 ± 14.44	0.060
Clinical				
Diabetes	Yes	9 (10.6%)	11 (8.3%)	0.563
	No	76 (89.4%)	122 (91.7%)	
Hypertension	Yes	26 (30.6%)	33 (24.8%)	0.349
	No	59 (69.4%)	100 (75.2%)	
Previous spine surgery	Yes	13 (15.3%)	6 (4.5%)	0.006
	No	72 (84.7%)	127 (95.5%)	
Trauma or sprain	Yes	6 (7.1%)	19 (14.3%)	0.102
	No	79 (92.9%)	114 (85.7%)	
Duration of symptoms	weeks	60.75 ± 79.14	16.53 ± 48.01	0.000
	Chronic	45 (52.9%)	17 (12.8%)	
	Subacute	15 (17.6%)	30 (22.6%)	0.000
	Acute	25 (29.4%)	86 (64.7%)	
Low back or buttock pain	Yes	50 (58.8%)	92 (69.2%)	0.118
	No	35 (41.2%)	41 (30.8%)	
Neurogenic claudication	Yes	19 (22.4%)	15 (11.3%)	0.028
	No	66 (77.6%)	118 (88.7%)	
SLR test	Full	73 (86.9%)	94 (74.0%)	0.024
	Positive	11 (13.1%)	33 (26.0%)	

Table 1. Cont.

Variables		Values		p-Value
		Poor Responders (n = 85)	Good Responders (n = 133)	
Motor exam	Normal	77 (90.6%)	109 (82.0%)	0.079
	Abnormal	8 (9.4%)	24 (18.0%)	
Sensory exam	Normal	72 (84.7%)	109 (82.0%)	0.598
	Abnormal	13 (15.3%)	24 (18.0%)	
MRI				
No. of HNP levels	1	14 (18.7%)	35 (28.7%)	
	2	22 (29.3%)	39 (32.0%)	0.160
	>2	39 (52.0%)	48 (39.3%)	
Root compression or contact	Yes	58 (77.3%)	101 (82.8%)	0.346
	No	17 (22.7%)	21 (17.2%)	
Foraminal stenosis	Yes	43 (57.3%)	79 (64.8%)	0.298
	No	32 (42.7%)	43 (35.2%)	
Central canal stenosis	Yes	34 (45.3%)	33 (27.0%)	0.009
	No	41 (54.7%)	89 (73.0%)	
EDx				
EDx diagnosis	Normal	22 (35.5%)	26 (29.5%)	0.443
	Radiculopathy	40 (64.5%)	62 (70.5%)	
PSW/Fib	Yes	10 (16.1%)	32 (36.4%)	0.007
	No	52 (83.9%)	56 (63.6%)	
MUAP change	Yes	37 (59.7%)	50 (56.8%)	0.727
	No	25 (40.3%)	38 (43.2%)	
No. of levels of TFESI		2.15 ± 0.60	2.04 ± 0.41	0.093

Data are expressed as mean ± standard deviation or absolute number (percentage). Abbreviations: EDx, electrodiagnosis; HNP, herniated nucleus pulposus; NRS, numerical rating scale; TFESI, transforaminal epidural steroid injection; PSW, positive sharp wave; Fib, fibrillation; MUAP, motor unit action potential.

The results of univariate and multivariate logistic regression analyses are listed in Table 2. In the univariate regression analysis, history of lumbar surgery, duration of symptoms, neurogenic claudication, the SLR test, PSW/Fib on EDx, and central canal stenosis on MRI findings were associated with good response. The multivariate regression analysis demonstrated that only a shorter duration of symptoms and PSW/Fib findings on EDx were predictors of a favorable response to TFESI. In addition, the absence of past spine surgery and central canal stenosis findings on MRI was also associated with a good response in the multivariate regression analysis, even though the association was not statistically significant.

Table 2. Univariate and multivariate analysis of variables.

		Univariate		Multivariate	
		OR (95%CI)	*p*-Value	OR (95%CI)	*p*-Value
Demographic					
Sex	Male	1			
	Female	0.956 (0.553–1.654)	0.874		
Age		0.982 (0.964–1.001)	0.061		
Clinical					
Diabetes	Yes	1			
	No	1.313 (0.520–3.317)	0.564		
Hypertension	Yes	1			
	No	1.335 (0.728–2.449)	0.350		
Previous spine surgery	Yes	1			
	No	3.822 (1.392–10.489)	0.009	3.496 (0.568–21.528)	0.177
Trauma or sprain	Yes	1			
	No	0.456 (0.174–1.192)	0.109		
Duration of symptoms	Chronic	1		1	
	Subacute	5.294 (2.299–12.189)	0.000	6.772 (2.034–22.546)	0.002
	Acute	9.106 (4.459–18.594)	0.000	7.080 (2.582–19.413)	0.000
Low back or buttock pain	Yes	1			
	No	0.637 (0.361–1.123)	0.119		
Neurogenic claudication	Yes	1			
	No	2.265 (1.079–4.751)	0.031	1.462 (0.489–4.289)	0.489
SLR test	Full	1			
	Positive	2.330 (1.103–4.921)	0.027	1.358 (0.413–4.464)	0.614
Motor exam	Normal	1			
	Abnormal	2.119 (0.904–4.967)	0.084		
Sensory exam	Normal	1			
	Abnormal	1.219 (0.583–2.550)	0.598		
MRI					
No. of HNP levels	1	1			
	2	0.709 (0.315–1.595)	0.406		
	>2	0.492 (0.233–1.042)	0.064		
Root compression or contact.	Yes	1			
	No	0.709 (0.347–1.452)	0.347		
Foraminal stenosis	Yes	1			
	No	0.731 (0.406–1.139)	0.298		
Central canalStenosis	Yes	1			
	No	2.237 (1.221–4.096)	0.009	2.291 (0.908–5.780)	0.079
EDx					
EDx diagnosis	Normal	1			
	Radiculopathy	1.312 (0.656–2.623)	0.443		
PSW/Fib	No	1			
	Yes	2.971 (1.330–6.641)	0.008	3.889 (1.359–11.133)	0.011
MUAP change	Yes	1			
	No	0.889 (0.460–1.720)	0.727		

Abbreviations: EDx, electrodiagnosis; Fib, fibrillation; HNP, herniated nucleus pulposus; MUAP, motor unit action potential; NRS, numerical rating scale; PSW, positive sharp wave; TFESI, transforaminal epidural steroid injection.

4. Discussion

In this study, we measured short-term outcomes 2–4 weeks after TFESI. Previous studies reported that epidural steroid injections may result in improvement in lumbosacral radicular pain between two and six weeks, which may relate to the duration of the therapeutic effect of corticosteroid [33,34]. All the procedures were extraepineural in this study, because extraepineural injections are less painful and more effective than intraepineural injections [16,33]. The patients from traffic accidents or injuries at industrial sites were excluded, as they were covered by auto-insurance and worker's compensation in South Korea. The treatment response may be affected by secondary gain [12].

The first finding was that shorter symptom duration was the strongest factor associated with a good response. Having acute symptoms or subacute symptoms increased the odds of significant improvement 2–4 weeks after TFESI compared with manifesting chronic symptoms. These results are consistent with previous studies. Ahilan et al. [28] reported that symptom duration for over a year decreased the odds of improvement 3 months after epidural lumbar steroid injection; however, they did not describe which medication was injected. Copper et al. [13] reported that patients with chronic symptoms tend to display worse outcomes than those with acute symptoms. A study by Cyteval et al. [15] also showed that the symptom duration before periradicular steroid injection for lumbar radiculopathy was highly correlated with pain relief outcomes at two weeks and at the one-year follow-up. Corticosteroid and local anesthetics were used in the above two studies.

A longer duration of symptoms results in chronic inflammation, including fibrosis and necrosis of nerve root fibers [35,36]. These results suggest that corticosteroids are less effective in chronic inflammation. In this study, we added hyaluronidase to steroid and lidocaine for injections, but the outcome was the same as in previous studies. This implies that the previously discussed mechanism of local anesthetics and hyaluronidase, which more likely targets chronic inflammation, is not as effective as the anti-inflammatory effect of corticosteroids.

Various management strategies have been suggested as chronic back pain and radicular pain do not well respond to various approaches. As seen in this study, TFESI is less effective for chronic low back pain. Therefore, we should emphasize non-pharmacologic treatment, such as exercise therapy, especially in chronic low back pain [37].

Whether EDx findings can be a predictor of response to epidural steroid injection has been challenged by several studies. A few studies [20,24,26] reported that radiculopathy in EDx was associated with a favorable outcome to epidural steroid injection, whereas other studies [12,21,22] reported a lack of association. In this study, the diagnosis of lumbosacral radiculopathy by EDx was not a predictive factor of response to TFESI. However, PSW/Fib findings related to limb muscles in patients diagnosed with lumbosacral radiculopathy by EDx increased the odds of improvement with TFESI. When PSW/Fib was detected only in the paravertebral muscle without limb muscles, the findings were not considered as radiculopathy in this study. Similar findings have been detected in 15–42% of asymptomatic individuals, and this increased with the age of the examined population [38,39].

Several explanations are possible. First, the diagnosis of radiculopathy by EDx is limited to motor neuron axonal damage in most cases. It is impossible to diagnose radiculopathy by EDx in the presence of only mild injury at the nerve root, such as focal demyelination without damage to the motor axons. The patients who were diagnosed with radiculopathy but exhibited normal findings on EDx also responded well to TFESI. This hypothesis explains the absence of association between EDx diagnosis and TFESI outcomes. Second, membrane instability characterized by PSW/Fib is generally detected in limb muscles within three weeks after acute neural insult and continues until the muscle fiber is reinnervated or atrophied completely. When the patient was diagnosed with radiculopathy without PSW/Fib, EDx was performed after reinnervation, because completely atrophied muscle would have been excluded from this study due to severe motor weakness. It is reported that the limb muscles are reinnervated about three months after symptom onset. In contrast to PSW/Fib, most of the MUAP changes, including polyphasic, large, and long duration, were found in chronic and static radiculopathy, even though polyphasic MUAP was detected at an early stage [40,41]. Thus, the duration of PSW/Fib correlated with good response to TFESI. Third, the diagnosis of radiculopathy based on MUAP changes alone may involve older and stable lesions, which may not be associated with recent symptoms. The absence of a significant difference between good and poor response groups based on EDx radiculopathy suggests the possibility of diagnosis unrelated to recent symptoms. Fourth, the growth of a bony spur may gradually compress the nerve root, resulting in relatively mild damage to the nerve fibers. In this case, collateral sprouting and denervation may occur at a similar rate with hard-to-observe PSW/Fib initially. The effect of TFESI is limited in this case, because the majority of mechanisms involved mechanical compression by bony spur.

The absence of spine surgery could be associated with favorable response to TFESI, even though the association was only present in the univariate analysis. This result can be explained by postoperative scar formation. Epidural scar from low back surgery probably induced soft tissue adhesion and mechanical compression of the nerve root, which is resistant to the anti-inflammatory effects of corticosteroid. The scar also mechanically prevents delivery into the epidural space and eventually decreases the effectiveness of injection. Previous studies report conflicting results. Sivaganesan et al. [28] reported that back surgery was associated with a poor response to epidural steroid injection, whereas Tong et al. [12] found no significant correlation between them. Neither of these two studies described the type of back surgery included. In this study, any type of back surgery, such as discectomy or posterior lumbar interbody fusion, was included. The degree of scarring is determined by the type of back surgery. Therefore, the association is also influenced by the proportion of various types of back surgeries and requires appropriate classification in future studies.

We were unable to determine the association between MRI findings and a good response to the TFESI in the multivariate regression analysis. However, a central canal stenosis observed on MRI may be associated with increased odds of a positive response, even though the association was not statistically significant in multivariate analysis. These associations have been disputed in previous studies [19,22,23,27,28]. Other variables, including age, sex, the presence of trauma or sprain, the location of pain, neurogenic claudication and findings of physical examination, cannot be considered as predictors of short-term outcome after a TFESI.

In this study, the short-term success rate of a TFESI at 2–4 weeks was 61%. Previous studies have reported that the success rate is about 34–78% and the success rate of the short-term effect is about 50%, which is similar to our study [8,42]. One systemic review [42] reported that the level of evidence in support of epidural steroid injections is moderate. However, many studies [9,43] have shown controversial results about the long-term effects of the procedure.

This study has several limitations. First, the outcome was only evaluated by a change in NRS. There are specific tools designed for evaluation of function and pain in patients with low back pain, such as the Oswestry Disability Index and the Pain Disability Questionnaire. Because it is difficult to objectively assess response to treatment, these tools can be also used simultaneously to assess pain, function, or emotion in a variety of ways. This is a limitation of retrospective studies analyzing data derived from pre-existing medical records. Second, the predictive factors suggested in this study are limited to short-term response to TFESIs. It was impossible to accurately and reliably predict long-term treatment response to lumbar TFESIs based on short-term pain relief [44]. Additional studies investigating long-term response are needed. Third, the location of the TFESI was not standardized. In our clinic, the most frequently targeted levels of TFESI were L4/L5, L5/S1, and S1 foramens, while L2/3 or L3/4 were rarely targeted. About two levels of TFESI were administered to both good and poor responders. However, the details of the injection level were not described in this study. Fourth, the difference between good and poor responders could be attributable to the natural course of the condition in the patients, such as chronicity of pain. Future studies comparing the natural course between two groups will be needed. Fifth, the patients were re-assessed in a 2–4 week range after the injection. Although 2–4 weeks is a short period of time compared to other studies [42], the pain response at two weeks after injection can be different to the response at four weeks.

5. Conclusions

The short duration of symptoms and the presence of PSW/Fib findings in lower limb muscles in EDx diagnosis are likely to predict a favorable response 2–4 weeks after a TFESI in patients diagnosed with lumbar disk herniation on MRI and who present with radiating leg pain. Clinicians should consider these factors in the risk–benefit analysis of TFESIs. The results should be validated via randomized prospective studies in the future.

Author Contributions: Conceptualization, J.H.P. and D.Y.P.; Methodology, S.K. and D.Y.P.; Formal analysis, D.Y.P. and S.K.; Investigation, D.Y.P. and S.K.; Writing—original draft preparation, D.Y.P.; Supervision, J.H.P.

Funding: This research received no external funding.

Conflicts of Interest: There are no conflicts of interest in relation to this paper.

References

1. Wickström, G.; Hänninen, K.; Lehtinen, M.; Riihimäki, H. Previous back syndromes and present back symptoms in concrete reinforecment workers. *Scand. J. Work Environ. Health* **1978**, *4*, 20–28. [CrossRef] [PubMed]
2. Videman, T.; Nurminen, T.; Tola, S.; Kuorinka, I.; Vanharanta, H.; Troup, J. Low-back pain in nurses and some loading factors of work. *Spine* **1984**, *9*, 400–404. [CrossRef] [PubMed]
3. Riihimaki, H.; Wickström, G.; Hanninen, K.; Luopajarvi, T. Predictors of sciatic pain among concrete reinforcement workers and house painters—A five-year follow-up. *Scand. J. Work Environ. Health* **1989**, *15*, 415–423. [CrossRef] [PubMed]
4. Abram, S.; Hopwood, M. What factors contribute to outcome with lumbar epidural steroids. In *Proceedings of the 6th World Congress on Pain*; Elsevier: Amsterdam The Netherlands, 1991; pp. 491–496.
5. Kraemer, J.; Ludwig, J.; Bickert, U.; Owczarek, V.; Traupe, M. Lumbar epidural perineural injection: A new technique. *Eur. Spine J.* **1997**, *6*, 357–361. [CrossRef] [PubMed]
6. Manchikanti, L.; Bakhit, C.E.; Pakanati, R.R.; Fellows, B. Fluoroscopy is medically necessary for the performance of epidural steroids. *Anesthesia Analg.* **1999**, *89*, 1330.
7. Roberts, S.T.; Willick, S.E.; Rho, M.E.; Rittenberg, J.D. Efficacy of lumbosacral transforaminal epidural steroid injections: A systematic review. *PM R* **2009**, *7*, 657–668. [CrossRef]
8. Bui, J.; Bogduk, N. A systematic review of the effectiveness of CT-guided, lumbar transforaminal injection of steroids. *Pain Med.* **2013**, *14*, 1860–1865. [CrossRef] [PubMed]
9. Shamliyan, T.A.; Staal, J.B.; Goldmann, D.; Sands-Lincoln, M. Epidural steroid injections for radicular lumbosacral pain: A systematic review. *Phys. Med. Rehabil. Clin.* **2014**, *25*, 471–489.e50. [CrossRef]
10. Fredman, B.; Nun, M.B.; Zohar, E.; Iraqi, G.; Shapiro, M.; Gepstein, R.; Jedeikin, R. Epidural steroids for treating" failed back surgery syndrome": Is fluoroscopy really necessary? *Anesthesia Analg.* **1999**, *88*, 367–372.
11. Candido, K.D. Transforaminal versus interlaminar approaches to epidural steroid injections: A systematic review of comparative studies for lumbosacral radicular pain. *Pain Physician* **2014**, *17*, E509–E524.
12. Tong, H.; Williams, J.; Haig, A.; Geisser, M.; Chiodo, A. Predicting outcomes of transforaminal epidural injections for sciatica. *Spine J.* **2003**, *3*, 430–434. [CrossRef]
13. Cooper, G.; Lutz, G.E.; Boachie-Adjei, O.; Lin, J. Effectiveness of transforaminal epidural steroid injections in patients with degenerative lumbar scoliotic stenosis and radiculopathy. *Pain Physician* **2004**, *7*, 311–318. [PubMed]
14. Inman, S.L.; Faut-Callahan, M.; Swanson, B.A.; Fillingim, R.B. Sex differences in responses to epidural steroid injection for low back pain. *J. Pain* **2004**, *5*, 450–457. [CrossRef]
15. Cyteval, C.; Fescquet, N.; Thomas, E.; Decoux, E.; Blotman, F.; Taourel, P. Predictive factors of efficacy of periradicular corticosteroid injections for lumbar radiculopathy. *Am. J. Neuroradiol.* **2006**, *27*, 978–982. [PubMed]
16. Lee, J.W.; Kim, S.H.; Lee, I.S.; Choi, J.A.; Choi, J.Y.; Hong, S.H.; Kang, H.S. Therapeutic effect and outcome predictors of sciatica treated using transforaminal epidural steroid injection. *AJR Am. J. Roentgenol.* **2006**, *187*, 1427–1431. [CrossRef]

17. Campbell, M.J.; Carreon, L.Y.; Glassman, S.D.; McGinnis, M.D.; Elmlinger, B.S. Correlation of spinal canal dimensions to efficacy of epidural steroid injection in spinal stenosis. *Clin. Spine Surg.* **2007**, *20*, 168–171. [CrossRef] [PubMed]
18. Jeong, H.S.; Lee, J.W.; Kim, S.H.; Myung, J.S.; Kim, J.H.; Kang, H.S. Effectiveness of transforaminal epidural steroid injection by using a preganglionic approach: A prospective randomized controlled study. *Radiology* **2007**, *245*, 584–590. [CrossRef] [PubMed]
19. Kapural, L.; Mekhail, N.; Bena, J.; McLain, R.; Tetzlaff, J.; Kapural, M.; Mekhail, M.; Polk, S. Value of the magnetic resonance imaging in patients with painful lumbar spinal stenosis (LSS) undergoing lumbar epidural steroid injections. *Clin. J. Pain* **2007**, *23*, 571–575. [CrossRef] [PubMed]
20. Fish, D.E.; Shirazi, E.P.; Pham, Q. The use of electromyography to predict functional outcome following transforaminal epidural spinal injections for lumbar radiculopathy. *J. Pain* **2008**, *9*, 64–70. [CrossRef]
21. Marchetti, J.; Verma-Kurvari, S.; Patel, N.; Ohnmeiss, D.D. Are electrodiagnostic study findings related to a patient's response to epidural steroid injection? *PM R* **2010**, *2*, 1016–1020. [CrossRef] [PubMed]
22. Cosgrove, J.L.; Bertolet, M.; Chase, S.L.; Cosgrove, G.K. Epidural steroid injections in the treatment of lumbar spinal stenosis efficacy and predictability of successful response. *Am. J. Phys. Med. Rehabil.* **2011**, *90*, 1050–1055. [CrossRef] [PubMed]
23. Ghahreman, A.; Bogduk, N. Predictors of a favorable response to transforaminal injection of steroids in patients with lumbar radicular pain due to disc herniation. *Pain Med.* **2011**, *12*, 871–879. [CrossRef] [PubMed]
24. Annaswamy, T.M.; Bierner, S.M.; Chouteau, W.; Elliott, A.C. Needle electromyography predicts outcome after lumbar epidural steroid injection. *Muscle Nerve* **2012**, *45*, 346–355. [CrossRef]
25. Park, C.-H.; Lee, S.-H. Correlation between severity of lumbar spinal stenosis and lumbar epidural steroid injection. *Pain Med.* **2014**, *15*, 556–561. [CrossRef] [PubMed]
26. McCormick, Z.; Cushman, D.; Caldwell, M.; Marshall, B.; Ghannad, L.; Eng, C.; Patel, J.; Makovitch, S.; Chu, S.K.; Babu, A.N. Does electrodiagnostic confirmation of radiculopathy predict pain reduction after transforaminal epidural steroid injection? A multicenter study. *J. Nat. Sci.* **2015**, *1*, e140. [PubMed]
27. Ekedahl, H.; Jonsson, B.; Annertz, M.; Frobell, R.B. Three week results of transforaminal epidural steroid injection in patients with chronic unilateral low back related leg pain: The relation to MRI findings and clinical features. *J. Back Musculoskelet. Rehabil.* **2016**, *29*, 693–702. [CrossRef]
28. Sivaganesan, A.; Chotai, S.; Parker, S.L.; Asher, A.L.; McGirt, M.J.; Devin, C.J. Predictors of the efficacy of epidural steroid injections for structural lumbar degenerative pathology. *Spine J.* **2016**, *16*, 928–934. [CrossRef] [PubMed]
29. Johansson, A.; Hao, J.; Sjölund, B. Local corticosteroid application blocks transmission in normal nociceptive C-fibres. *Acta Anaesthesiol. Scand.* **1990**, *34*, 335–338. [CrossRef]
30. Pasqualucci, A.; Varrassi, G.; Braschi, A.; Peduto, V.A.; Brunelli, A.; Marinangeli, F.; Gori, F.; Colò, F.; Paladini, A.; Mojoli, F. Epidural local anesthetic plus corticosteroid for the treatment of cervical brachial radicular pain: Single injection versus continuous infusion. *Clin. J. Pain* **2007**, *23*, 551–557. [CrossRef]
31. Poupak Rahimzadeh, M.; Sharma, V.; Farnad Imani, M.; Reza, H. Adjuvant hyaluronidase to epidural steroid improves the quality of analgesia in failed back surgery syndrome: A prospective randomized clinical trial. *Pain Physician* **2014**, *17*, E75–E82.
32. Racz, G.B.; Heavner, J.E.; Trescot, A. Percutaneous lysis of epidural adhesions—Evidence for safety and efficacy. *Pain Pract.* **2008**, *8*, 277–286. [CrossRef] [PubMed]
33. Pfirrmann, C.W.; Oberholzer, P.A.; Zanetti, M.; Boos, N.; Trudell, D.J.; Resnick, D.; Hodler, J. Selective nerve root blocks for the treatment of sciatica: Evaluation of injection site and effectiveness—A study with patients and cadavers. *Radiology* **2001**, *221*, 704–711. [CrossRef] [PubMed]
34. Armon, C.; Argoff, C.E.; Samuels, J.; Backonja, M.-M. Assessment: Use of epidural steroid injections to treat radicular lumbosacral pain Report of the Therapeutics and Technology Assessment Subcommittee of the American Academy of Neurology. *Neurology* **2007**, *68*, 723–729. [CrossRef] [PubMed]
35. Delamarter, R.B.; Bohlman, H.; Dodge, L.E.A.; Biro, C. Experimental lumbar spinal stenosis. Analysis of the cortical evoked potentials, microvasculature, and histopathology. *J. Bone Jt. Surg. Am. Vol.* **1990**, *72*, 110–120. [CrossRef]
36. Olmarker, K.; Holm, S.; Rosenqvist, A.-L.; Rydevik, B. Experimental nerve root compression. A model of acute, graded compression of the porcine cauda equina and an analysis of neural and vascular anatomy. *Spine* **1991**, *16*, 61–69. [CrossRef] [PubMed]

37. Foster, N.E.; Anema, J.R.; Cherkin, D.; Chou, R.; Cohen, S.P.; Gross, D.P.; Ferreira, P.H.; Fritz, J.M.; Koes, B.W.; Peul, W. Prevention and treatment of low back pain: Evidence, challenges, and promising directions. *Lancet* **2018**, *391*, 2368–2383. [CrossRef]
38. Date, E.S.; Mar, E.Y.; Bugola, M.R.; Teraoka, J.K. The prevalence of lumbar paraspinal spontaneous activity in asymptomatic subjects. *Muscle Nerve Off. J. Am. Assoc. Electrodiagn. Med.* **1996**, *19*, 350–354. [CrossRef]
39. Nardin, R.A.; Raynor, E.M.; Rutkove, S.B. Fibrillations in lumbosacral paraspinal muscles of normal subjects. *Muscle Nerve Off. J. Am. Assoc. Electrodiagn. Med.* **1998**, *21*, 1347–1349. [CrossRef]
40. Wilbourn, A. The value and limitations of electromyographic examination in the diagnosis of lumbosacral radiculopathy. In *Lumbar Disc Disease*; Raven Press: New York, NY, USA, 1982; pp. 65–109.
41. Wilbourn, A.J.; Aminoff, M.J. AAEM minimonograph 32: The electrodiagnostic examination in patients with radiculopathies. *Muscle Nerve Off. J. Am. Assoc. Electrodiagn. Med.* **1998**, *21*, 1612–1631. [CrossRef]
42. Manchikanti, L.; Benyamin, R.M.; Falco, F.J.; Kaye, A.D.; Hirsch, J.A. Do epidural injections provide short-and long-term relief for lumbar disc herniation? A systematic review. *Clin. Orthop. Relat. Res.* **2015**, *473*, 1940–1956. [CrossRef] [PubMed]
43. Bhatia, A.; Flamer, D.; Shah, P.S.; Cohen, S.P. Transforaminal epidural steroid injections for treating lumbosacral radicular pain from herniated intervertebral discs: A systematic review and meta-analysis. *Anesthesia Analg.* **2016**, *122*, 857–870. [CrossRef] [PubMed]
44. Joswig, H.; Neff, A.; Ruppert, C.; Hildebrandt, G.; Stienen, M.N. The Value of Short-Term Pain Relief in Predicting the Long-Term Outcome of Lumbar Transforaminal Epidural Steroid Injections. *World Neurosurg.* **2017**, *107*, 764–771. [CrossRef] [PubMed]

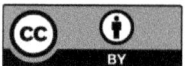

© 2019 by the authors. Licensee MDPI, Basel, Switzerland. This article is an open access article distributed under the terms and conditions of the Creative Commons Attribution (CC BY) license (http://creativecommons.org/licenses/by/4.0/).

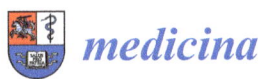

Article

Prediction of Chronic Lower Back Pain Using the Hierarchical Neural Network: Comparison with Logistic Regression—A Pilot Study

Yutaka Owari [1,2,*] and Nobuyuki Miyatake [2]

1. Shikoku Medical College, Utazu, Kagawa 769-0205, Japan
2. Department of Hygiene, Faculty of Medicine, Kagawa University, Miki, Kagawa 761-0793, Japan; miyarin@med.kagawa-u.ac.jp
* Correspondence: owari@med.kagawa-u.ac.jp; Tel.: +81-87-41-2321

Received: 31 March 2019; Accepted: 4 June 2019; Published: 9 June 2019

Abstract: *Background:* Many studies have reported on the causes of chronic lower back pain (CLBP). The aim of this study is to identify if the hierarchical neural network (HNN) is superior to a conventional statistical model for CLBP prediction. Linear models, which included multiple regression analysis, were executed for the analysis of the survey data because of the ease of interpretation. The problem with such linear models was that we could not fully consider the influence of interactions caused by a combination of nonlinear relationships and independent variables. *Materials and Methods:* The subjects in our study were 96 people (30 men aged 72.3 ± 5.6 years and 66 women aged 71.9 ± 5.4 years) who participated at a college health club from 20 July 2016 to 20 March 2017. The HNN and the logistic regression analysis (LR) were used for the prediction of CLBP and the accuracy of each analysis was compared and examined by using our previously reported data. The LR verified the fit using the Hosmer–Lemeshow test. The efficiencies of the two models were compared using receiver performance analysis (ROC), the root mean square error (RMSE), and the deviance (−2 log likelihood). *Results:* The area under the ROC curve, the RMSE, and the −2 log likelihood for the LR were 0.7163, 0.2581, and 105.065, respectively. The area under the ROC curve, the RMSE, and the log likelihood for the HNN were 0.7650, 0.2483, and 102.787, respectively (the correct answer rates were HNN = 73.3% and LR = 70.8%). *Conclusions:* On the basis of the ROC curve, the RMSE, and the −2 log likelihood, the performance of the HNN for the prediction probability of CLBP is equal to or higher than the LR. In the future, the HNN may be useful as an index to judge the risk of CLBP for individual patients.

Keywords: chronic lower back pain; hierarchical neural network; logistic regression analysis

1. Introduction

The prevalence of lower back pain (LBP) in an adult is approximately 12% [1]. In Japan, in 2013, the proportion of LBP patients was reported as 9.2% (male) and 11.8% (female) [2]. In the Brazilian older population, the prevalence of chronic LBP (CLBP) was 25.4% [3]. CLBP not only brings about a surge in medical expenses, but also results in enormous economic loss in each country because patients are prevented from participating in society. Therefore, researching the cause of CLBP is an urgent task.

Many researchers have reported on the causes of CLBP. For this study, the analysis of survey data was performed using linear models, which included multiple regression analysis, because of the ease of interpretation. The problem with such linear models was that we could not sufficiently consider the influence of nonlinear relations and interactions caused by combinations between independent variables. Needless to say, we introduced previously used nonlinear regression models such as variable transformation, polynomials, and so on. However, during actual analysis, it was difficult to sufficiently assume such requirements in advance.

In this study, we verified that nonlinear coupling using the hierarchical neural network (HNN) [4,5] is superior for predicting the possibility of CLBP as compared with predictions by a conventional statistical model.

2. Materials and Methods

2.1. Study Design

We performed a neural network simulation study and adopted the following hypothesis: The HNN is superior for predicting the possibility of CLBP as compared with predictions using a conventional statistical model. The subjects for our study were 96 people (30 men aged 72.3 ± 5.6 years and 66 women aged 71.9 ± 5.4 years) who were members at a college health club, as well as prior subjects from a previous investigation [6]. We excluded subjects with specific lower back pain.

Ethical approval for the study was obtained from the Shikoku Medical College Ethics Screening Committee, Japan (approval number: H28-8, 25 May 2016). The decision date of the ethics committee was 25 May 2016.

2.2. Clinical Parameters and Measurements

The data included age, gender, sleeping time, spouse, steps, BMI, and excluding ≤1.5 metabolic equivalents (METs). We collected for 3 consecutive days during each week over the study period. Stiff shoulder was defined as pain in the neck, shoulder, or back, and chronic stiff shoulder was pain lasting longer than 3 months. In addition, chronic stiff shoulder was considered as a variable affecting psychological distress. We used a visual analog scale as a measurement tool to investigate the degree of pain experienced by each subject. The scale consisted of a straight line where the degree of pain was expressed (scored) as a numerical value from 0 to 10 points. The left end of the straight line was "painless", and the right end was "the most severe pain that can be imagined". Subjects were asked to place a cross on the line at a point that seemed to be the degree of pain they were feeling. Assuming that the total length of the straight line was 10, the distance from the left end to the cross indicated the degree of pain. The closer the number was to 10, the stronger the pain. The subjects were requested to respond by choosing either "experienced" (1, other than 0), or "not experienced" (0) [6].

2.3. Psychological Distress

For the data from a previous investigation, we used the K6 scale. The K6 is a self-written questionnaire developed by Kessler as a screening test for psychological distress that could effectively discriminate psychological distress [7]. It is valid and reliable. Subjects answered six items on a 5-point Likert scale, and responses for each item were transformed to scores ranging from 0 to 4 points. The questionnaire consisted of the following six questions: Over the last month, about how often did you feel: (1) nervous, (2) hopeless, (3) restless or fidgety, (4) so sad that nothing could cheer you up, (5) that everything was an effort, or (6) worthless? For each of the questions, the subjects were requested to choose from the following responses: All of the time (4 points), most of the time (3 points), some of the time (2 points), a little of the time (1 point), and none of the time (0 point). The total of the responses was the evaluation level [8]. Thus, the score range was 0–24. A higher total score corresponded to higher psychological distress.

2.4. Chronic Lower Back Pain (CLBP)

Chronic lower back pain was defined as pain localized between the 12th rib and the inferior gluteal folds [9] lasting longer than 3 months [10]. The subjects were shown the location of the pain and requested to respond to chronic lower back pain entered on the questionnaire by choosing from the following: "experienced" (1), "not experienced" (0) [6]. In addition, the subjects received a definitive diagnosis of orthopedic surgery.

2.5. Social Participation

Using the data from a previous investigation, we evaluated social participation as established by Haeuchi et al. [11]. The respondents were asked whether they participated in eight types of social activities. These types were as follows: (1) local events and festivals; (2) resident and neighborhood associations; (3) circle activities, i.e., a group activity based on a hobby or an interest such as history; (4) golden age club; (5) volunteer activities; (6) religious activities; (7) paid work; and (8) learning in a social environment within the past year from the date of the survey. The subjects were requested to respond by choosing either "some kind of social activity or more than one within the past month, once or more per week" (1) or "participates in no activities" (0) [6].

2.6. Models

2.6.1. HNN

Variables: For this study, there were two dependent variables for CLBP, i.e., absence (0, experienced) and presence (1, not experienced). In order to carry out the comparison with the logistic regression analysis, the number of independent variables was set to four. There were 10 possible candidates for the independent variables which included gender [12], age [13], spouse (presence or none), BMI (kg/m^2) [14], chronic stiff shoulder (presence or none), social participation (presence or none) [15–17], sleeping time (hours/day), the K6 scores [18–20], a rate of 1.5 METs or less [21], and number of steps (steps/day). The relationship among these ten independent variables, in a conventional study, and the dependent variables was discussed, and the four variables with high correlation were taken as the independent variables. Therefore, the four independent variables selected were age, body mass index (BMI), social participation and the K6 score.

Structure of HNN: The neural network consisted of multiple layers (input layer, hidden layer, and output layer). The number of nodes of the input layer was the number of nodes of data 4. Moreover, by changing the number of layers in the hidden layer and the number of nodes in each layer, we identified how the accuracy changed. We adopted the number of layers of the hidden layer and the number of the nodes of each layer which were higher in the system. Here, we adopted a sigmoid function as the activation function of the hidden layer. This was the function to output by deforming the input data (transform). For the prediction of CLBP, we determined the number of output layers to be two (2 nodes, onset as 1 = with CLBP and non-onset as 0 = without CLBP). The learning of the neural network was conducted 10,000 times using the back-propagation method.

2.6.2. Logistic Regression Analysis (LR)

We used LR to compare with HNN, using the four independent variables discussed above.

2.7. Statistical Analyses

First, we used the HNN to determine the number of hidden layers and the number of nodes in each layer by trial and error. Second, the HNN was used to verify the prediction rate of the onset of CLBP. Third, the efficiencies of the two models were compared using the receiver performance analysis (ROC), the root mean square error (RMSE), and the deviance (−2 log likelihood). In addition, we compared the prediction accuracy rates of the two models. And finally, we increased the independent variables to 10 by adding gender, spouse (presence or absence), shoulder stiffness, sleeping time, rate of 1.5 METs or less, and steps. We verified the prediction rate of CLBP onset with the HNN using the software SPSS ver. 24.0 (IBM SPSS Inc., Chicago, IL, USA) and Python 3.6.4 (Python Software Foundation, Delaware, United States).

3. Results

The subject characteristics are summarized in Table 1. First, the model had the highest accuracy when the number of hierarchical layers was one and the number of nodes was seven (Figure 1). Second, Table 2 compares the HNN and the LR. Using the case for learning, of the 33 with CLBP, 18 were accurately predicted, and of the 33 without CLBP, 31 were accurately predicted. Of the total 66, 49 were accurately predicted. In learning, the result was accurately predicted overall (74.2%). When the learning model was applied to the testing model, the accuracy answer rate was 73.3% and the accuracy rates obtained for the HNN and the LR were 73.3% and 70.8%, respectively. Third, the area under the ROC curve, the RMSE, and the −2 log likelihood for the LR were 0.7163, 0.2581, and 105.065, respectively, and for HNN they were 0.7650, 0.2483, and 102.787, respectively (Table 3 shows the area under the ROC between HNN and LR in detail). And finally, the predictive value rate increased from 73.3% to 84.6% using 10 variables (Table 4).

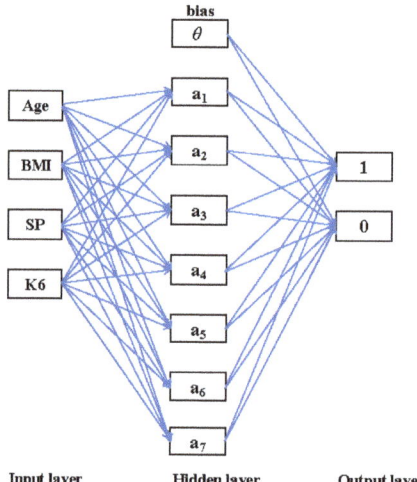

Figure 1. Structure of the hierarchical neural network

SP, social participation; K6, K6 scores.
1, with chronic low back pain; 0, without chronic low back pain.

Figure 1. The rectangles indicate nodes, and weights are indicated by arrows (→) between nodes. The number of nodes in the input layer is 4 (age, BMI, social participation (SP), and K6 scores), the number of nodes in the hidden layer is 7 (7 hidden neurons), and the number of nodes in the output layer is 2 (1: With chronic lower back pain, 0: Without chronic lower back pain).

Table 1. Clinical characteristics of the enrolled subjects in a college health club in the Kagawa Prefecture (Japan).

	Total					Men					Women				
	Mean	±	SD	Min	Max	Mean	±	SD	Min	Max	Mean	±	SD	Min	Max
Number of Subjects	96					30					66				
Age (year)	72.0	±	5.4	65	85	72.3	±	5.6	65	85	71.9	±	5.4	65	85
BMI (kg/m^2)	22.7	±	2.9	14.9	30.2	23.4	±	2.9	17.6	29.1	22.4	±	2.8	14.9	30.2
Number of Steps (steps/day)	5692.8	±	2527.2	569.9	12230.1	5881.5	±	2413.8	1585.4	11049.1	5615.5	±	2587.7	569.9	12230.1
Sleep Time (hours/day)	6.5	±	1.1	4	10	6.7	±	0.9	5	9	6.5	±	1.1	4	10
≤1.5 METs (%/day)	55.9	±	10.0	35.4	79.9	59.5	±	11.6	36.8	79.9	54.3	±	8.9	35.4	75.7
K6 Scores	2.7	±	3.3	0	14	3.1	±	3.6	0	13	2.5	±	3.2	0	14
Spouse (Present) (%)	75.5					96.0					67.2				
Social Participation (Participates) (%)	83.3					76.7					86.4				
Chronic Stiff Shoulder (Present) (%)	26.0					16.7					30.3				
Chronic Low Pack Pain (Present) (%)	47.9					50.0					47.0				

Min: Minimum; Max: Maximum; BMI: Body mass index (kg/m^2), METs: Metabolic equivalents.

Table 2. Comparison between the hierarchical neural network (HNN) and logistical regression (LR). Classification of the results (HNN): 66 learning data, 49 (18 + 31) accurately predicted, and 30 testing data, 22 (14 + 8) accurately predicted.

	Actual		Predicted	
		Non-Default	Default	Accuracy (%)
Learning	Non-Default	31	2	93.9
	Default	15	18	54.5
	Total			74.2
Testing	Non-Default	14	3	82.4
	Default	5	8	61.5
	Total			73.3
LR				
	Actual		Predicted	
		Non-Default	Default	Accuracy (%)
	Non-Default	38	12	76.0
	Default	16	30	65.2
	Total			70.8

HNN: Hierarchical neural network; LR: Logistic regression; Non-Default: Without CLBP, Default: with CLBP; HNN: $N = 30$; testing; LR: $N = 96$.

Table 3. Comparison between HNN and LR by the area under the ROC curve.

	Area	Standard error	Lower Bound	Upper Bound	p
HNN	0.7650	0.0492	0.6552	0.8315	<0.001
LR	0.7163	0.0557	0.6070	0.8255	<0.001

HNN: Hierarchical neural network; LR: Logistic regression.

Table 4. Relationship between each independent variable.

	Gender	Age	Spouse	BMI	CSS	SP	Sleep Time	K6 Scores	1.5METs or Less	Steps
Gender	1.0000	0.2000	0.2957	0.0949	0.1426	0.2372	0.0980	0.0458	0.2896	0.0265
Age		1.0000	0.0728	0.0344	0.1725	0.0959	−0.0956	0.0392	0.2285	−0.3479
Spouse			1.0000	0.0509	0.0426	0.1176	0.2946	0.1091	0.0547	0.0624
BMI				1.0000	0.0994	0.0224	0.0509	−0.0334	0.2848	−0.1740
CSS					1.0000	0.2372	0.0100	0.0721	0.1077	0.1889
SP						1.0000	0.0883	0.1034	0.0728	0.0616
Sleep Time							1.0000	0.0025	−0.2184	0.0054
K6 Scores								1.0000	0.1020	−0.2173
1.5METs or Less									1.0000	−0.2956
Steps										1.0000

CSS: Chronic stiff shoulder; SP: Social participation; Correlation coefficient: Quantitative variable vs. quantitative variable; Correlation ratio (η): Quantitative variable vs. qualitive variable; Coefficient of association: Qualitative variable vs. qualitative variable.

4. Discussion

The HNN showed prediction ability equal to or greater than the LR. In the future, the HNN is expected to be useful as an index to judge the risk of CLBP for individual patients. First, in the input layer, when the order of the inputting variables was changed, the initial values of various patterns were assigned, and therefore the result might be affected. Therefore, the order of various variables was changed, and the stability of a specific solution was evaluated. We found the most accurate model by changing the total number of hidden layers. As a result, when looking at the accuracy with the verification data, the model with one layer of a hidden layer has the highest accuracy. Moreover, we examined the number of nodes with the highest accuracy with the model of the selected hidden layer being one layer. In this case, if the number of nodes in the hidden layer increased, the accuracy with respect to the learning data increased, but the accuracy of estimation with the testing data was not necessarily high. As a result, seven nodes had the highest accuracy (Figure 1). Secondly, the HNN did not require specifying a prior model and could predict from patterns learned in the data [21]. In addition, even if there was a process with a large unexpected influence in advance, the influence could be effectively found and detected [21,22]. Therefore, it was possible to predict more accurately than the LR model. Finally, the independent variables were increased to 10 by adding gender, spouse (presence or absence), shoulder stiffness, sleeping time, rate of 1.5 METs or less, and steps. The predictive value rate increased from 73.3% to 84.6%. Improvement of the prediction rate also depended on the height of the correlation coefficient between the dependent and independent variables.

The potential limitations of this study are as follows: First, the responses reported by the individual participants with respect to their response of chronic lower back pain were not always accurate, and therefore an orthopedic surgeon was contacted to act as an adviser for the health club. Although factors such as work history, education, income, etc., are considered to be important causes of chronic lower back pain, they could not be considered. Second, due to the small sample size, verification of this survey was somewhat difficult. When the number of samples is small, the results obtained become unstable. For this study, the number of samples was 96, which is considered small, and therefore the following countermeasures were taken: Samples were randomly classified into model learning and verification and random numbers were changed and performed 10,000 times. The average value of each sample, which was plurality estimated, may not represent an appropriate estimated value. Future investigations will need to increase the number of samples and conduct rigorous verification. Third, although the HNN has high prediction ability, it cannot explain the mutual relationship between dependent and independent variables [23]. Empirical research is necessary to explain the mutual relationship.

5. Conclusions

On the basis of the ROC curve, the RMSE, and the −2 log likelihood, the prediction probability performance of the HNN for predicting CLBP is equal to or higher than the LR. In the future, the HNN is expected to be useful as an index to judge the risk of CLBP for individual patients.

Author Contributions: Y.O., writing-original draft preparation; N.M., supervision.

Funding: This research received no external funding.

Conflicts of Interest: The authors declare that they have no conflict of interest.

References

1. Manchikanti, L.; Singh, V.; Falco, F.J.; Benyamin, R.M.; Hirsch, J.A. Epidemiology of Low Back Pain in Adults. *Neuromodulation* **2014**, *2*, 3–10. [CrossRef] [PubMed]
2. Ministry of Health Labour and Welfare. Comprehensive Survey of Living Condition 2017. Available online: http://www.mhlw.go.jp/toukei/saikin/hw/k-tyosa/k-tyosa13/dl/04.pdf (accessed on 30 March 2019).
3. Rodrigo, D.M.; Anaclaudia, G.F.; Neice, M.X.F. Prevalence of chronic low back pain: Systematic review. *Rev. Saude Publica* **2015**, *49*, 73.
4. Rosenblatt, F. The perceptron: A probabilistic model for information storage and organization in the brain. *Psychol. Rev.* **1958**, *65*, 386–408. [CrossRef] [PubMed]
5. Rumelhart, D.E.; Hinton, G.E.; Williams, R.J. Learning representations by back propagating errors. *Nature* **1986**, *323*, 533–536. [CrossRef]
6. Owari, Y.; Miyatake, N. Relationship between chronic low back pain, social participation, and psychological distress in elderly people: A pilot mediation analysis. *Acta Med. Okayama* **2018**, *72*, 337–342. [PubMed]

7. Kessler, R.C.; Andrews, G.; Colpe, L.J.; Hiripi, E.; Mroczek, D.K.; Normand, S.L.; Walters, E.E.; Zaslavsky, A.M. Short screening scales to monitor population prevalences and trends in non-specific psychological distress. *Psychol. Med.* **2002**, *32*, 959–976. [CrossRef] [PubMed]
8. Furukawa, T.A.; Kawakami, N.; Saitoh, M.; Ono, Y.; Nakane, Y.; Nakamura, Y.; Tachimori, H.; Iwata, N.; Uda, H.; Nakane, H.; et al. The performance of the Japanese version of the K6 and K10 in the World Mental Health Survey Japan. *Int. J. Methods Psychiatr. Res.* **2008**, *17*, 152–158. [CrossRef] [PubMed]
9. Krismer, M.; van Tulder, M. Strategies for prevention and management of musculoskeletal condition, Low back pain (non-specific). *Best Pract. Res. Clin. Rheumatol.* **2007**, *21*, 77–91. [CrossRef]
10. The Japanes Orthopedic Association and the Japanese Society for the Study of Low Back Pain. *Definition; in Back Pain Examination Guidelines*, 1st ed.; The Japanese Orthopedic Association: Nankodo, Tokyo; The Japanese Society for the Study of Low Back Pain: Nankodo, Tokyo, 2012; pp. 11–14. (In Japanese)
11. Haeuchi, Y.; Honda, T.; Chen, T.; Narazaki, K.; Chen, S.; Kumagai, S. Association between participation in social activity and physical fitness in community-dwelling older Japanese adults. *Jpn. Soc. Public Health* **2016**, *63*, 727–737. (In Japanese)
12. Gayle, D.W.; Yong-Fang, K.; Mukaila, A.R.; Soham, A.I.S.; Laura, R.; Elizabeth, T.; Kenneth, J.O. Pain and Disability in Mexican American Older Adults. *J. Am. Geriatr. Soc.* **2009**, *57*, 992–999.
13. Heikki, F.; Svetlana, S.; Pertti, M.; Harri, P.; Markku, H.; Eira, V.J. Role of overweight and obesity in low back disorders among men: A longitudinal study with a life course approach. *BMJ Open.* **2015**, *5*, e007805.
14. Florian, B.; Violaine, F.; Sylvie, R.; Bruno, F.; Laure, G. The impact of chronic low back pain is partly related to loss of social role: A qualitative study. *Jt. Bone Spine* **2015**, *82*, 437–441.
15. Amagasa, S.; Fukushima, N.; Kikuchi, H.; Oka, K.; Takamiya, T.; Odagiri, Y.; Inoue, S. Types of social participation and psychological distress in Japanese older adults: A five-year cohort study. *PLoS ONE* **2017**, *7*, e0175392. [CrossRef] [PubMed]
16. Samantha, A.; Maureen, F.; Simon, R. The Impact of Chronic Low Back Pain on Leisure Participation: Implications for Occupational Therapy. *Br. J. Occup. Ther.* **2012**, *75*, 503–508.
17. Stubbs, B.; Koyanagi, A.; Thompson, T.; Veronese, N.; Carvalho, A.F.; Solomi, M.; Mugisha, J.; Schofield, P.; Cosco, T.; Wilson, N.; et al. The epidemiology of back pain and its relationship with depression, psychosis, anxiety, sleep disturbances, and stress sensitivity: Data from 43 low- and middle-income countries. *Gen. Hosp. Psychiatry* **2016**, *43*, 63–70. [CrossRef] [PubMed]
18. Angelo, C.; Paolo, M.; Cristina, Z. Risk Factors Linked to Psychological Distress, ProductivityLosses and Sick Leave in Low-Back-Pain Employees: A Three-Year Longitudinal Cohort Study. *Pain Res. Treat.* **2016**, 3797493.
19. Eric, L.; Hurwitz, D.C.; Hal, M.; Chi, C. Effects of Recreational Physical Activity and Back Exercises on Low Back Pain and Psychological Distress: Finding from the UCLA Low Back Pain Study. *Am. J. Public Health* **2005**, *95*, 1817–1824.
20. Naugle, K.M.; Fillingim, R.B.; Riley, J.L., 3rd. A meta-analysis review of the hypoalgesic effects of exercise. *J. Pain* **2012**, *13*, 1139–1150. [CrossRef]
21. Eken, C.; Bilge, U.; Kartal, M.; Eray, O. Artificial neural network, genetic algorithm and logistic regression applications for predicting renal colic in emergency settings. *Int. J. Emerg. Med.* **2009**, *2*, 99–105. [CrossRef]
22. Mehdi, S.; Hashemi, S.; Kazemnejad, A.; Lucas, C.; Badie, K. Predicting the type of pregnancy using artificial neural networks and multinomial logistic regression: A comparison study. *Neural Comput. Appl.* **2005**, *14*, 198–202.
23. Eftekhar, B.; Mohammad, K.; Eftekhar, H.A.; Ghodsi, M.; Ketabchi, E. Comparison of artificial neural network and logistic regression models for prediction of mortality in head trauma based on initial clinical data. *BMC Med. Inform. Decis. Mak.* **2005**, *5*, 3. [CrossRef] [PubMed]

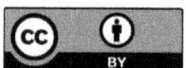

© 2019 by the authors. Licensee MDPI, Basel, Switzerland. This article is an open access article distributed under the terms and conditions of the Creative Commons Attribution (CC BY) license (http://creativecommons.org/licenses/by/4.0/).

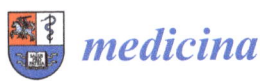

Review

Movement Control Impairment and Low Back Pain: State of the Art of Diagnostic Framing

Soleika Salvioli, Andrea Pozzi * and Marco Testa

Department of Neuroscience, Rehabilitation, Ophthalmology, Genetics, Maternal and Child Health, University of Genova, Campus of Savona, 17100 Savona, Italy
* Correspondence: andreapozzi1987@gmail.com

Received: 21 June 2019; Accepted: 26 August 2019; Published: 29 August 2019

Abstract: *Background and objectives:* Low back pain is one of the most common health problems. In 85% of cases, it is not possible to identify a specific cause, and it is therefore called Non-Specific Low Back Pain (NSLBP). Among the various attempted classifications, the subgroup of patients with impairment of motor control of the lower back (MCI) is between the most studied. The objective of this systematic review is to summarize the results from trials about validity and reliability of clinical tests aimed to identify MCI in the NSLBP population. *Materials and Methods:* The MEDLINE, Cochrane Library, and MedNar databases have been searched until May 2018. The criteria for inclusion were clinical trials about evaluation methods that are affordable and applicable in a usual clinical setting and conducted on populations aged > 18 years. A single author summarized data in synoptic tables relating to the clinical property; a second reviewer intervened in case of doubts about the relevance of the studies. *Results:* 13 primary studies met the inclusion criteria: 10 investigated inter-rater reliability, 4 investigated intra-rater reliability, and 6 investigated validity for a total of 23 tests (including one cluster of tests). Inter-rater reliability is widely studied, and there are tests with good, consistent, and substantial values (waiter's bow, prone hip extension, sitting knee extension, and one leg stance). Intra-rater reliability has been less investigated, and no test have been studied for more than one author. The results of the few studies about validity aim to discriminate only the presence or absence of LBP in the samples. *Conclusions:* At the state of the art, results related to reliability support the clinical use of the identified tests. No conclusions can be drawn about validity.

Keywords: low back pain; motor control impairment; movement control disease; movement test; reliability; validity

1. Introduction

Low Back Pain (LBP) is one of the most frequent health problems causing absenteeism and disability, and it is the most expensive diagnosis in the Western World [1–3]. LBP is defined as pain "strong enough to limit normal activities for more than one day" [4] in the lower part of the column, between the 12th thoracic vertebra and the 1st sacral, with possible projection to the lower limb [5].

Temporal staging defines LBP acute when an episode occurred not more than 6 weeks previously, subacute between 6 and 12 weeks, and chronic beyond 3 months [6].

Smoking and obesity have shown a significant association for developing LBP [7], while sedentary lifestyle, low aerobic capacity [8], and psychological factors related to personal or professional discomfort [9] have been indicated as highly related.

Patients with LBP generally improve in the first 6 weeks after an acute episode [10], but approximately 70% of patients show a recurrence in the following year [11,12] while 40% develop chronic LBP [13].

Only in 10–15% of patients with LBP is it possible to identify the triggering factor (root compressions, vertebral fractures, tumors, infections, inflammatory diseases, spondylolisthesis and vertebral stenosis, or proclaimed instability [14]); in the remaining 85–90%, it is difficult to recognize the source of pain. In these cases, the term Non-specific Low Back Pain (NSLBP) is generally used [15–17].

Since there is no clear detrimental mechanism identifiable as the source of the disorder, in the last years, researchers focused on identification of subcategories with the aim of developing targeted interventions. The heterogeneity of the samples of study seems to be the basis of the disappointing results obtained in clinical trials that have investigated the management of LBP in the past [18].

The subgroup of patients with motor control impairment (MCI) was proposed for the first time by O'Sullivan [19]. In the literature, different synonyms are used, including movement control dysfunction, movement system impairment or clinical instability, and segmental instability [20].

Patients with MCI tend to experience pain during motor tasks that load the spine mainly in one plane of space. They performed it with unconscious compensation strategies or with the adoption of postures traceable to typical patterns. In order to allow for a more detailed classification and targeted treatment, patients are categorized according to the type of posture and the direction of provocative movement (e.g., flexion pattern and extension pattern) [21].

Strategies for conducting the objective examination are based mainly on the interpretation of the quality of execution of specific tasks or on the use of technology through motion analysis tools. Several tests have been proposed to diagnose MCI, but diagnostic properties have not been thoroughly and conclusively investigated. In order for a classification system to be useful, examiners must be able to determine a valid and reliable individual's classification.

Reliability is the degree of agreement between a series of measurements of the same occurrence when the measurements are made by changing one or more conditions; validity is the ability of a test to actually measure what the author intended to measure [22].

To date, only two systematic reviews are available, limited purely to the reliability parameters [23,24].

The aim of this review is to summarize the results derived from diagnostic accuracy studies and to update the knowledge about reproducibility in order to provide an exhaustive overview of the state of the art of the diagnostic procedures useful to identify MCI.

2. Materials and Methods

No protocol has been previous registered. In order to ensure transparency and reproducibility of the research results, the indications from the PRISMA statement [25] and the COSMIN checklist have been integrated [26].

2.1. Eligibility Criteria

2.1.1. Study Design

Primary studies investigating the clinical properties of tests developed to detect MCI have been included. The study design did not influence the decision to include it in this review. Only papers published in English or Italian were considered, with no filters on the date of publication.

2.1.2. Participants Characteristics

The studied population is defined by the presence of NSLBP (with or without lower limb pain) and age > 18 years, without gender distinction.

2.1.3. Test

Only evaluation methods that are easy to use in clinical practice have been considered, excluding examinations that require complex and expensive technological instrumentation.

2.1.4. Diagnostic Values

Properties of tests taken into consideration in the synthesis are validity and reliability, described through the typical coefficients of biomedical statistics.

2.1.5. Data Sources and Search

A systematic search was conducted on the Medline, Cochrane Library, and MedNar (grey or unpublished literature) databases without time filters. The selection of articles can be considered updated to 13 May 2018. Table 1 summarizes the strategy used.

Table 1. Search strategy used for every database.

Database	Search Strategy
MEDLINE—Clinical queries	Low Back Pain AND motor control
	(Impairment AND (motor control OR movement OR movement control OR movement coordination OR movement system OR muscle control OR trunk motor control)) OR (Dysfunction AND (movement control OR movement OR stability)) OR (deficit AND (movement precision OR trunk muscle timing OR trunk movement control)) OR MCI OR altered sensory function OR segmental instability) AND (Low Back Pain OR LBP OR non-specific low back pain OR NSLBP)
Cochrane Library—Simple Search	Low Back Pain AND motor control
MedNar—Simple Search	Low back pain AND motor control

2.2. Data Synthesis and Analysis

2.2.1. Study Selection

The studies obtained were initially reported in a comprehensive database, and double reports were excluded. Only one reviewer performed the first screening following the reading of the title and abstracts. Relevance was then assessed by reading the full text: any doubts were resolved with the intervention of a second reviewer. The inclusion process is summarized graphically in a flowchart in the results section (Figure 1). Hand searching has been conducted checking bibliographies of included articles.

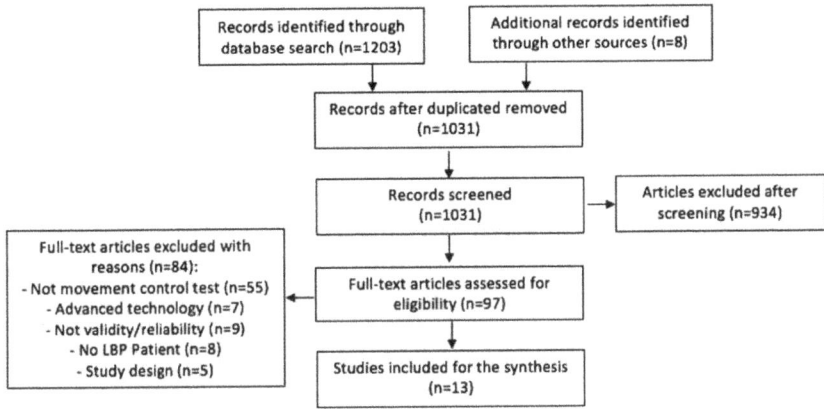

Figure 1. Study selection process.

2.2.2. Data Extraction and Synthesis

The relevant data were organized in a synoptic tables (Tables A1–A4) which shows author and year of publication, objectives of the study, the characteristics of the participants (number, sex, age, and condition), the characteristics of the examiners, the diagnostic test/examination and the procedure followed, the statistical values, and the main results. No meta-analysis of the collected data was performed, but a narrative synthesis in accordance with the emerging evidence was performed.

2.2.3. Risk of Bias Assessment

The quality of each study was assessed for methodological rigor and risk of bias by one reviewer using the tool described by Brink and Louw [27] (Table A5) and developed for the analysis of validity and reliability studies. Doubtful opinions have been resolved with the help of a second reviewer. This appraisal tool does not incorporate a quality score, but instead, the impact of each item on the study design should be considered individually. This tool contains 13 items, which should be considered according to the nature of the study: 4 are useful only for the evaluation of reliability studies, 4 are useful only for validity studies, and 9 are useful for both. The results were summarized in a synoptic table (Table A1), and a critical discussion of the strengths and weaknesses of the studies included was drafted.

3. Results

The database research identified 1203 articles, while 8 others have been identified with free research in the bibliographies of relevant studies for a total of 1211 articles; 180 articles were deleted because they were duplicated, resulting in 1031 basic articles as a partial result. Following the reading of the title, 386 articles were discarded; following the reading of abstract, 548 remained. Following the reading of the full text, 13 studies were included in the review and 84 studies were excluded as not relevant. The steps related to the selection of articles are outlined in the flow-diagram below (Figure 1). Of the 13 studies included, 10 investigated inter-rater reliability [28–37], 4 investigated intra-rater reliability [31–33,38], and only 6 studies analyzed validity [28,29,31,32,39,40]. Overall, the tests showed reliability ranging from fair to excellent (K value between 0.32 and 1.00) for the inter-rater and from moderate to excellent for the intra-rater (K value from 0.42 to 1.00). The ICC also varied from 0.41 to 0.98, indicating a range from poor to very good (Table A1). A meta-analysis of collected data was not conducted due to the small number of studies that have investigated the same test. In addition to this, the highly heterogeneous nature of the descriptions and the small samples make the calculation superfluous.

3.1. Inter-Rater Reliability

The results for inter-observer reliability are shown in Table A2.

Seventeen tests were investigated by a single author [28,30–33,36,37]. In the remaining 6 evaluated by multiple studies, only 4 (waiter's bow, one leg stance, sitting knee extension, and prone hip extension) showed agreement between reliability values [29,33,34,36], while for the other 2 (bent knee fall out and active straight leg raising), this did not happen [29,30,33,35–37].

3.1.1. Tests Described by More Than One Study that Did Not Give Consistent Results

Bent knee fall out was studied by 3 authors out of 132 patients. It was identified as having modest reliability by Luomajoki et al. [33] ($K = 0.38$) and as poor-excellent by Roussel et al. [36] (ICC = 0.61–0.91) and Enoch et al. [30] (ICC = 0.94). Active straight leg raising has been described in 3 studies on 158 total subjects. Roussel et al. [35] and Bruno et al. [29] showed good reliability (K from 0.70 left leg to 0.71 right leg for the first study and 0.79 for the second). Also, Roussel et al. in the study of 2009 [36] provide more variable values, with an ICC from poor to excellent (ICC = 0.41–0.91).

3.1.2. Tests Described by More Than One Study that Showed Agreement between the Results

Substantial reproducibility was found for both waiter's bow (investigated in 2 studies [33,36], 92 subjects, $K = 0.62$ and 0.78) and prone hip extension (investigated in 2 studies [29,34], with 112 total subjects, $K = 0.72$–0.76). The Sitting knee extension was analyzed in 2 studies for a total of 80 subjects. It provided a good K in the study by Luomajoki et al. [33] ($K = 0.72$) and was excellent in the study by Enoch et al. [30] (ICC = 0.95). The one leg stance was described in 3 studies for a total of 95 participants. Only Luomajoki et al. [33] identified a moderate-good reliability ($K = 0.43$–0.65), while both Roussel et al. [35] and Tidstrand and Horneij [37] obtained good-excellent values (K from 0.75 to 1.00).

3.1.3. Tests Described by a Single Study

Excellent reliability has been identified for joint position sense [30], sitting forward lean [30], and leg lowering [30]. Substantial reliability was identified for pelvic tilt [33], rocking pelvis forwards [33], standing back extension test [31], static lunge test [32], and dynamic lunge test [32]. Moderate reliability was identified for knee lift abdominal test [36], rocking pelvis backwards [33], prone active knee flexion [33], and standing knee-lift test [32]. The unilateral pelvic lift showed moderate reliability for the left side ($K = 0.47$) and substantial for the right side ($K = 0.61$) [37]. The sitting-on-a-ball test, on the other hand, was substantial for the right ($K = 0.79$) but excellent for the left ($K = 0.88$) [37]. The trunk forward bending and return to upright test, described by Biely et al. [28], showed K values from 0.35 to 0.89, depending on the criterion used to define the positivity of the test. Also, static lunge test [32], dynamic lunge test [32], and standing knee-lift test [32] showed different reliability values depending on each component observed during the execution of the test.

3.2. Intra-Rater Reliability

A total of 13 tests were investigated for intra-examiner reliability (Table A3), all by a single author. Waiter's bow, pelvic tilt, one leg stance, sitting knee extension, rocking backwards, rocking forwards, prone active knee flexion, and crook lying hip abduction were investigated by Luomajoki et al. [33] on 40 subjects; the standing back extension test was investigated by Gondhalekar et al. [31] on 50 subjects; and the knee-lift abdominal test was investigated by Ohe et al. [38] on 60 subjects. The K value is between 0.51 and 0.95, indicating moderate to excellent reliability; it is the same for the good ICC value for Knee lift abdominal test (KLAT) (0.71–0.79). Standing knee-lift test, static lunge test, and dynamic lunge test were studied by Granström et al. [32] and showed good to poor reliability (ICC from 0.54 to 0.87). In the same study, the intra-examiner reliability of different aberrant movements analyzed during the execution of the above 3 tests was also investigated, and in this case, an extreme variability in the results also emerged (K from 0.42 to 1.00).

3.3. Validity

A total of 10 tests (including batteries) have been reported with indicating their validity, represented in Table A4 and all investigated by a single author. The battery of Luomajoki et al. [39], the knee-lift abdominal test, the bent knee fall out, the prone hip extension, and the active straight leg raise showed significant relationships between test positivity and the presence of LBP compared to healthy subjects (all $p < 0.05$). The use of Judder/shake/instability catch (JUD), deviation from sagittal plane (DEV) and aberrant movement score (AMS) as positive criteria in anterior trunk flexion movement and return to upright position also showed significant correlations with the presence of LBP. On the contrary, for the standing back extension test, standing knee-lift test, static lunge test, and dynamic Lunge, test there were not enough high values of diagnostic power (AUC from 0.47 to 0.78).

3.4. Risk of Bias in Included Studies

All studies included reported a complete description of the selected sample (Table 2). In several [29,34,37,38], however, there was no method for calculating the sample size, so we do not know with certainty the statistical power of the results obtained. The presence of an adequate method for calculating the sample size was not described as a parameter to be evaluated in criterion 1, and for this reason, it was considered satisfied in all the studies. Three studies [36,38,40] did not clarify the characteristics of the evaluators. The main source of risk of bias in 8 out of 11 studies dealing with reproducibility was the simultaneous evaluation by the observers [34,37]. Three studies did not clarify or carry out the randomization of the order of the patients evaluated [33,36,39]. Four did not randomized the order of the tests administered [30,33,37,39], and one did not clarify it [36].

In addition, in 2 studies, the blindness of the evaluators to the results between them was not clearly explained [36,37]. In studies dealing with intra-operator reproducibility, the concealment of patients or an adequate time gap between the two observations was adopted, except for 1 study [38], where the assessments were re-performed in a matter of minutes. In the studies that dealt with validity, they were not met or it was not possible to judge the criteria (3,7,9,11) because there is no shared reference in the literature. Analyses of diagnostic accuracy were developed with respect to the presence of LBP or not. Only 1 study [31] gave a description of the reference standard used, but in our opinion, the choice was not appropriate. The choice of statistical methods was considered appropriate for all studies; only 1 study [34] introduced a possible distortion of the effect of the results because it presented data of a nonparametric nature by inserting the standard deviation.

Table 2. Risk of bias summary.

Question and Nature of the Study	[34]	[33]	[35]	[39]	[36]	[37]	[30]	[40]	[28]	[29]	[38]	[31]	[32]
1. Human subjects and detailed description of the sample (validity and reliability studies)	Y	Y	Y	Y	Y	Y	Y	Y	Y	Y	Y	Y	Y
2. Qualification or competence of rater/s clarified (validity and reliability studies)	Y	Y	Y	Y	N	Y	Y	N	Y	Y	N	Y	Y
3. Reference standard explained (validity studies)	N/A	N/A	N/A	N	N/A	N/A	N/A	N	N	N	N/A	Y	N
4. Blinding of raters to the findings of other raters (inter-rater reliability studies)	Y	Y	Y	N/A	N	N	Y	N/A	Y	Y	N/A	Y	Y
5. Blinding of raters to their own prior findings (intra-rater reliability studies)	N/A	Y	N/A	N/A	N/A	N/A	N/A	N/A	N/A	N/A	N	Y	Y
6. Variation in order of examination (reliability studies)	N	N	Y	N	N	N	Y	N/A	N	N	N	Y	Y
7. Latency between application of reference and index test reasonably (validity studies)	N/A	N/A	N/A	N/A	N/A	N/A	N/A	N	N	N	N/A	Y	N
8. Stability of the variable considered before repeated measures (reliability studies)	Y	Y	Y	N/A	Y	Y	Y	N/A	Y	Y		Y	Y
9. Reference standard independent of the index test (validity studies)	N/A	N/A	N/A	N	N/A	N/A	N/A	N	N	N	N/A	Y	N
10. Detailed description of index test (validity and reliability studies)	Y	Y	Y	Y	Y	Y	Y	Y	Y	Y	Y	Y	Y
11. Detailed execution of reference standard (validity studies)	N/A	N/A	N/A	N	N/A	N/A	N/A	N	N	N	N/A	Y	N
12. Explanation of the withdrawals (validity and reliability studies)	Y	Y	Y	Y	Y	Y	Y	N	Y	Y	N	Y	Y
13. Appropriateness of statistical methods (validity and reliability studies)	N	Y	Y	Y	Y	Y	Y	Y	Y	Y	Y	Y	Y

4. Discussion

This review is the first to include and summarize results from reliability (inter- and intra-rater) and validity studies of tests designed to detect MCI in subjects with NSLBP.

In 2013, Carlsson and Rasmussen-Barr [23] studied the reliability of tests to diagnose MCI and found it difficult to identify consistent results because they were investigated by studies with a high risk of bias. At the time (with a research updated to October 2011) only prone knee bend and the one leg stance were indicated by the author as useful because they were presented in one study with a low risk of bias. Recently, Denteneer et al. [24] identified a greater number of tests (specifically 30) but the limit of his research were the inclusion criteria. Studies included populations classified with functional lumbar instability or MCI or with the association of both. This leads to sampling limits with difficult interpretation and comparison of results.

In the present research, 15 tests have shown good inter-examiner reliability in at least one study, but only waiter's bow, one leg stance, sitting knee extension, and prone hip extension had almost overlapping values in at least 2 studies.

As is well known, inter-rater reliability is just a component of the reliability of a test and take greater importance when its context of use is characterized by the alternation of operators. NSLBP rehabilitation process is in most cases managed by a single therapist; nevertheless, the number of studies that have dealt with intra-rater reliability is far less than those of the inter-rater reliability.

From the few data available, there seems to be a good degree of agreement in the case of repeated measurements by the same therapist for almost all tests. The summary of results about intra- and inter-rater reliability shows that observing abnormal movement strategies in patients with NSLBP seems to be possible through simple tests; anyway, positivity criteria and execution modalities need to be standardized with precise protocols, as suggested by Enoch et al. [30].

The clinical use of the tests has to be based on consistent evidence both for the intra/inter-rater reliability, and these conclusions must derive from at least 2 studies of good quality.

Compared to knowledge set by Carlsson and Rasmussen-Barr [23], we can still recommend the use of the one leg stance, but we add also waiter's bow and sitting knee extension for the low risk of bias of the studies. These 3 tests are the only ones to have been studied both for inter-rater and intra-rater reliability. The use of prone knee bend suggested by Carlsson and Rasmussen-Barr [23] is less corroborated because, to date, it remains investigated only by one author and values of inter-rater reliability are moderate. Prone hip extension cannot be recommended due to high risk of bias in one of the two studies in which it is investigated. Moreover, there are no studies available about intra-rater reliability for prone hip extension.

Since 2011, the literature did not add much to previous knowledge, because of both the number of studies published and the quality of them.

As well as for the intra-rater reliability, the studies that have dealt with the validity are few in number. There is not a single test that has been evaluated by more than one author. The studies included in this review show that most tests are able to distinguish only subjects with LBP from healthy subjects (knee-lift abdominal test, bent knee fall out, and trunk forward bending and return to upright) [28,40]. This means that they do not provide any additional information to that which may result from a well-conducted medical history. It must be said that, in general, there is a higher sensitivity of the tests [39] towards subjects with chronic LBP, suggesting an association between the duration of symptoms and MCI, which would require observational studies to be demonstrated. At the same time, more patients with a history of LBP than healthy subjects [28] were positive, indicating the possibility that MCI may persist over time despite the resolution of symptoms. Again, only the design of ad hoc cohort studies could demonstrate the relationship between MCI and recurrence due to possible overloading of the tissues of the lower spine.

The validity data also shows the small number of researches that dealt with the diagnostic procedures aimed at identifying directional patterns of MCI [31]. The most important barrier to the development of validity research is the absence of a golden standard to compare the same outcome with different methods of investigation. Considering that tests for MCI evaluate the performance of certain motor tasks, the use and validation of motion capture tools seems to be the most appropriate strategy to make the evaluation as objective as possible. To date, only Wattananon et al. [41] has tried to establish reference values for the interpretation of clinical trials through comparison between the observation of examiners and the digital data collected.

Summarizing, only waiter's bow, sitting knee extension, and one leg stance are assessed across studies of good quality with good-excellent values both for intra-rater and inter-rater reliability; therefore, their use in clinical practice may be considered. However, the main problem remains the lack of clarity about the validity, which today, does not allow conclusions on the accuracy of the subgrouping procedure.

5. Conclusions

Implications for clinical practice:

- Inter-rater reliability is widely studied. Waiter's bow, prone hip extension, sitting knee extension, and one leg stance showed good values confirmed by at least two studies;
- Intra-rater reliability is not largely investigated. From the few studies available, good repeatability values seem to emerge;
- Only waiter's bow, sitting knee extension, and one leg stance are assessed across studies of good quality with good-excellent values both for intra-rater and inter-rater reliability;
- There is a lack of evidence regarding the validity of MCI tests, which results from diagnostic accuracy analyses aimed at discriminating only the presence or absence of LBP in the study samples;
- Final conclusions regarding the clinical and scientific use of the identified tests can be drawn only when consistent values of reliability and validity can be found in the literature.

Review limitations:

- Processes of identification, selection, evaluation, and data collection were carried out by a single author, contrary to the indications contained in the PRISMA statement. Intervention of a second author was required only in case of doubt;
- Inclusion of studies published only in Italian and English;
- Absence of protocol registration procedure.

Review strengths:

- Inclusion of grey literature.

Implications for research and future research:

- Investigate further intra-rater reliability of MCI tests in patients with NSLBP;
- Indicate subgroups of patients with NSLBP having salient characteristics related to MCI and deductibles in history. Develop an analysis of diagnostic accuracy of tests for motor control as a function of them;
- Identify a gold standard to evaluate the diagnostic accuracy of individual tests;
- Standardize protocols for the preparation, execution, and evaluation of the tests in order to allow a comparison between them and the generalization of the results.

Author Contributions: Conceptualization, A.P. and S.S.; methodology, A.P.; investigation S.S.; writing—original draft preparation, S.S.; writing—review and editing, A.P. and M.T.; supervision, M.T.

Funding: This research received no external funding.

Acknowledgments: The papers were obtained through the NILDE library network system through the University of Genoa.

Conflicts of Interest: The authors declare that there are no conflicts of interest.

Appendix A

Table A1. Characteristics of included studies.

Study	Aim	Population Characteristics	Examiners Characteristics	Methods	Outcomes	Results
Murphy et al. [34]	To investigate whether the finding of deviation of the lumbar spine during the hip extension test could be detected reliably by clinicians trained in the performance of the test	$N = 42$ (31 W) with LBP >7 weeks Average age 37.8 (range 19–60). Patients from spinal center.	Two chiropractic physicians: (1 with 13 years of experience and 1 with <1 year of experience) and a training period pre-study of 1 h.	Hip extension test for each hip. Max 3 repetitions. Observers evaluate the patient at the same time and are "blind" to the results of the colleague's evaluation.	Dichotomous judgment (Test +/−) K coefficient for inter-operator reliability	$K = 0.72$ (L)–0.76 (R)
Luomajoki et al. [33]	To determine the inter- and intra-operator reliability of 10 MCI tests of the lumbar spine.	$N = 40$ (26 D, 14 U). 13 LBP + 27 healthy. Average age: 52.1. Patients from private physiotherapy practice.	4 examiners with 3-day of intensive course on MCI prior to assessment. 2 examiners were specialists in MCI and had postgraduate degrees in manual therapy, with 25 years of working experience. The 2 raters were PTs with 5 years of experience.	10 MCI tests: Waiter's bow, pelvic tilt, one leg stance L, one leg stance R, sitting knee extension, rocking backwards, rocking forwards, dorsal tilt of pelvis, prone active knee-flexion, and crook lying. Raters were blinded to the diagnosis of patients and the colleagues' evaluation results. The performances were recorded (anonymously), and raters watched each video only once. Reviewed after 2 weeks.	Dichotomous judgment (Test +/−); K coefficient for inter-and intra-operator reliability	Inter-rater: $K = 0.38–0.72$ Intra-rater: $K = 0.51–0.95$
Roussel et al. [35]	To investigate reliability and internal consistency of 2 clinical tests that analyze motor control mechanisms.	$N = 36$ (21 W) with LBP Average age (mean ± SD): 37.4 ± 11.6 (range 21–62) Patients from a private clinic and 2 outpatient physiotherapy clinics.	2 examiners: 1 with master's degree and 1 Pt with 4 years of clinical experience. Training of 2 h × 2 days by an expert + evaluation of 10 pre-study patients.	Trendelenburg Active straight leg raise Evaluation by examiner 1, 10' rest (in which the patient was asked to complete questionnaires), then evaluation by examiner 2. Order of the tests randomly assigned. Both examiners were blinded to the others' scores and the patients' medical history.	Dichotomous judgment (Test +/−) weighted K for inter-operator reliability	$K = 0.70–0.83$ for Trendelenburg and ASLR.
Luomajoki et al. [39]	To evaluate the performance of 6 MCI tests in LBP and healthy patients.	$N = 210$ (130 W, 80 M) 102 healthy, 108 LBP: 29 with LBP <6 weeks, 30 with LBP 6–12 weeks, 46 with LBP >12 weeks. Patients from 5 physiotherapy clinics.	12 examiners with 7 years of average working experience, all with OMT specialization. Raters were trained using instruction, patient cases, and rating of videotaped tests.	Cluster of 6 tests: Waiter's bow, pelvic tilt, one leg stance, sitting knee extension, rocking 4 point kneeling, and prone knee bend. The order of the tests was always the same. Pt were not blinded to the patient's group.	Dichotomous judgment (Test +/−) N° of test + Effect size for the difference between group	N° of positive tests: 2.21 in LBP group and 0.75 in healthy controls. Effect size between-group: 1.18 (95% CI: 1.02–1.34), $p < 0.001$.
Roussel et al. [36]	To determine inter-ex reliability and internal consistency of the 4 clinical tests examining lumbopelvic MCI in patients with and without LBP.	$N = 52$ 25 healthy, 27 with LBP (>3 months).	With three 1-h training sessions, 2 examiners were trained in performing the tests under supervision of 2 manual therapists.	MCI evaluation with PBU: -Active straight leg raising, bent knee fall out, knee lift abdominal test, and standing bow. Observation examiner 1 → 10-min rest → observation examiner 2. Assessors were blinded to the medical history of the patients.	ICC K coefficient Chronbach α for internal consistency	ICC = 0.41–0.91 $K = 0.78$ (healthy) e 0.80 (LBP) Chronbach $\alpha = 0.83$ (LBP) e 0.65 (healthy).

Table A1. Cont.

Study	Aim	Population Characteristics	Examiners Characteristics	Methods	Outcomes	Results
Tidstrand and Horneij [37]	To determine inter-examiner reliability of 3 tests of muscular functional coordination of the lumbar spine in patient with LBP.	$N = 19$ (9 W, 10 M) 13 with LBP. Average age ± SD: 42 years ± 12. Patients from a private physiotherapy clinic.	2 experienced PTs, both trained in orthopedic manual therapy and in the McKenzie method. Both had more than 5 years of experience of treating patients with lumbar instability. Pre-study trial on 10 patients.	The 2 examiners evaluated individually but simultaneously the patients in the following tests: 1e-Single limb stance, sitting on Bobath ball with one leg lifted, and unilateral pelvic lift. Each test was performed once on both sides, and each test position was maintained for 20 s. Tests were administered in the same order to all patients. Examiners were blinded to the patient's symptoms. Detected the VAS score before each test: VAS > 7/10 was an exclusion criterion.	Dichotomous judgment (Test +/−) - K of Cohen for inter-ex reliability. % of agreement	K range = 0.47–1.00 mean K = 0.77.
Enoch et al. [30]	To determine inter-operator reliability of MCI tests on patients with and without LBP.	$N = 40$ (26 W, 14 M). LBP 25 + 15 healthy. Age range: 20–82. Patients from 3 private clinics of physical therapy.	2 examiners with 20 years of clinical experience, teachers at the Danish Manual Therapy Society. Pre-study trial on 10 patients.	Each patient was evaluated by each operator independently in two separate rooms. Both examiners performed the tests in the same order on each subject. 5 tests for MCI: Joint position sense, sitting forward lean, sitting knee extension, bent knee fall out, and leg lowering. Max 10 repetitions of each test.	total mean + standard deviation for each test. ICC for inter-ex reproducibility	ICC = 0.90–0.98 Mean ICC = 0.95
Roussel et al. [40]	To compare lumbopelvic motor control between dancers with and without a history of LBP.	$N = 40$ (38 W, 2 M) Age 17–26. Mean age 20.3 (SD 2.4). 16 patients with LBP (at least 2 consecutive days in the last year). Patients from the Department of Dance of a Conservatoire in Belgium.		2 tests were used for evaluation of MCI: Knee lift abdominal test, Bent knee fall out. The tests were performed in supine position and monitored with a PBU.	mmHg pressure on PBU and difference between groups	$p = 0.048$ KLAT $p = 0.049$ BKFO
Biely et al. [28]	To investigate the inter-examiner reliability of observation of aberrant movement patterns and whether each pattern is associated with current LBP.	$N = 102$ (48–57% D) Average age: 41.1–44.4 35 without LBP, 31 with current LBP, 36 with history of LBP. Patients from 2 physiotherapy clinics.	5 examiners with experience from 5 to 25 years in orthopaedic examination of the low back, including 2 certified orthopaedic clinical specialists. 2 h of pre-study training and a study manual.	2 therapists simultaneously observed the patient perform 3 repetitions of trunk forward bending and return to upright for the presence of the following 3 aberrant movement patterns: Altered lumbo-pelvic rhythm (including Gower's sign), deviation from the sagittal plane (DEV), instability catch (JUD). Examiner blinded to group membership. Each therapist's observations were recorded on a separate clinical observation of aberrant movement form. No discussion between raters.	Dichotomous judgment (Test +/−) K value for inter-examiner reliability p value as correlation index for construct validity.	$K = 0.35$–1.00 Construct validity: LBP vs no LBP: $p = 0.004$ DEV $p = 0.002$ JUD LBP vs LBP history: $p = 0.001$ JUD No LBP vs history LBP: $p = 0.001$ DEV AMS; $p < 0.001$ for LBP No LBP vs LBP LBP vs history LBP $p = 0.021$ for No LBP vs history LBP

Table A1. Cont.

Study	Aim	Population Characteristics	Examiners Characteristics	Methods	Outcomes	Results
Bruno et al. [29]	To investigate: the difference between LBP subjects and healthy in reported perception of difficulty in the test execution and; participant difference in reported perception of difficulty between subjects rated as positive or negative.	$N = 70$ (40 W, 30 M) Average age 27.7 years old. 30 with LBP; 40 healthy.	2 chiropractors with over 30 years of clinical experience.	The participants performed 3–5 repetitions of each test, while the examiners simultaneously observed the performances. Prone hip extension (PHE), Active straight leg raise (ASLR). The order of the test and leg lifted first were randomized.	Dichotomous judgment (Test +/−) score 0–5 for the participant-reported perception of difficulty K for inter-ex reliability Sensitivity and specificity	PHE: K = 0.72 ASLR: K = 0.79 Participant scores (average): PHE: 1.33 (0.11) LBP 0.38 (0.07) healthy. ASLR: 0.85 (0.11) LBP 0.25 (0.05) healthy. PHE and ASLR: $p < 0.001$ for group status and participant scores. Not between group and examiner classification. Not between examiner classification and participant scores. LBP group perceived significant difficulty compared to the control group. PHE: Sn: 0.82–Sp: 0.69 ASLR: Sn: 0.60–Sp: 0.76. (in cut-off 0–1).
Ohe et al. [35]	To quantify the characteristics of the trunk control during active limb movement in LBP patients with different types of LBP manifestation based on direct mechanical stress to the lumbar spine.	Patients from local medical, chiropractic, physiotherapy, and massage therapy clinics. $N = 60$ (33 W, 27 M). Age 20–58 30 LBP; 30 healthy. Patients from the outpatient department of the local hospital.	Pre-study: 1 meeting and 3 training session to achieve a consensus. 1 examiner which instructs the patient to perform the test.	The examiners were blinded to the group status and to the colleague's score. Patient were blinded to the evaluation of the examiners, and they were asked to express a score on a scale of 0–5 after the observer had left the room. During the unilateral leg-raising movement in crook-lying position (for 3 times), pressure changes produced by the movement of the lumbar lordotic curve were measured by a PBU. Data collection was executed 4 times. These 4 trials provided 4 repetitive sets of data of back pressure. Each trial was performed with 30 s rest.	ICC were calculated to confirm the relative reliability	ICC = 0.71–0.79
Gondhalekar et al. [31]	To determine the intra- and inter-rater reliability and concurrent validity of the standing back extension test for detecting MCI of the lumbar spine.	$N = 50$. 25 with NS-LBP; 25 healthy controls. Age 32.6–33.5	2 examiners with OMT specialization.	All patients were assessed in two observations that were 24 to 48 h apart at the same time of day by both operators separately. Both the raters took two readings for each subject in two different visits. Finally, they underwent evaluation by ultrasound as a gold standard. Order of examination was varied. Both raters were blinded to the findings of the other rater and to their own prior findings. Raters were not blinded to the subject's disease status.	Dichotomous judgment (Test +/−) For reliability: % agreement K coefficient. For validity: Test +/− Area under the curve (AUC) Sn and Sp LR	Intra-rater: K = 0.87 % agreement: 96 Inter-es: K = 0.78 % agreement: 94 AUC 0.785 for ADIM 0.780 for ASLRs

Table A1. Cont.

Study	Aim	Population Characteristics	Examiners Characteristics	Methods	Outcomes	Results
Granström et al. [32]	To evaluate inter- and intra-examiner reliability and discriminative validity of 3 movement control tests.	$N = 38$ (24 W, 14 M). Average age 37.5 years (19–58). 21 NSLBP, 17 healthy. Patients with LBP from private physiotherapy clinics, the healthy selected from university students and acquaintances.	4 examiners with 13–32 years' work experience, all were qualified orthopedic manual therapists. Pre-study: one-day course in evaluating the tests + training session and test trial on video clips.	Patients performed 3 tests in a standardized order: Standing knee lift (SKL), static lunge (SL), and dynamic lunge (DL). They were video recorded on the frontal and sagittal planes. The examiners (blinded to the subjects' health status and each other's results) individually scored the tests and calculated a composite score for each test based on the number of incorrect test components (0 or 1). For inter-observer reliability, the observers received the numbered video clips (a random-drawn number showing which of the video clips to begin with). They were instructed to study each video clip no more than five times. The same procedure was repeated after 2 weeks.	For inter and intra-ex reliability: ICC For validity: ROC curves AUC	Inter-observer: ICC = 0.68–0.80. Intra-observer: ICC = 0.54–0.82 Validity ranged between 0.47 and 0.56. SKL not-informative, SL and DL are less accurate than the effect of chance alone in discriminating subjects into healthy or NS-LBP group.

Table A2. Inter-rater reliability of clinical tests.

Test	Authors	Reproducibility INTER-ES	Percentage of Agreement	Description	Positivity Criteria
Active Straight Leg Raising (ASLR)	Bruno et al. [29] ***	$K = $ L: 0.70 R: 0.71		In supine position, hip flexion with fully extended knee required.	* Expressed the perceived difficulty on a scale of 0–5 ** Observation of the difference in mmHg from the starting phase, through the PBU positioned behind the column. *** The examiner determines the positivity/negative of the test according to the subject's ability to maintain neutral alignment.
	Roussel et al. [35] *	ICC = 0.41–0.91 Cronbach α = 0.83			
	Roussel et al. [36] **	$K = 0.79$			
Crook lying hip abduction/bent knee fall out (BKFO)	Luomajoki et al. [33] *	$K = 0.38$	P1 = 78.6	Supine with hip and knee flexed, required abduction/extra rotation of hip	* Execution evaluated as qualitatively correct by the examiner after careful observation. ** A pressure biofeedback (PBU) was placed behind the column and evaluated the pressure variation. *** A 5-cm tape is placed between the two antero-superior iliac spine, with a laser pointer on the right end of the line. After 5 movements, the distance between the laser pointer and the extremity 0 of the tape (in cm) is measured.
	Enoch et al. [30] ***	ICC = tra 0.61 e 0.91 Cronbach α = 0.83	P2 = 65.0		
	Roussel et al. [36] **	ICC = 0.94	88		
Dynamic lunge test (DL)	Granström et al. [32]	ICC = 0.80 (0.68–0.89) $K = 0.45$ (0.16–0.73) for trunk lateral flexion (TLF) $K = 0.50$ (0.22–0.78) for knee moving inwards (KMI) $K = 0.54$ (0.28–0.81) for pelvic tilt (PT) $K = 0.46$ (0.18–0.75) for hips moving backwards (HMB) $K = 0.55$ (0.29–0.82) for trunk moving forwards (TMF) $K = 0.77$ (0.57–0.97) for shoulders moving backwards (SMB)		In an upright position, required the functional movement of front lunge and evaluated the dynamic execution with upper limbs in full elevation. TLF: Trunk lateral flexion to either side. KMI: The front knee moves inwards and not aligned with the hip and foot PT: The pelvis tilts to either side and not horizontally aligned. HMB: The hips move backwards instead of downwards. The back seems to arch. TMF: The trunk moves forwards and falls over the front leg. SMB: The shoulders move backwards when returning back to start position.	Appearance of compensation. Assess each of the 6 components of the test as correct (1 point) or incorrect (0). A final score is obtained by combining the individual components.

Table A2. Cont.

Test	Authors	Reproducibility INTER-ES	Percentage of Agreement	Description	Positivity Criteria
Knee lift abdominal test (KLAT)	Roussel et al. [36]	ICC > 0.85 Cronbach α = 0.83		In supine position, with flexion of knees and hips, flexion of a hip is required.	Difference in the pressure variation between the performance carried out with the two lower limbs
Leg lowering (LL)	Enoch et al. [30]	ICC = 0.98		Required to maintain constant pressure on the PBU during repeated lowering of the leg towards the support surface, starting with hips flexed at 90 degrees and knee extended as much as possible.	Difference in the pressure variation between the performance carried out with the two lower limbs.
One leg stance/Trendelenburg	Luomajoki et al. [33] *	K = R: 0.43 L: 0.65	P1 = R/L: 88.0	One leg balance required	* Lateral displacement of the asymmetrical navel and difference of >2 cm between the two sides
	Roussel et al. [35] **	K = R: 0.75 L: 0.83	P2 = R: 97.5 L: 92.5		** Appearance of pelvic tilt or rotation or inability to maintain position for 30 s
	Tidstrand and Horneij [37] **	K = R: 1.00 L: 0.88	R: 100 L: 95		
Pelvic tilt	Luomajoki et al. [33]	K = 0.65	P1 = 80.0 P2 = 92.5	Request for anti and retroversion of pelvis	Presence of compensatory movements in others anatomical districts or inability to do the task required
Prone active knee flexion/prone knee bending	Luomajoki et al. [33]	K(Est) = 0.47 K(Rot) = 0.58	P1 = (Est) 97.6 (Rot) 90.5 P2 = (Est/Rot) 87.5	Keeping the lumbar spine in neutral position lying prone, knee flexion required	Loss of neutral position before 90° knee flexion
Prone hip extension (PHE)	Bruno et al. [29] *	K = L: 0.72 R: 0.76		Patient in prone position, hip extension with fully extended knee required	* Appearance of rotation, hyperextension, or inclination of the lower spine or pelvic tract. Considered also the difficulty perceived during the execution indicating a score from 0 to 5 (where 0 indicates no difficulty and 5 impossibility to perform) in the overall assessment
	Murphy et al. [34]	K = 0.72			
Repositioning (RPS)/joint position sense	Enoch et al. [30]	ICC = 0.90		In an upright position, the patient is asked to search for the neutral lumbar position, following a maximum antiversion and retroversion of the pelvis.	A 5-cm tape positioned vertically starting from S1 (point 0) on which a laser is pointed. The patient moves the pelvis twice in anti and retroversion, finally returning to the starting position. The distance in cm between the laser pointer and S1 is measured.
Rocking backwards	Luomajoki et al. [33]	K = 0.57	P1 = 88.0 P2 = 90.0	Keeping the lumbar spine in neutral position, knees and hips flexion required starting from quadrupedic position	Loss of neutral position or appearance of compensation
Rocking forwards	Luomajoki et al. [33]	K = 0.68	P1 = 92.8 P2 = 92.5	Keeping the lumbar spine in neutral position, knees and hips extension required starting from quadrupedic position	Loss of neutral position or appearance of compensation
Sitting forward lean (SFL)	Enoch et al. [30]	ICC = 0.96		Required flexion of the trunk in a seated position, without losing neutral position of the lumbar spine. The distance measured between two points marked on the patient's skin (point 0 on S1 and point 1 placed 10 cm above).	Increased distance between the two points from the starting position
Sitting knee extension (SKE)	Enoch et al. [30] **	K = 0.72	P1 = 90.4	Required to maintain neutral lumbar spine position during knee extension with patient sitting on the edge of the cot	* Capable of maintaining the neutral position of the lumbar spine up to 30–50° knee flexion.
	Luomajoki et al. [33]	ICC = 0.95	P2 = 95.0		** A 5-cm tape is placed on the lumbar area starting from S1, on which a laser pointer is placed. After 5 full knee extensions, the distance in cm between the laser pointer and S1 is measured.
Sitting on a ball	Tidstrand and Horneij [37]	K = R: 0.79 L: 0.88	R: 89 L: 95	Sitting on a Bobath ball, required to lift one foot off the ground by at least 5 cm.	Occurrence of compensatory movements at the level of the pelvis and trunk or loss of the neutral position of the lumbar spine
Standing back extension test	Gondhalekar et al. [31]	K = 0.78	94	Request for extension hip with fully extended knee in an upright position	Occurrence of ipsilateral superior anterior iliac spine forward translation or compensatory movements.

Table A2. Cont.

Test	Authors	Reproducibility INTER-ES	Percentage of Agreement	Description	Positivity Criteria
Standing knee-lift test (SKL)	Granström et al. [32]	ICC = 0.68 (0.47–0.82) $K = 0.32$ (0.02–0.63) for hip hitch (HH) $K = 0.67$ (0.43–0.90) for lateral sway (LS) $K = 0.77$ (0.57–0.97) for trunk lateral flexion (TLF) $K = 0.48$ (0.20–0.76) for knee not lifted straight up (KNLSU) $K = 0.83$ (0.66–1.00) for arm lowering (AL) $K = 0.91$ (0.78–1.00) for back extension (BE) $K = 0.68$ (0.44–0.91) for back flexion (BF)		In an upright position, required flexion of hip and knee at 90°, remaining in monopodal balance, with upper limbs abducted at 90 degrees and elbows extended. Hip hitch (HH): instead of lifting the thigh up in the sagittal plane, the pelvis tilts in the frontal plane. LS is a lateral sway of the pelvis on the stance leg. TLF: Trunk lateral flexion to either side. KNLSU: Knee is not lifted straight up. AL: One arm is lower on one side. BE: The back extends during the movement. BF: The back flexes during the movement.	Appearance of compensation. Assess each of the 7 components of the test as correct (1 point) or incorrect (0) A final score is obtained by combining the individual components.
Static lunge test (SL)	Granström et al. [32]	ICC = 0.79 (0.65–0.88) $K = 0.61$ (0.35–0.86) for trunk lateral flexion (TLF) $K = 0.91$ (0.78–1.00) for arm lowering (AL) $K = 0.59$ (0.33–0.84) for knee moving inwards (KMI) $K = 0.67$ (0.43–0.90) for pelvic tilt (PT) $K = 0.49$ (0.21–0.77) for hips backwards (HMB)		In an upright station, required the functional movement of the front lunge and evaluated the ability to maintain it with upper limbs abducted at 90° and elbows extended. TLF: Trunk lateral flexion to either side. AL: One arm is lower on one side. KMI: The front knee moves inwards and not aligned with the hip and foot. PT: The pelvis tilts to either side and not horizontally aligned. HMB: The hips move backwards instead of downwards. The back seems to arch.	Appearance of compensation. Assess each of the 5 components of the test as correct (1 point) or incorrect (0) A final score is obtained by combining the individual components.
Unilateral pelvic lift	Tidstrand and Horneij [37]	K: R: 0.61 L: 0.47	R: 79 L: 74	In supine position, with hips and knees bent, required to lift pelvis from the cot, supporting it on just one foot.	Occurrence of compensatory movements at the level of the pelvis and trunk or loss of the neutral position of the lumbar spine
Waiter's bow/standing bow (SB)	Luomajoki et al. [33] * Roussel et al. [36] **	$K = 0.62$ $K = 0.78$	P1 = 85.7 P2 = 75.0	Required hip flexion with lumbar spine in neutral position.	Loss of neutral position of the lumbar spine a: * 50–70° flexion of the hips. ** Approx. 50° hip flexion.
Trunk forward bending and return to upright	Biely et al. [28]	For JUD: $K = 0.35$ (0.00–0.71) * $K = 0.46$ (0.31–0.61) ** For DEV: $K = 0.68$ (0.34–1.00) * $K = 0.60$ (0.50–0.69) ** For altered LPR: $K = 0.89$ (0.69–1.00) * $K = 0.83$ (0.73–0.93) ** For battery: $K = 0.65$ (0.00–1.00) * $K = 0.53$ (0.43–0.64) **	96 96 87 80 96 96 96 80	During forward bending of the patient and return to upright standing, the examiner observes any aberrant movement pattern: JUD = Judder/shake/instability catch. In an attempt to return from flexion, the patient flexes their knees or moves their pelvis anteriorly before reaching the upright position of the trunk. DEV = Deviation from sagittal plane. Considered positive if any deviation from the sagittal plane appears during movement. LPR = Reversal of lumbopelvic rhythm (including Gower's sign). In an attempt to return from flexion, the patient flexes their knees and moves their pelvis anteriorly before reaching the upright position of the trunk. Battery test considered positive for the presence of at least 1 out of 3 of the aberrant movements between JUD, altered LPR and DEV.	* Result calculated considering the test as positive if at least 1 movement on 3 repetitions is altered ** Result calculated considering the test as positive only if the movement is altered in each repetition

Table A3. Intra-rater Reliability of clinical tests.

Test	Authors	INTRA-RATER Reliability	Percentage Agreement/Description
Crook lying hip abduction/lateral rotation	Luomajoki et al. [33]	K = 0.86	O1/O2 = 97.5
Dynamic lunge test (DL)	Granström et al. [32]	ICC = 0.54–0.82 K = 0.47–0.79 for Trunk Lateral Flexion K = 0.63–0.74 for Knee moving inwards K = 0.68–0.89 for Pelvic Tilt K = 0.47–0.90 for Hips moving backwards K = 0.64–0.95 for shoulders moving forwards K = 0.79–0.95 for shoulders moving backwards	The trunk moves forwards (TMF) and falls over the front of the leg. The shoulders move backwards (SMB) when returning back to the start position.
Knee lift abdominal test (KLAT)	Ohe et al. [38]	ICC = 0.71–0.79	
One leg stance/Trendelenburg	Luomajoki et al. [33]	K = R:0.67 L: 0.84	O1 = R: 92.5 L: 87.5 O2 = R/L:100
Pelvic tilt	Luomajoki et al. [33]	K = 0.80	O1/O2 = 95.0
Prone active knee flexion/prone knee bending	Luomajoki et al. [33]	K(Ext) = 0.70 K(Rot) = 0.78	O1 = (Ext/Rot) 92.5 O2 = (Ext) 92.5—(Rot) 100
Rocking backwards	Luomajoki et al. [33]	K = 0.72	O1/O2 = 97.5
Rocking forwards	Luomajoki et al. [33]	K = 0.51	O1 = 95.0 O2 = 100
Sitting knee extension	Luomajoki et al. [33]	K = 0.95	O1/O2 = 100
Standing back extension test	Gondhalekar et al. [31]	K = 0.87	96
Standing knee-lift test (SKL)	Granström et al. [32]	ICC = 0.57–0.75 K = 0.42–0.79 for hip hitch K = 0.63–0.95 for lateral sway K = 0.79–0.89 for trunk lateral flexion K = 0.42–0.84 for knee not lifted straight up K = 0.76–1.00 for arm lowering K = 0.89–1.00 for back extension K = 0.61–1.00 for back flexion	Hip hitch (HH): Instead of lifting the thigh up in the sagittal plane, the pelvis tilts in the frontal plane. Lateral sway (LS) of the pelvis on the stance leg. Trunk lateral flexion (TLF) to either side. Knee is not lifted straight up (KNLSU). One arm is lower (AL) on one side. The back extends (BE) during the movement. The back flexes (BF) during the movement.
Static lunge test (SL)	Granström et al. [32]	ICC = 0.54–0.87 K = 0.42–0.89 for trunk lateral flexion K = 0.95–1.00 for arm lowering K = 0.63–0.74 for knee moving inwards K = 0.63–0.95 for pelvic tilt K = 0.53–0.89 for hips backwards	The front knee moves inwards (KMI) and not aligned with the hip and foot. The pelvis tilts (PT) to either side and not horizontally aligned. The hips move backwards (HMB) instead of downwards. The back seems to arch.
Waiter's bow/trunk flexion	Luomajoki et al. [33]	K = 0.88	O1 = 97.5 O2 = 100

NB: Tests are described in the table "Inter-examiner reliability". Legend: O = Observation, R = Right, L = Left, Ext = Extension, Rot = Rotation.

Table A4. Validity of clinical tests.

Test	Authors	Validity	Notes and Summary of Results
6 tests battery:	Luomajoki et al. [39]	Effect size (ES) for the difference between the groups: 1.18 (CI 95%: 1.02–1.34).	Physiotherapists valued the performance of the subjects on the six movement control tests resulting in a score of 0–6 positive tests.
Waiter's bow		$p < 0.001$ LBP vs healthy controls.	Authors compared the mean number of positive tests in the two groups. The differences between the groups were analyzed by the effect size (ES).
Pelvic tilt		Between all the group: $p < 0.02$	The statistical test showed that this was a significant difference ($p < 0.001$).
One leg stance		$p < 0.01$ acute vs chronic	A subgroup analysis was performed of the number of positive tests depending on LBP.
Sitting knee extension		$p < 0.03$ subacute vs chronic	A statistically significant difference was also found between acute and chronic ($p < 0.01$) as well as between subacute and chronic ($p < 0.03$). No difference between acute and subacute patient groups ($p > 0.7$).
Rocking 4 points kneeling			
Prone lying active knee flexion		$p > 0.7$ acute and subacute.	
Knee lift abdominal test (KLAT)	Roussel et al. [40]	$p = 0.048$ (R/L)	The tests were performed in supine position and monitored with a pressure biofeedback unit (PBU): maximal pressure deviation from baseline was recorded during each test. The aim was to have as little deviation as possible.
Bent knee fall out (BKFO)	Roussel et al. [40]	$p = 0.049$ (L), 0.304 (R)	Significant differences were observed between dancers with and without a history of LBP (p value <0.05 bilaterally for KLAT and on the left leg for the BKFO).
Prone hip extension (PHE)	Bruno et al. [29]	$p < 0.001$ LBP group-patient score $p = 0.30$ patient score-examiner classification $p = 0.96$ LBP group—ex classification. Sn = 0.82 Sp = 0.69 (cut-off 0–1)	The following analyses were performed: → exam of the effects of group status (LBP/control) and examiner classification (positive/negative) on the participant-reported perception of difficulty scores (0–5) → The sensitivity (LBP group) and specificity (control group) were calculated for different cut-offs used to distinguish "positive" and "negative" participant scores.
Active straight leg raise (ASLR)	Bruno et al. [29]	$p < 0.001$ LBP group-patient score $p = 0.54$ patient score-examiner classification $p = 0.89$ LBP group—ex classification Sn = 0.60 Sp = 0.76 (cut-off 0–1)	For both PHE and ASLR tests, a significant difference ($p < 0.001$) was found between the groups (LBP group perceived significant difficulty compared to the control group) but not for examiner classification. Not significant For both tests, the sum of sensitivity and specificity was highest with a cut-off of 0–1: Values are reported beside.

Table A4. Cont.

Test	Authors	Validity	Notes and Summary of Results
Trunk forward bending and return to upright	Biely et al. [28]	For altered lumbo-pelvic rhythm (LPR): * $p = 0.07$ ** $p = 0.52$ *** $p = 0.23$ For deviation from sagittal plane (DEV): * $p = 0.004$ ** $p = 0.75$ *** $p = 0.001$ For instability catch (IUD): * $p = 0.002$ ** $p = 0.001$ *** $p = 0.95$ For aberrant movement score (AMS): No LBP: 0.8 ± 0.63 History of LBP: 1.3 ± 0.61 LBP: 2.5 ± 0.96 * $p < 0.001$ ** $p < 0.001$ *** $p = 0.021$	Two different approaches for construct validity: (1) The ability of each individual aberrant movement to distinguish between patients with LBP, with history of LBP and without LBP. * → LBP vs No LBP ** → LBP vs history of LBP *** → No LBP vs history of LBP p values expressed indicate the association between the presence of aberrant movement and the presence/absence/history of low back pain. (2) AMS: The average Aberrant Movement Score (AMS) score was calculated to provide a description. Considering the 4 aberrant movements LPR, DEV, JUD, and painful arc of motion, the mean AMS has been calculated for each group, showing how the group that currently complains about LBP has the highest value. The p values show a statistically significant difference between all groups ($p < 0.05$).
Standing back extension test	Gondhalekar et al. [31]	AUC: 0.785 for abdominal drawing-in maneuver (ADIM), 0.780 for ASLR	To establish validity, results of movement test from the first rater were compared with the difference in thickness during ASLR and ADIM results. Area Under the Curve (AUC) was used for assessing the validity of the standing back extension test with respect to reference standard of ultrasound measurements during ADIM and ASLR maneuvers. It can be between 0 and 1: the closer the curve is to the top of the graph (i.e., to 1), the greater the discriminating power of the test. For AUC = 0.785 and 0.780, standing back extension test can be considered moderately accurate.
Standing knee-lift test (SKL)	Granström et al. [32]	AUC: 0.47	The ability of the tests to classify the subjects into the healthy or NSLBP group was analyzed using the ROC curve quantified by using the area under the curve.
Static lunge Test (SL)	Granström et al. [32]	AUC: 0.56	Compared to the previous one, in this study, the AUC values are of lower accuracy. The authors considered an AUC of <0.5 as non-informative; 0.5 < AUC < 0.7 less accurate than chance alone; 0.7 < AUC < 0.9 moderately accurate; 0.9 < AUC < 1.0 highly accurate; and AUC = 1.0 like a perfect test.
Dynamic lunge test (DL)	Granström et al. [32]	AUC: 0.52	

Legend: Sn = Sensitivity, Sp = Specificity, ROC = Receiver Operator Characteristic. For description and criteria of tests, see table "Inter-rater reliability".

Table A5. Critical appraisal tool for validity and reliability studies of objective clinical tools as described by Brink and Louw [27].

N Item	Type of Question	Nature of the study
1	If human subjects were used, did the authors give a detailed description of the sample of subjects used to perform the (index) test?	Validity and reliability studies
2	Did the authors clarify the qualification, or competence of the rater(s) who performed the (index) test?	Validity and reliability studies
3	Was the reference standard explained?	Validity studies
4	If interrater reliability was tested, were raters blinded to the findings of other rathers?	Reliability studies
5	If intrarater reliability was tested, were raters blinded to their own prior findings of the test under evaluation?	Reliability studies
6	Was the order of examination varied?	Reliability studies
7	If human subjects were used, was the time period between the reference standard and the index test short enough to be reasonably sure that the target condition did not change between the two tests?	Validity studies
8	Was the stability (or theoretical stability) of the variable being measured taken into account when determining the suitability of the time interval between repeated measures?	Reliability studies
9	Was the reference standard independent of the index test?	Validity studies
10	Was the execution of the reference standard described in sufficient detail to permit its replication?	Validity and reliability studies
11	Was the execution of the (index) test described in sufficient detail to permit replication of the test?	Validity studies
12	Were withdrawals from the study explained	Validity and reliability studies
13	Were the statistical methods appropriate for the purpose of the study?	Validity and reliability studies

References

1. Airaksinen, O.; Brox, J.I.; Cedraschi, C.; Hildebrandt, J.; Klaber-Moffett, J.; Kovacs, F.; Zanoli, G. Chapter 4 European guidelines for the management of chronic nonspecific low back pain on behalf of the COST B13 Working Group on Guidelines for Chronic Low Back Pain. *Eur. Spine. J.* **2006**, *15*, 192–300. [CrossRef] [PubMed]
2. Dagenais, S.; Caro, J.; Haldeman, S. A systematic review of low back pain cost of illness studies in the United States and internationally. *Spine J.* **2008**, *8*, 8–20. [CrossRef] [PubMed]
3. Katz, R.T. Impairment and disability rating in low back pain. *Phy. Med. Rehabil. Clin. N. Am.* **2001**, *12*, 681–694. [CrossRef]
4. Dionne, C.E.; Dunn, K.M.; Croft, P.R.; Nachemson, A.L.; Buchbinder, R.; Walker, B.F.; Von Korff, M. A Consensus Approach Toward the Standardization of Back Pain Definitions for Use in Prevalence Studies. *Spine* **2008**, *33*, 95–103. [CrossRef] [PubMed]
5. Waddell, G. *The Back Pain Revolution*; Churchill Livingstone: London, UK, 2004.
6. van Tulder, M.; Becker, A.; Bekkering, T.; Breen, A.; Gil del Real, M.T.; Hutchinson, A.; COST B13 Working Group on Guidelines for the Management of Acute Low Back Pain in Primary Care. Chapter 3 European guidelines for the management of acute nonspecific low back pain in primary care. *Eur. Spine J.* **2006**, *15*, s169–s191. [CrossRef] [PubMed]
7. Shiri, R.; Karppinen, J.; Leino-Arjas, P.; Solovieva, S.; Viikari-Juntura, E. The association between smoking and low back pain: A meta-analysis. *Am. J. Med.* **2010**, *123*, 87.e7–87.e35. [CrossRef] [PubMed]
8. Smeets, R.J.E.M.; Wittink, H.; Hidding, A.; Knottnerus, J.A. Do patients with chronic low back pain have a lower level of aerobic fitness than healthy controls? Are pain, disability, fear of injury, working status, or level of leisure time activity associated with the difference in aerobic fitness level? *Spine* **2006**, *31*, 90–97, discussion 98. [CrossRef] [PubMed]
9. Nachemson, A.L. Work related low back pain treatment outcomes: The experience in Gothenburg, Sweden. *Bulletin* **1996**, *55*, 203.
10. Actis, J.A.; Honegger, J.D.; Gates, D.H.; Petrella, A.J.; Nolasco, L.A.; Silverman, A.K. Validation of lumbar spine loading from a musculoskeletal model including the lower limbs and lumbar spine. *J. Biomech.* **2008**, *68*, 107–114. [CrossRef]
11. Hestbaek, L.; Leboeuf-Yde, C.; Manniche, C. Low back pain: What is the long-term course? A review of studies of general patient populations. *Eur. Spine J. Off. Publ. Eur. Spine Soc. Eur. Spin Deform. Soc. Eur. Sect. Cerv. Spine Res. Soc.* **2003**, *12*, 149–165. [CrossRef]
12. Pengel, L.H.M.; Herbert, R.D.; Maher, C.G.; Refshauge, K.M. Acute low back pain: Systematic review of its prognosis. *BMJ (Clin. Res. Ed.)* **2003**, *327*, 323. [CrossRef] [PubMed]
13. Costa, L.C.M.; Maher, C.G.; Hancock, M.J.; McAuley, J.H.; Herbert, R.D.; Costa, L.O.P. The prognosis of acute and persistent low-back pain: A meta-analysis. *CMAJ Can. Med. Assoc. J. (J. de l'Assoc. Med. Can.)* **2002**, *184*, E613–E624. [CrossRef] [PubMed]
14. Wieser, S.; Horisberger, B.; Schmidhauser, S.; Eisenring, C.; Brügger, U.; Ruckstuhl, A.; Müller, U. Cost of low back pain in Switzerland in 2005. *Eur. J. Health Econ. HEPAC Health Econ. Prev. Care* **2001**, *12*, 455–467. [CrossRef] [PubMed]
15. Hancock, M.J.; Maher, C.G.; Latimer, J.; Spindler, M.F.; McAuley, J.H.; Laslett, M.; Bogduk, N. Systematic review of tests to identify the disc, SIJ or facet joint as the source of low back pain. *Eur. Spine J.* **2003**, *16*, 1539–1550. [CrossRef] [PubMed]
16. Niemisto, L.; Rissanen, P.; Sarna, S.; Lahtinen-Suopanki, T.; Lindgren, K.-A.; Hurri, H. Cost-effectiveness of combined manipulation, stabilizing exercises, and physician consultation compared to physician consultation alone for chronic low back pain: A prospective randomized trial with 2-year follow-up. *Spine* **2005**, *30*, 1109–1115. [CrossRef] [PubMed]
17. Panjabi, M.M. Clinical spinal instability and low back pain. *J. Electromyogr. Kinesiol.* **2003**, *13*, 371–379. [CrossRef]
18. Fritz, J.M.; Cleland, J.A.; Childs, J.D. Subgrouping patients with low back pain: Evolution of a classification approach to physical therapy. *J. Orthop. Sports Phy. Ther.* **2007**, *37*, 290–302. [CrossRef]
19. O'Sullivan, P. Diagnosis and classification of chronic low back pain disorders: Maladaptive movement and motor control impairments as underlying mechanism. *Man. Ther.* **2007**, *10*, 242–255. [CrossRef]

20. Luomajoki, H. Movement Control Impairment as a Sub-Group of Non-Specific Low Back Pain. Evaluation of Movement Control Test Battery as a Practical Tool in the Diagnosis of Movement Control Impairment and Treatment of This Dysfunction. Ph.D. Thesis, University of Eastern Finland, Kuopio, Finland, 2010.
21. O'sullivan, P.B. Masterclass: Lumbar segmental 'instability': Clinical presentation and specific stabilizing exercise management. *Man. Ther.* **2000**, *5*, 1–12. [CrossRef]
22. Molina, K.M.; Molina, K.M.; Goltz, H.H.; Kowalkouski, M.A.; Hart, S.L.; Latini, D.; Gidron, Y. Reliability and Validity. In *Encyclopedia of Behavioral Medicine*; Springer: New York, NY, USA, 2003; pp. 1643–1644. [CrossRef]
23. Carlsson, H.; Rasmussen-Barr, E. Clinical screening tests for assessing movement control in non-specific low-back pain. A systematic review of intra- and inter-observer reliability studies. *Man. Ther.* **2013**, *18*, 103–110. [CrossRef] [PubMed]
24. Denteneer, L.; Stassijns, G.; De Hertogh, W.; Truijen, S.; Van Daele, U. Inter- and Intrarater Reliability of Clinical Tests Associated with Functional Lumbar Segmental Instability and Motor Control Impairment in Patients with Low Back Pain: A Systematic Review. *Arch. Phy. Med. Rehabil.* **2017**, *98*, 151–164.e6. [CrossRef] [PubMed]
25. Moher, D.; Liberati, A.; Tetzlaff, J.; Altman, D.G.; Group, T.P. Linee guida per il reporting di revisioni sistematiche e meta-analisi: Il PRISMA Statement. *Evidence* **2015**, *7*, e1000114.
26. Mokkink, L.B.; Terwee, C.B.; Patrick, D.L.; Alonso, J.; Stratford, P.W.; Stratford, P.W.; Knol, D.L.; Bouter, L.M.; de Vet, H.C. The COSMIN checklist for assessing the methodological quality of studies on measurement properties of health status measurement instruments: An international Delphi study. *Qual. Life Res.* **2010**, *19*, 539–549. [CrossRef] [PubMed]
27. Brink, Y.; Louw, Q.A. Clinical instruments: Reliability and validity critical appraisal. *J. Eval. Clin. Pract.* **2012**, *18*, 1126–1132. [CrossRef] [PubMed]
28. Biely, S.A.; Silfies, S.P.; Smith, S.S.; Hicks, G.E. Clinical Observation of Standing Trunk Movements: What Do the Aberrant Movement Patterns Tell Us? *J. Orthop. Sports Phy. Ther.* **2014**, *44*, 262–272. [CrossRef] [PubMed]
29. Bruno, P.A.; Goertzen, D.A.; Millar, D.P. Patient-reported perception of difficulty as a clinical indicator of dysfunctional neuromuscular control during the prone hip extension test and active straight leg raise test. *Man. Ther.* **2014**, *19*, 602–607. [CrossRef] [PubMed]
30. Enoch, F.; Kjaer, P.; Elkjaer, A.; Remvig, L.; Juul-Kristensen, B. Inter-examiner reproducibility of tests for lumbar motor control. *BMC Musculoskelet. Disord.* **2011**, *12*, 114. [CrossRef] [PubMed]
31. Gondhalekar, G.A.; Kumar, S.P.; Eapen, C.; Mahale, A. Reliability and Validity of Standing Back Extension Test for Detecting Motor Control Impairment in Subjects with Low Back Pain. *J. Clin. Diagn. Res.* **2016**, *10*, KC07-11. [CrossRef] [PubMed]
32. Granström, H.; Äng, B.O.; Rasmussen-Barr, E. Movement control tests for the lumbopelvic complex. Are these tests reliable and valid? *Physiother. Theory Pract.* **2017**, *33*, 386–397. [CrossRef]
33. Luomajoki, H.; Kool, J.; Kool, J.; de Bruin, E.D.; Airaksinen, O. Reliability of movement control tests in the lumbar spine. *BMC Musculoskelet. Disord.* **2007**, *8*, 90. [CrossRef]
34. Murphy, D.R.; Byfield, D.; McCarthy, P.; Humphreys, K.; Gregory, A.A.; Rochon, R. Interexaminer Reliability of the Hip Extension Test for Suspected Impaired Motor Control of the Lumbar Spine. *J. Manip. Physiol. Ther.* **2006**, *29*, 374–377. [CrossRef] [PubMed]
35. Roussel, N.A.; Nijs, J.; Truijen, S.; Smeuninx, L.; Stassijns, G. Low Back Pain: Clinimetric Properties of the Trendelenburg Test, Active Straight Leg Raise Test, and Breathing Pattern During Active Straight Leg Raising. *J. Manip. Physiol. Ther.* **2007**, *30*, 270–278. [CrossRef] [PubMed]
36. Roussel, N.A.; Nijs, J.; Mottram, S.; Van Moorsel, A.; Truijen, S.; Stassijns, G. Altered lumbopelvic movement control but not generalized joint hypermobility is associated with increased injury in dancers. A prospective study. *Man. Ther.* **2009**, *14*, 630–635. [CrossRef] [PubMed]
37. Tidstrand, J.; Horneij, E. Inter-rater reliability of three standardized functional tests in patients with low back pain. *BMC Musculoskelet. Disord.* **2009**, *10*, 58. [CrossRef] [PubMed]
38. Ohe, A.; Kimura, T.; Goh, A.-C.; Oba, A.; Takahashi, J.; Mogami, Y. Characteristics of trunk control during crook-lying unilateral leg raising in different types of chronic low back pain patients. *Spine* **2015**, *40*, 550–559. [CrossRef] [PubMed]
39. Luomajoki, H.; Kool, J.; de Bruin, E.D.; Airaksinen, O. Movement control tests of the low back; evaluation of the difference between patients with low back pain and healthy controls. *BMC Musculoskelet. Disord.* **2008**, *9*, 170. [CrossRef] [PubMed]

40. Roussel, N.; De Kooning, M.; Schutt, A.; Mottram, S.; Truijen, S.; Nijs, J.; Daenen, L. Motor Control and Low Back Pain in Dancers. *Int. J. Sports Med.* **2012**, *34*, 138–143. [CrossRef] [PubMed]
41. Wattananon, P.; Ebaugh, D.; Biely, S.A.; Smith, S.S.; Hicks, G.E.; Silfies, S.P. Kinematic characterization of clinically observed aberrant movement patterns in patients with non-specific low back pain: A cross-sectional study. *BMC Musculoskelet. Disord.* **2017**, *18*, 455. [CrossRef]

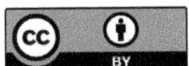

© 2019 by the authors. Licensee MDPI, Basel, Switzerland. This article is an open access article distributed under the terms and conditions of the Creative Commons Attribution (CC BY) license (http://creativecommons.org/licenses/by/4.0/).

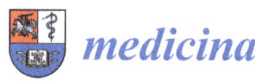

Article

Somatosensory and Motor Differences between Physically Active Patients with Chronic Low Back Pain and Asymptomatic Individuals

Juan Nieto-García [1], Luis Suso-Martí [2,3], Roy La Touche [1,2,4,5,*] and Mónica Grande-Alonso [1,2]

1. Departamento de Fisioterapia, Centro Superior de Estudios Universitarios La Salle, Universidad Autónoma de Madrid, 28023 Madrid, Spain
2. Motion in Brains Research Group, Institute of Neuroscience and Sciences of the Movement (INCIMOV), Centro Superior de Estudios Universitarios La Salle, Universidad Autónoma de Madrid, 28023 Madrid, Spain
3. Department of Physiotherapy, Universidad CEU Cardenal Herrera, CEU Universities, 46115 Valencia, Spain
4. Instituto de Neurociencia y Dolor Craneofacial (INDCRAN), 28023 Madrid, Spain
5. Instituto de Investigación Sanitaria del Hospital Universitario La Paz (IdiPAZ), 28046 Madrid, Spain
* Correspondence: roylatouche@yahoo.es; Tel.: +34-91-740-19-80; Fax: +34-91-357-17-30

Received: 30 June 2019; Accepted: 20 August 2019; Published: 23 August 2019

Abstract: *Background and Objectives*: Chronic low back pain (CLBP) is the most common occupational disorder due to its associated disability and high risk of recurrence and chronicity. However, the mechanisms underlying physical and psychological variables in patients with CLBP remain unclear. The main objective of this study was to assess whether there were differences between physically active patients with nonspecific CLBP compared with asymptomatic individuals in sensorimotor and psychological variables. *Materials and Methods*: This was an observational cross-sectional design with a nonprobabilistic sample. The sample was divided into two groups: individuals with nonspecific CLBP ($n = 30$) and asymptomatic individuals as a control (n = 30). The psychological variables assessed were low back disability, fear of movement, pain catastrophizing, and self-efficacy. The sensorimotor variables assessed were two-point discrimination, pressure pain threshold, lumbopelvic stability, lumbar flexion active range of motion, and isometric leg and back strength. *Results*: Statistically significant differences between the groups in terms of catastrophizing levels ($p = 0.026$) and fear of movement ($p = 0.001$) were found, but no statistically significant differences between groups were found in self-efficacy ($p > 0.05$). No statistically significant differences between the groups in any of the sensorimotor variables were found ($p > 0.05$). *Conclusion*: No sensorimotor differences were found between patients with asymptomatic and chronic low back pain, but differences were found in the psychological variables of catastrophizing and fear of movement.

Keywords: chronic low back pain; psychological variables; sensorimotor variables; pain catastrophizing; fear of movement

1. Introduction

Low back pain (LBP) is the most prevalent musculoskeletal problem and one of the most common reasons for medical consultations [1,2]. Research studies have determined that LBP is the most common occupational disorder due to its associated disability and multifactorial character as well as its high risk of recurrence and chronicity. Chronic LBP (CLBP) not determined by any previous pathology is called nonspecific CLBP and is defined as " ... tension, soreness and/or stiffness in the lower back region for which it is not possible to identify a specific cause of the pain. Several structures in the back, including the joints, discs and connective tissues, may contribute to symptoms" [3]. In addition, according to the World Health Organization (WHO), CLBP comprises approximately 85–90% of LBP cases [3].

Previous studies have determined that the chronicity of the symptoms could involve, at the neurophysiological level, a processing alteration at the central level. This alteration contributes to the generation of neuroplastic maladaptive changes at the medullary and the supramedullar levels in which psychological, somatosensory, and motor factors can be affected. [4,5]. It has been observed that patients with nonspecific CLBP present somatosensory alterations, such as a decrease in sensitivity or a lower pain pressure threshold [6]. The presence of tissue hyperalgesia is also common in these patients, suggesting that central sensitization mechanisms are involved [7]. It has been suggested that ongoing nociception is associated with cortical and subcortical reorganization and might play an important role in the process of LBP chronification [8]. Previous studies have suggested that such alterations could be determined by neurochemical changes produced during central sensitization processes in addition to a potential body schema distortion at the cortical level that might lead to alterations in tactile sensitivity [9,10]. These neurophysiological changes at the central level could be related to motor disorders present in patients with CLBP and poorer treatment responses [11].

In addition, central sensitization mechanisms could be associated with psychosocial factors, which play a significant role in patients with CLBP. Regarding the influence of psychosocial factors in individuals with nonspecific CLBP, there is an important body of evidence demonstrating that negative psychosocial attributes are strongly associated with a greater perception of pain and disability [12]. Thus, individuals with low levels of self-efficacy have greater fear of movement, which, at the same time, might lead to a greater perception of pain and disability [13,14]. Similarly, it has been observed that negative cognitive factors such as rumination correlate with a lower level of self-efficacy and, together with fear of movement and catastrophism, predict symptom recurrence [12,14,15]. In addition, it has been previously reported that motor and functional factors could be affected, such as extensor muscle strength, which influences motor control, dynamic stability, and range of motion [16]. Along these lines, it has been shown that patients who tend towards fear avoidance behaviors perceive greater disability levels and have less range of motion in lumbar flexion [17]. Similarly, higher levels of pain intensity, anxiety, depression, and fear avoidance result in negative outcomes in physical functioning [18]. Current research findings suggest neurophysiological mechanisms to explain why fear of pain is such a strong predictor of disability [19].

In recent years, new lines of research have emerged to identify the mechanisms underlying the associations between physical and psychological variables in patients with nonspecific CLBP [20]. Traditionally, physical inactivity has been associated with the appearance and the onset of CLBP. Previously, it has been shown that physical inactivity is associated with high-intensity low back pain and disability in a dose-dependent manner [21]. Therefore, one of the most commonly used therapeutic approaches in patients with CLBP today is therapeutic exercise and increased levels of physical activity [22]. However, it has been suggested that patients with CLBP are no less active than asymptomatic individuals, and that levels of physical activity are not associated with pain intensity or disability in a direct manner [23,24]. Thus, it remains uncertain which factors beyond activity levels participate in CLBP. Our hypothesis is that physically active patients with CLBP have differences in both psychological and sensorimotor variables related to the onset of CLBP compared with asymptomatic individuals.

Therefore, the main objective of this study was to assess differences between physically active patients with nonspecific CLBP compared with asymptomatic individuals in terms of sensorimotor and psychological variables, with both groups composed of physically active people currently participating in a general exercise program. The secondary objective was to analyze the association between sensorimotor variables and psychological variables in both groups.

2. Materials and Methods

2.1. Design

An observational cross-sectional study with a nonprobabilistic sample was designed. Participants were allocated into two groups, with the first group composed of patients with nonspecific CLBP, and asymptomatic individuals comprising the control group (CG). The procedures were planned following the ethical considerations of the Helsinki Declaration. The study was approved by the Local Ethics Committee of the La Salle University Centre for Advanced Studies, Madrid, Spain (Project identification code: CSEUL-PI-126/2016; Date: January 2016). This study followed the Strengthening the Reporting of Observational Studies in Epidemiology statement guidelines [25]. All participants completed the informed consent document prior to the study.

2.2. Setting and Participants

A consecutive, nonprobabilistic convenience sample of 30 patients with nonspecific CLBP and 30 asymptomatic individuals for the CG were recruited between April 2017 and July 2017. The sample was recruited from clients of a physical fitness center and patients of a physical therapy clinic, both located in Pozuelo de Alarcón, Spain.

The inclusion criteria for the CLBP group were (a) low back pain in at least the prior 6 months; (b) low back pain of a nonspecific nature; (c) men and women older than 18 years; and (d) participating in at least 1 moderate exercise session per week. The exclusion criteria were as follows: (a) neurological signs; (b) specific spinal pathology (e.g., inflammatory joint or bone diseases); (c) having had back surgery; and (d) signs of acute inflammation.

The CG was recruited from among the clients of the previously mentioned fitness center using posters, email newsletters, and social media. Asymptomatic individuals were examined and included in the study if they met the following criteria: (a) individuals who had not had low back pain in the last 6 months; (b) men and women older than 18 years; (c) participating in at least 1 moderate exercise session per week.

There were common exclusion criteria for both groups: (a) cognitive deficiencies that impede correct execution of the tests; (b) illiteracy; (c) understanding or communication difficulties or no comprehension of the Spanish language.

2.3. Outcomes

2.3.1. Psychological Variables

Low Back Disability

The Spanish version of the Roland Morris Disability Questionnaire (RMDQ) has demonstrated acceptable psychometric properties in measuring the perceived limitation of daily activities as a result of low back pain, and it has a Cronbach's alpha ranging between 0.84 and 0.93 [26,27]. The RMDQ is a 24-item self-administered questionnaire. Its total score ranges from 0 to 24, where higher scores indicate greater disability [28].

Fear of Movement

Fear of movement was assessed using the Spanish version of the Tampa Scale for Kinesiophobia (TSK-11), whose reliability and validity have been demonstrated (internal consistency, Cronbach's alpha = 0.78) [29]. The TSK-11 is a reduced version (11-item) of the TSK-11 questionnaire that eliminates psychometrically poor items from the original version of the TSK-11 and offers the advantage of brevity [30]. Higher scores indicate greater fear of pain and reinjury due to movement.

Pain Catastrophizing

Pain catastrophizing was assessed using the Spanish version of the Pain Catastrophizing Scale (PCS). The PCS has demonstrated good psychometric properties [31]. This scale is composed of 13 items divided into 3 domains: rumination, magnification, and helplessness. Higher scores indicate greater catastrophizing [32].

Self-Efficacy

The Spanish version of the Chronic Pain Self-Efficacy Scale (CPSS) has acceptable psychometric properties [33] in assessing perceived self-efficacy (SE) and an ability to cope with the consequences of chronic pain. The CPSS consists of 19 items and 3 domains that assess SE for pain management (PSE), physical function (FSE), and coping with symptoms (SSE). Higher scores indicate greater SE for managing pain [34]. The CPSS presented a reliability of 0.88, 0.87, and 0.90 for PSE, FSE, and SSE, respectively [34].

2.3.2. Sensorimotor Variables

Two-Point Discrimination

Research has shown that individual clinicians can reliably assess the 2-point discrimination (TPD) threshold at the neck, the back, the hand, and the foot using mechanical callipers [35]. Participants were positioned in prone decubitus, and the evaluator marked 1 cm lateral of the spinous apophysis of L3 towards the dominant side [36]. The test commenced with callipers set at 70 mm, and the evaluator decreased the distance by 10 mm until the participant was able to perceive only 1 point instead of 2 [35]. This test presented an intraclass correlation coefficient (ICC) of 0.81 (95% confidence interval) [36].

Pressure Pain Threshold

Algometers are devices that can be used to identify the pressure and/or the force eliciting a pressure pain threshold (PPT). Participants were positioned in prone decubitus, and the evaluator marked at 2 different points: the tibia and the erector spinae muscle. The evaluator then pressed against the tissue vertically, increasing the force at a constant rate of 1 kg/cm^2. The researcher instructed the individuals to express pain by saying "yes". This procedure has shown excellent reliability for the low back (ICC 0.86 to 0.99) and moderate to excellent reliability for the tibia (ICC 0.53–0.90). The evaluator took 3 measurements, and the mean was employed in the data analysis [37,38].

Lumbopelvic Stability

To assess the ability of the participants to voluntarily control the motion of the lower back, we selected the Hip Flexion Test measured with a "Pressure Biofeedback Unit" (PBU). A validation study concluded that trained examiners can reliably perform PBU measurements for patients with chronic LBP [39].

For this test, the participant lay supine with the hips and knees extended, and the PBU was positioned under the lumbar spine so that the inferior border of the device was aligned with the posterior superior iliac spine marks. After the participant was positioned, the PBU was inflated to 40 mm Hg pressure. The participant was then asked to flex their dominant hip, moving the knee towards the chest without touching the table with the foot. Once the maximum hip flexion was achieved, the pressure registered in the PBU was recorded by the assessor. The mean of 3 measurements was used in the analysis.

Lumbar Flexion Active Range of Motion

To collect this measurement, a mobile device goniometer called "Goniometer Records" was used. It has shown high intrarater reliability with an ICC greater than 0.80 (95% confidence interval) [40]. It can be used to assess the range of motion of spinal flexion, representing uniplanar movement [41].

The clinician held the mobile device over the participant's sacrum and maintained a slight pressure while the participant performed a "waiter's bow" movement. The mean of 3 measurements was employed in the data analysis.

Isometric Leg and Back Strength

To measure the isometric strength (IS) of the leg and the back extensor muscles, a portable dynamometer was used. The reliability of this device has been validated and can be used for determining leg and back strength in maintained positions, provided that the measurement protocol is standardized [42]. It is a valid and reliable test to measure muscular strength.

For the measurement, the participants let their arms hang straight down to hold the bar with both hands with the palms facing towards the body. The chain was then adjusted so that the knees were bent at approximately 110 degrees. Then, without bending the back, the participant pulled against the weight steadily as much as possible, trying to straighten their legs and keeping the arms straight. The evaluator took 3 measurements, and the mean was employed in the data analysis.

2.3.3. Physical Activity Level

The participants' levels of physical activity were measured by using the International Physical Activity Questionnaire (IPAQ), which divided the participants into 3 groups according to their level of activity: high, moderate, and low or inactive [43]. This questionnaire has shown acceptable validity and psychometric properties to measure total physical activity.

2.4. Procedure

For this study, both patients with nonspecific CLBP and the CG performed the same procedure following the same instructions. The assessor delivering the physical tests ignored whether the participant performing the test was from the CG or the CLBP group.

Once the participants signed the informed consent document, they received a sociodemographic questionnaire, which collected sex, date of birth, education level, and work situation. In addition, physical activity levels were assessed using the Spanish version of the IPAQ [44]. Once the sociodemographic and the IPAQ questionnaires were completed, the participants completed all 4 psychological questionnaires (RMDQ, PCS, TSK-11, and CPSS) in the same order for all the participants.

Following the completion of the self-reported measures, the participants were instructed to perform the sensorimotor tests in the same order (TPD, PPT, lumbopelvic stability (LS), lumbar flexion active range of motion (LF-AROM) and IS).

2.5. Data Analysis

The sociodemographic and the clinical variables of the participants were analyzed. The data were summarized using frequency counts, descriptive statistics, summary tables, and figures.

The data analysis was performed using the Statistics Package for Social Sciences (SPSS 20.00, IBM Inc., Armonk, NY, USA). The categorical variables are shown as frequencies and percentages. The quantitative results are represented by descriptive statistics (confidence interval, mean, and standard deviation). For all variables, the z-score was assumed to follow a normal distribution based on the central limit theorem because all the groups had more than 30 participants [45,46]. Student's t-test was used for the group comparisons. Cohen's d effect sizes were calculated for multiple comparisons of the outcome variables. According to Cohen's method, the magnitude of the effect was classified as small (0.20–0.49), medium (0.50–0.79), or large (0.80).

The relationships between psychological measures as well as between physical measurements were examined using Pearson's correlation coefficients. A Pearson's correlation coefficient greater than 0.60 indicated a strong correlation, a coefficient between 0.30 and 0.60 indicated a moderate correlation, and a coefficient below 0.30 indicated a low or very low correlation [47].

3. Results

Table 1 shows the baseline characteristics of the sociodemographic and the activity level variables. The total sample was 60 participants (27 women and 33 men). No statistically significant differences between groups in relation to sociodemographic or activity variables were found ($p > 0.05$) except for weight ($p = 0.016$). There were no statistically significant differences in age, sex, height, education, or physical activity levels ($p > 0.05$).

Table 1. Descriptive demographic data and control variables.

	CLBP ($n = 30$)	CG ($n = 30$)	p-Value
Age (years) [a]	49.3 ± 11.36	48 ± 10.74	0.65
Sex [b]			0.438
Female (%)	14 (46.7)	13 (43.3)	
Male (%)	16 (53.3)	17 (56.7)	
Height (cm) [a]	172.03 ± 7.55	169.57 ± 6.83	0.19
Weight (kg) [a]	73 ± 12.88	65.07 ± 11.80	0.016
Educational level [b]			0.64
No studies (%)	0 (0)	0 (0)	
Primary education (%)	0 (0)	0 (0)	
Secondary education (%)	3 (10)	2 (6,7)	
College education (%)	27 (90)	28 (93.3)	
IPAQ [b]			0.24
Low level (%)	6 (20)	2 (6.7)	
Moderate level (%)	13 (43.3)	18 (60)	
High level (%)	11 (36.7)	10 (33.3)	

Values are presented as mean ± standard deviation or number (%). CLBP: chronic low back pain; CG: control group; IPAQ: International Physical Activity Questionnaire. [a] Independent Student's t-test. [b] Chi-squared test.

3.1. Psychological Variables

Table 2 shows statistically significant differences between groups in catastrophizing levels ($p = 0.026$), including helplessness ($p = 0.036$) and magnification ($p = 0.01$) subscales of the PCS questionnaire and fear of movement ($p = 0.001$) in both subscales of the TSK-11 (activity avoidance and harm) ($p < 0.01$). No statistically significant differences between groups were found in any of the subscales of the CPSS, showing high levels of self-efficacy in both groups ($p > 0.05$).

Table 2. Comparative data for the psychological variables (Student's *t*-test and Cohen's *d*).

	CLBP (n = 30)	CG (n = 30)	Mean Difference (95% CI); Effect Size (d)
RMDQ	4.467 ± 2.97	-	-
PCS	12.13 ± 8.5	7.67 ± 6.48	4.47 (0.55 to 8.38) * d = 0.59
PCS-H	4.5 ± 2.85	3 ± 2.56	1.5 (0.1 to 2.9) * d = 0.55
PCS-M	3.57 ± 2.46	2.07 ± 1.84	1.5 (0.38 to 2.62) * d = 0.69
PCS-R	4.07 ± 4.05	2.6 ± 2.7	1.47 (−0.32 to 3.25) d = 0.43
TSK-11	25.57 ± 5.65	20.30 ± 5.40	5.27 (2.4 to 8.12) ** d = 0.95
TSK-AA	15.67 ± 3.74	12.37 ± 3.42	3.3 (1.45 to 5.15) ** d = 0.92
TSK-H	9.9 ± 2.82	7.93 ± 2.86	1.97 (0.49 to 3.44) * d = 0.69
CPSS	149.17 ± 21.40	153.4 ± 22.45	−4.23 (−15.57 to 7.10) d = −0.19
PSE	33.97 ± 10.70	35.83 ± 13.77	−1.87 (−8.25 to 4.52) d = −0.15
SSE	59.77 ± 12.44	61.10 ± 10.85	−1.33 (−7.37 to 4.70) d = −0.11
FSE	55.43 ± 5.09	56.47 ± 3.71	−1.03 (−3.34 to 1.27) d = −0.23

CLBP: chronic low back pain; CG: control group. RMDQ: Roland-Morris Disability Questionnaire; PCS: Pain Catastrophizing Scale; PCS-H: helplessness subscale of the PCS; PCS-M: magnification subscale of the PCS; PCS-R: rumination subscale of the PCS; TSK-11: Tampa Scale of Kinesiophobia; TSK-AA: activity avoidance subscale of the TSK-11; TSK-H: harm subscale of the TSK-11; CPSS: Chronic Pain Self-Efficacy Scale; PSE: self-efficacy in pain management; SSE: self-efficacy in coping with symptoms; FSE: self-efficacy in function. * p-value < 0.05; ** p-value < 0.01.

3.2. Sensorimotor Variables

Table 3 shows no statistically significant differences between groups in any of the sensorimotor variables ($p > 0.05$).

Table 3. Comparative data for the sample of sensorimotor variables (Student's *t*-test and Cohen's d).

	CLBP (n = 30)	CG (n = 30)	Mean Difference (95% CI); Effect Size (d)
PPT-T	4.95 ± 2.43	5.84 ± 1.9	−0.89 (−2.02 to 0.24) d = −0.41
PPT-LB	4.62 ± 2.23	5.1 ± 1.94	−0.47 (−1.55 to 0.60) d = −0.23
TPD	40.6 ± 14.89	38.17 ± 12.24	2.43 (−4.61 to 9.48) d = 0.18
IS	82.17 ± 35	77.31 ± 28.05	4.86 (−11.55 to 21.27) d = 0.15
LF-AROM	58.34 ± 14.92	63.94 ± 16.44	−5.60 (−13.71 to 2.51) d = −0.36
LS	8.76 ± 6.33	6.36 ± 3.15	2.4 (−0.20 to 5) d = 0.48

CLBP: chronic low back pain; CG: control group. PPT-T: pressure-pain threshold in tibia; PPT-T: pressure-pain threshold in low back; TDP: 2-point discrimination; IS: isometric strength; LF-AROM: lumbar flexion active range of motion; LS: lumbopelvic stability.

3.3. Correlation Analysis

Table 4 shows the results of the correlation analysis examining the bivariate relationships among sensorimotor and psychological measures. The strongest correlations found in the analysis were for the CG between fear of movement and LS. Less ability to control lumbopelvic motion was strongly correlated with higher scores on the TSK-11 (r = 0.524; $p < 0.01$). In the CG, a positive correlation was also found between higher FSE and higher LF-AROM (r = 0.406; $p < 0.05$) and low back pressure pain threshold (PPT-LB) (r = 0.412; $p < 0.05$). In the nonspecific CLBP group, a higher SSE was positively correlated with higher PPT both in the tibia (r = 0.382; $p < 0.05$) and the low back (r = 0.415; $p < 0.05$). Finally, a positive correlation between higher scores in the PPT-LB and the RMDQ was found (r = 0.368; $p < 0.05$).

Table 4. Pearson correlation analysis.

	PPT-T	PPT-LB	TPD	IS	LF-AROM	LS
RMDQ						
CLBP	0.329	0.368 *	0.078	−0.228	0.123	0.010
CG	−0.312	−0.090	−0.016	−0.260	0.191	0.052
PCS						
CLBP	0.035	−0.161	0.267	0.019	−0.130	−0.120
CG	−0.232	−0.307	0.116	−0.120	−0.268	−0.002
PCS-H						
CLBP	0.072	−0.133	0.209	0.038	−0.062	−0.181
CG	−0.159	−0.223	0.230	−0.036	−0.222	−0.014
PCS-M						
CLBP	0.004	−0.140	0.245	0.026	−0.257	0.045
CG	−0.172	−0.272	0.001	−0.224	−0.309	−0.002
PCS-R						
CLBP	0.019	−0.159	0.265	−0.002	−0.074	−0.152
CG	−0.289	−0.340	0.059	−0.100	−0.223	0.009
TSK-11						
CLBP	0.037	−0.058	0.335	0.030	−0.194	−0.014
CG	−0.128	−0.165	0.199	0.204	−0.207	0.524 **
TSK-AA						
CLBP	0.015	−0.047	0.301	−0.007	−0.230	0.005
CG	−0.107	−0.102	0.204	0.190	−0.187	0.406 *
TSK-H						
CLBP	0.054	−0.053	0.273	0.069	−0.085	−0.035
CG	−0.114	−0.189	0.130	0.157	−0.166	0.502 **
CPSS						
CLBP	0.221	0.149	−0.061	−0.001	−0.014	−0.076
CG	0.044	−0.091	0.135	0.038	0.276	0.030
PSE						
CLBP	−0.045	−0.175	−0.136	−0.028	−0.175	0.114
CG	−0.077	−0.165	0.199	−0.106	0.104	0.040
SSE						
CLBP	0.382 *	0.415 *	−0.060	−0.044	0.114	−0.224
CG	0.077	−0.120	0.072	0.098	0.300	0.059
FSE						
CLBP	0.091	−0.020	0.178	0.163	0.032	−0.010
CG	0.328	0.412 *	−0.132	0.337	0.406 *	−0.138

CLBP: chronic low back pain; CG: control group. RMDQ: Roland-Morris Disability Questionnaire; PCS: Pain Catastrophizing Scale; PCS-H: helplessness subscale of the PCS; PCS-M: magnification subscale of the PCS; PCS-R: rumination subscale of the PCS; TSK-11: Tampa Scale of Kinesiophobia; TSK-AA: activity avoidance subscale of the TSK-11; TSK-H: harm subscale of the TSK-11; CPSS: Chronic Pain Self-Efficacy Scale; PSE: self-efficacy for pain management; SSE: self-efficacy for coping with symptoms; FSE: self-efficacy for function. PPT-T: pressure-pain threshold in tibia; PPT-T: pressure-pain threshold in low back; TDP: 2-point discrimination; IS: isometric strength; LF-AROM: lumbar flexion active range of motion; LS: lumbopelvic stability. * $p < 0.05$. ** $p < 0.01$.

4. Discussion

The primary objective of this study was to determine the differences between psychological and sensorimotor measures between two physically active populations, one group with nonspecific CLBP and another group that was asymptomatic. Our results suggest no significant differences in somatosensory and functional variables. There were statistically significant differences in catastrophism and kinesiophobia but not in self-efficacy.

Numerous studies support the influence of various psychological factors in patients with chronic pain conditions. Among the most influential is the fear of movement, which, according to the fear avoidance model, is associated with catastrophic conditions and disability. Thus far, it has been determined that physical activity can act as a mediator, reducing disability and pain and therefore the fear of movement. Previous studies have shown that interventions based on physical activity can lead to changes in the fear of movement variable, despite the fact that the size of the effect has been small to medium. [48,49] On the other hand, other authors show that there are no significant changes in fear avoidance after an active intervention model, but instead in pain and disability. [50,51]. These results might suggest why the active population with nonspecific CLBP presents significant differences in psychological variables compared with asymptomatic individuals. In fact, Marshall et al. (2017) indicated that the best option for an intervention in the psychological factors that are not modified by regular physical activity is probably therapeutic education. [52].

Our results showed no significant differences between groups for the psychological variable of self-efficacy or for somatosensory and functional variables. This unusual characteristic of the nonspecific CLBP group can be explained by the socioeconomic context of the participants. Our sample reflects an active population with higher sociocultural and economic levels and patients who did not seek help for their condition. A higher socioeconomic status has been associated with lower disability in patients with CLBP [53]. The sample was recruited from among the clients of a physical activity facility where the individuals participate in two to four supervised exercise classes every week. There has been a considerable increase in the body of evidence showing the beneficial effects of physical activity and exercise in the management of CLBP in terms of certain psychological variables and, above all, on sensorimotor variables, which could justify our results, given both groups performed regular therapeutic exercise every week. [54,55].

According to our findings, patients with various conditions of chronic musculoskeletal pain who seek help present an external locus of control, which could be correlated with a lack of self-efficacy [56]. In addition, it has been shown that lack of self-efficacy correlates with greater pain intensity and greater disability, which is a predictive variable of chronic pain recovery [57–59]. This might be one of the reasons why our results did not provide significant differences between groups for the variable of self-efficacy and sensorimotor character, given we had patients with nonspecific CLBP who were not in active search of health care.

As for the results of the correlation analysis, only one large-magnitude association was found in our analysis. In healthy individuals, the greater the precision in controlling the lumbopelvic movement was, the less fear of movement existed. Physical activity, including motor control exercises, produces hypoalgesic effects [60]. The positive association between movement and psychological wellbeing in patients is key to reducing movement-related fear in patients with chronic pain. It is likely that the sense of stability and control in the lumbopelvic area in those patients facilitates positive behaviors that increase their confidence and reduce their fear of movement.

With respect to the nonspecific CLBP group, the strongest positive correlations were found between PPTs and lumbar disability and between PPTs and coping with symptoms subscales. Along these lines, Immura et al. found a correlation between PPTs in the lumbar region and the level of disability in patients with nonspecific CLBP [61]. In addition, a study performed by Falla et al. determined that the reduction in pain thresholds in patients with LBP was associated with different functional alterations, which suggests it could indirectly have an impact on perceived disability and level of self-efficacy [62].

Limitations

The most important limitation of this study is its cross-sectional design. Our findings are valid for suggesting new hypotheses but not for establishing causal relationships. In addition, no corrections have been made for multiple comparisons, which should be considered in the interpretation of the results. Future longitudinal research is recommended to confirm the hypothesis of this study. Therefore, other sensorimotor measures such as dynamic trunk movement, acceleration, or resistance would be necessary to obtain more consistent conclusions and to confirm these results. It would also be interesting to increase the sample size to confirm whether the obtained results could be extrapolated to larger populations.

5. Conclusions

The results of the present study suggest no sensorimotor differences between asymptomatic and physically active patients with CLBP. However, differences were found in the psychological variables of catastrophizing and fear of movement. No significant correlation was found between sensorimotor and psychological variables except for lumbopelvic stability and less fear of movement in healthy individuals. These results highlight the relevance of psychological variables in patients with CLBP and suggest that these variables should be considered clinically for the management of these patients.

Author Contributions: Conceptualization, J.N.-G., L.S.-M., R.L.T. and M.G.-A.; Data curation, J.N.-G., L.S.-M. and R.L.T.; Formal analysis, R.L.T. and M.G.-A.; Investigation, J.N.-G., L.S.-M., R.L.T. and M.G.-A.; Methodology, J.N.-G., R.L.T. and M.G.-A.; Resources, J.N.-G.; Supervision, R.L.T.; Validation, M.G.-A.; Writing—original draft, J.N.-G., L.S.-M., R.L.T. and M.G.-A.; Writing—review & editing, J.N.-G., L.S.-M., R.L.T. and M.G.-A.

Funding: This research received no external funding.

Conflicts of Interest: The authors declare no conflicts of interest.

References

1. Hoy, D.; Bain, C.; Williams, G.; March, L.; Brooks, P.; Blyth, F.; Woolf, A.; Vos, T.; Buchbinder, R. A systematic review of the global prevalence of low back pain. *Arthritis Rheum.* **2012**, *64*, 2028–2037. [CrossRef] [PubMed]
2. Rossignol, M.; Rozenberg, S.; Leclerc, A. Epidemiology of low back pain: What's new? *Joint Bone Spine* **2009**, *76*, 608–613. [CrossRef] [PubMed]
3. Savigny, P.; Watson, P.; Underwood, M. Guideline Development Group. Early management of persistent non-specific low back pain: Summary of NICE guidance. *BMJ* **2009**, *338*, b1805. [CrossRef] [PubMed]
4. Hashmi, J.A.; Baliki, M.N.; Huang, L.; Baria, A.T.; Torbey, S.; Hermann, K.M.; Schnitzer, T.J.; Apkarian, A.V. Shape shifting pain: Chronification of back pain shifts brain representation from nociceptive to emotional circuits. *Brain* **2013**, *136*, 2751–2768. [CrossRef] [PubMed]
5. Zusman, M. Forebrain-mediated sensitization of central pain pathways: "non-specific" pain and a new image for MT. *Man. Ther.* **2002**, *7*, 80–88. [CrossRef]
6. Imamura, M.; Chen, J.; Matsubayashi, S.R.; Targino, R.A.; Alfieri, F.M.; Bueno, D.K.; Hsing, W.T. Changes in Pressure Pain Threshold in Patients With Chronic Nonspecific Low Back Pain. *Spine (Phila Pa 1976)* **2013**, *38*, 2098–2107. [CrossRef] [PubMed]
7. O'Neill, S.; Manniche, C.; Graven-Nielsen, T.; Arendt-Nielsen, L. Generalized deep-tissue hyperalgesia in patients with chronic low-back pain. *Eur. J. Pain* **2007**, *11*, 415–420. [CrossRef]
8. Roussel, N.A.; Nijs, J.; Meeus, M.; Mylius, V.; Fayt, C.; Oostendorp, R. Central Sensitization and Altered Central Pain Processing in Chronic Low Back Pain. *Clin. J. Pain* **2013**, *29*, 625–638. [CrossRef]
9. Grachev, I.D.; Fredrickson, B.E.; Apkarian, A.V. Brain chemistry reflects dual states of pain and anxiety in chronic low back pain. *J. Neural Transm.* **2002**, *109*, 1309–1334. [CrossRef]
10. Lloyd, D.; Findlay, G.; Roberts, N.; Nurmikko, T. Differences in Low Back Pain Behavior Are Reflected in the Cerebral Response to Tactile Stimulation of the Lower Back. *Spine (Phila Pa 1976)* **2008**, *33*, 1372–1377. [CrossRef]
11. Sanzarello, I.; Merlini, L.; Rosa, M.A.; Perrone, M.; Frugiuele, J.; Borghi, R.; Faldini, C. Central sensitization in chronic low back pain: A narrative review. *J. Back Musculoskelet Rehabil.* **2016**, *29*, 625–633. [CrossRef] [PubMed]
12. Meyer, K.; Tschopp, A.; Sprott, H.; Mannion, A.F. Association between catastrophizing and self-rated pain and disability in patients with chronic low back pain. *J. Rehabil. Med.* **2009**, *41*, 620–625. [CrossRef] [PubMed]
13. Woby, S.R.; Urmston, M.; Watson, P.J. Self-efficacy mediates the relation between pain-related fear and outcome in chronic low back pain patients. *Eur. J. Pain* **2007**, *11*, 711–718. [CrossRef] [PubMed]
14. de Moraes Vieira, É.B.; de Góes Salvetti, M.; Damiani, L.P.; de Mattos Pimenta, C.A. Self-Efficacy and Fear Avoidance Beliefs in Chronic Low Back Pain Patients: Coexistence and Associated Factors. *Pain. Manag. Nurs.* **2014**, *15*, 593–602. [CrossRef] [PubMed]
15. Sullivan, M.J.; Thorn, B.; Haythornthwaite, J.A.; Keefe, F.; Martin, M.; Bradley, L.A.; Lefebvre, J.C. Theoretical perspectives on the relation between catastrophizing and pain. *Clin. J. Pain* **2001**, *17*, 52–64. [CrossRef] [PubMed]

16. Behennah, J.; Conway, R.; Fisher, J.; Osborne, N.; Steele, J. The relationship between balance performance, lumbar extension strength, trunk extension endurance, and pain in participants with chronic low back pain, and those without. *Clin. Biomech.* **2018**, *53*, 22–30. [CrossRef]
17. Basler, H.D.; Luckmann, J.; Wolf, U.; Quint, S. Fear-avoidance Beliefs, Physical Activity, and Disability in Elderly Individuals With Chronic Low Back Pain and Healthy Controls. *Clin. J. Pain* **2008**, *24*, 604–610. [CrossRef]
18. Guclu, D.G.; Guclu, O.; Ozaner, A.; Senormanci, O.; Konkan, R. The relationship between disability, quality of life and fear-avoidance beliefs in patients with chronic low back pain. *Turk. Neurosurg.* **2012**, *22*, 724–731. [CrossRef]
19. Sullivan, M.J.L.; Thibault, P.; Andrikonyte, J.; Butler, H.; Catchlove, R.; Larivière, C. Psychological influences on repetition-induced summation of activity-related pain in patients with chronic low back pain. *Pain* **2009**, *141*, 70–78. [CrossRef]
20. Karayannis, N.V.; Smeets, R.J.E.M.; van den Hoorn, W.; Hodges, P.W. Fear of Movement Is Related to Trunk Stiffness in Low Back Pain. *PLoS ONE* **2013**, *8*, e67779. [CrossRef]
21. Teichtahl, A.J.; Urquhart, D.M.; Wang, Y.; Wluka, A.E.; O'Sullivan, R.; Jones, G.; Cicuttini, F.M. Physical inactivity is associated with narrower lumbar intervertebral discs, high fat content of paraspinal muscles and low back pain and disability. *Arthritis Res. Ther.* **2015**, *17*, 114. [CrossRef] [PubMed]
22. Gordon, R.; Bloxham, S. A Systematic Review of the Effects of Exercise and Physical Activity on Non-Specific Chronic Low Back Pain. *Healthc (Basel Switz.)* **2016**, *4*, 22. [CrossRef] [PubMed]
23. Hendrick, P.; Milosavljevic, S.; Hale, L.; Hurley, D.A.; McDonough, S.; Ryan, B.; Baxter, G.D. The relationship between physical activity and low back pain outcomes: A systematic review of observational studies. *Eur. Spine J.* **2011**, *20*, 464–474. [CrossRef] [PubMed]
24. Griffin, D.W.; Harmon, D.C.; Kennedy, N.M. Do patients with chronic low back pain have an altered level and/or pattern of physical activity compared to healthy individuals? A systematic review of the literature. *Physiotherapy* **2012**, *98*, 13–23. [CrossRef] [PubMed]
25. von Elm, E.; Altman, D.G.; Egger, M.; Pocock, S.J.; Gøtzsche, P.C.; Vandenbroucke, J.P. The Strengthening the Reporting of Observational Studies in Epidemiology (STROBE) statement: Guidelines for reporting observational studies. *J. Clin. Epidemiol.* **2008**, *61*, 344–349. [CrossRef] [PubMed]
26. Roland, M.; Fairbank, J. The Roland-Morris disability questionnaire and the Oswestry disability questionnaire. *Spine (Phila Pa 1976)* **2000**, *25*, 3115–3124. [CrossRef]
27. Kovacs, F.M.; Llobera, J.; Gil Del Real, M.T.; Abraira, V.; Gestoso, M.; Fernández, C.; Primaria Group, K.A. Validation of the spanish version of the Roland-Morris questionnaire. *Spine (Phila Pa 1976)* **2002**, *27*, 538–542. [CrossRef]
28. Roland, M.; Morris, R. A study of the natural history of back pain. Part I: Development of a reliable and sensitive measure of disability in low-back pain. *Spine (Phila Pa 1976)* **1983**, *8*, 141–144. [CrossRef]
29. Gomez-Perez, L.; Lopez-Martinez, A.E.; Ruiz-Parraga, G.T. Psychometric Properties of the Spanish Version of the Tampa Scale for Kinesiophobia (TSK). *J. Pain* **2011**, *12*, 425–435. [CrossRef]
30. Woby, S.R.; Roach, N.K.; Urmston, M.; Watson, P.J. Psychometric properties of the TSK-11: A shortened version of the Tampa Scale for Kinesiophobia. *Pain* **2005**, *117*, 137–144. [CrossRef]
31. García Campayo, J.; Rodero, B.; Alda, M.; Sobradiel, N.; Montero, J.; Moreno, S. Validation of the Spanish version of the Pain Catastrophizing Scale in fibromyalgia. *Med. Clin. (Barc.)* **2008**, *131*, 487–492. [CrossRef] [PubMed]
32. Sullivan, M.J.L.; Bishop, S.R.; Pivik, J. The Pain Catastrophizing Scale: Development and validation. *Psychol. Assess.* **1995**, *7*, 524–532. [CrossRef]
33. Martín-Aragón, M.; Pastor, M.A.; Rodríguez-Marí, N.J.; March, M.J.; Lledó, A.L. pez-RS. Percepción de autoeficacia en dolor crónico: Adaptación y validación de la Chronic Pain Self-Efficacy Scale. *Rev. Psicol. La Salud* **1999**, *11*, 53–75.
34. Anderson, K.O.; Dowds, B.N.; Pelletz, R.E.; Edwards, W.T.; Peeters-Asdourian, C. Development and initial validation of a scale to measure self-efficacy beliefs in patients with chronic pain. *Pain* **1995**, *63*, 77–84. [CrossRef]
35. Catley, M.J.; Tabor, A.; Wand, B.M.; Moseley, G.L. Assessing tactile acuity in rheumatology and musculoskeletal medicine—how reliable are two-point discrimination tests at the neck, hand, back and foot? *Rheumatology* **2013**, *52*, 1454–1461. [CrossRef] [PubMed]

36. Nolan, M.F. Quantitative measure of cutaneous sensation. Two-point discrimination values for the face and trunk. *Phys. Ther.* **1985**, *65*, 181–185. [CrossRef] [PubMed]
37. Aweid, O.; Gallie, R.; Morrissey, D.; Crisp, T.; Maffulli, N.; Malliaras, P.; Padhiar, N. Medial tibial pain pressure threshold algometry in runners. *Knee Surg. Sport Traumatol. Arthrosc.* **2014**, *22*, 1549–1555. [CrossRef] [PubMed]
38. Balaguier, R.; Madeleine, P.; Vuillerme, N. Is One Trial Sufficient to Obtain Excellent Pressure Pain Threshold Reliability in the Low Back of Asymptomatic Individuals? A Test-Retest Study. *PLoS ONE* **2016**, *11*, e0160866. [CrossRef]
39. Azevedo, D.C.; Lauria, A.C.; Pereira, A.R.S.; Andrade, G.T.; Ferreira, M.L.; Ferreira, P.H.; Van Dillen, L. Intraexaminer and Interexaminer Reliability of Pressure Biofeedback Unit for Assessing Lumbopelvic Stability During 6 Lower Limb Movement Tests. *J. Manip. Physiol. Ther.* **2013**, *36*, 33–43. [CrossRef]
40. Kolber, M.J.; Mdt, C.; Pizzini, M.; Robinson, A.; Yanez, D.; Hanney, W.J. Original research the reliability and concurrent validity of measurements used to quantify lumbar spine mobility: An analysis of an iphone application. *Int. J. Sports Phys. Ther.* **2013**, *8*, 129–137.
41. Bedekar, N.; Suryavanshi, M.; Rairikar, S.; Sancheti, P.; Shyam, A. Inter and intra-rater reliability of mobile device goniometer in measuring lumbar flexion range of motion. *J. Back Musculoskelet. Rehabil.* **2014**, *27*, 161–166. [CrossRef] [PubMed]
42. Coldwells, A.; Atkinson, G.; Reilly, T. Sources of variation in back and leg dynamometry. *Ergonomics* **1994**, *37*, 79–86. [CrossRef] [PubMed]
43. Roman-Viñas, B.; Serra-Majem, L.; Hagströmer, M.; Ribas-Barba, L.; Sjöström, M.; Segura-Cardona, R. International Physical Activity Questionnaire: Reliability and validity in a Spanish population. *Eur. J. Sport Sci.* **2010**, *10*, 297–304. [CrossRef]
44. Rubio Castaneda, F.J.; Tomas Aznar, C.; Muro Baquero, C. Validity, Reliability and Associated Factors of the International Physical Activity Questionnaire Adapted to Elderly (IPAQ-E). *Rev. Esp. Salud Publica* **2017**, *91*, e201701004. [PubMed]
45. Mouri, H. Log-normal distribution from a process that is not multiplicative but is additive. *Phys. Rev. E* **2013**. [CrossRef] [PubMed]
46. Nixon, R.M.; Wonderling, D.; Grieve, R.D. Non-parametric methods for cost-effectiveness analysis: The central limit theorem and the bootstrap compared. *Health Econ.* **2010**, *19*, 316–333. [CrossRef]
47. Hinkle, D.E.; Wiersma, W.; Jurs, S.G. Applied Statistics for the Behavioral Sciences. *Source J. Educ. Stat.* **1990**, *15*, 84–87.
48. Henry, S.M.; Van Dillen, L.R.; Ouellette-Morton, R.H.; Hitt, J.R.; Lomond, K.V.; DeSarno, M.J.; Bunn, J.Y. Outcomes are not different for patient-matched versus nonmatched treatment in subjects with chronic recurrent low back pain: A randomized clinical trial. *Spine J.* **2014**, *14*, 2799–2810. [CrossRef]
49. da Luz, M.A.; Costa, L.O.P.; Fuhro, F.F.; Manzoni, A.C.T.; Oliveira, N.T.B.; Cabral, C.M.N. Effectiveness of Mat Pilates or Equipment-Based Pilates Exercises in Patients With Chronic Nonspecific Low Back Pain: A Randomized Controlled Trial. *Phys. Ther.* **2014**, *94*, 623–631. [CrossRef]
50. Marshall, P.W.M.; Kennedy, S.; Brooks, C.; Lonsdale, C. Pilates Exercise or Stationary Cycling for Chronic Nonspecific Low Back Pain. *Spine (Phila Pa 1976)* **2013**, *38*, E952–E959. [CrossRef]
51. Balthazard, P.; de Goumoens, P.; Rivier, G.; Demeulenaere, P.; Ballabeni, P.; Dériaz, O. Manual therapy followed by specific active exercises versus a placebo followed by specific active exercises on the improvement of functional disability in patients with chronic non specific low back pain: A randomized controlled trial. *BMC Musculoskelet. Disord.* **2012**, *13*, 162. [CrossRef] [PubMed]
52. Marshall, P.W.M.; Schabrun, S.; Knox, M.F. Physical activity and the mediating effect of fear, depression, anxiety, and catastrophizing on pain related disability in people with chronic low back pain. *PLoS ONE* **2017**, *12*, e0180788. [CrossRef] [PubMed]
53. Valencia, C.; Robinson, M.E.; George, S.Z. Socioeconomic status influences the relationship between fear-avoidance beliefs work and disability. *Pain Med.* **2011**, *12*, 328–336. [CrossRef] [PubMed]
54. Hayden, J.A.; van Tulder, M.W.; Tomlinson, G. Systematic review: Strategies for using exercise therapy to improve outcomes in chronic low back pain. *Ann. Intern. Med.* **2005**, *142*, 776–785. [CrossRef] [PubMed]
55. Searle, A.; Spink, M.; Ho, A.; Chuter, V. Exercise interventions for the treatment of chronic low back pain: a systematic review and meta-analysis of randomised controlled trials. *Clin. Rehabil.* **2015**, *29*, 1155–1167. [CrossRef] [PubMed]

56. Rollman, A.; Gorter, R.; Visscher, C.; Naeije, M. Why Seek Treatment for Temporomandibular Disorder Pain Complaints? A Study Based on Semi-structured Interviews. *J. Orofac. Pain* **2013**, *27*, 227–234. [CrossRef] [PubMed]
57. Esteve, R.; Ramírez-Maestre, C.; López-Marínez, A.E. Adjustment to chronic pain: The role of pain acceptance, coping strategies, and pain-related cognitions. *Ann. Behav. Med.* **2007**, *33*, 179–188. [CrossRef]
58. Dohnke, B.; Knäuper, B.; Müller-Fahrnow, W. Perceived self-efficacy gained from, and health effects of, a rehabilitation program after hip joint replacement. *Arthritis Rheum.* **2005**, *53*, 585–592. [CrossRef]
59. Brisson, N.M.; Gatti, A.A.; Stratford, P.W.; Maly, M.R. Self-efficacy, pain, and quadriceps capacity at baseline predict changes in mobility performance over 2 years in women with knee osteoarthritis. *Clin. Rheumatol.* **2018**, *37*, 495–504. [CrossRef]
60. Ellingson, L.D.; Koltyn, K.F.; Kim, J.S.; Cook, D.B. Does exercise induce hypoalgesia through conditioned pain modulation? *Psychophysiology* **2014**, *51*, 267–276. [CrossRef]
61. Imamura, M.; Alfieri, F.M.; Filippo, T.R.M.; Battistella, L.R. Pressure pain thresholds in patients with chronic nonspecific low back pain. *J. Back Musculoskelet. Rehabil.* **2016**, *29*, 327–336. [CrossRef] [PubMed]
62. Falla, D.; Gizzi, L.; Tschapek, M.; Erlenwein, J.; Petzke, F. Reduced task-induced variations in the distribution of activity across back muscle regions in individuals with low back pain. *Pain* **2014**, *155*, 944–953. [CrossRef] [PubMed]

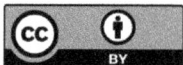

© 2019 by the authors. Licensee MDPI, Basel, Switzerland. This article is an open access article distributed under the terms and conditions of the Creative Commons Attribution (CC BY) license (http://creativecommons.org/licenses/by/4.0/).

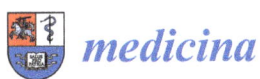

Article

Rehabilitation Program Combined with Local Vibroacoustics Improves Psychophysiological Conditions in Patients with ACL Reconstruction

Jung-Min Park [1], Sihwa Park [1] and Yong-Seok Jee [1,2,*]

1. Research Institute of Sports and Industry Science, Hanseo University, Seosan 31962, Korea; mine7728@hanmail.net (J.-M.P.); slim@korea.ac.kr (S.P.)
2. Department of Leisure Marine Sports, Hanseo University, Seosan 31962, Korea; jeeys@hanseo.ac.kr
* Correspondence: jeeys@hanseo.ac.kr; Tel.: +82-41-660-1028; Fax: +82-41-660-1088

Received: 10 July 2019; Accepted: 26 September 2019; Published: 30 September 2019

Abstract: *Background and objective*: This study investigated the therapeutic effect of applying local body vibration (LBV) with built-in vibroacoustic sound on patients who had an anterior cruciate ligament (ACL) reconstruction. *Materials and Methods*: Twenty-four participants were randomly classified into a LBV group (LBVG; n = 11) or a non-LBV group (nLBVG; n = 13). Both groups received the same program; however, the LBVG received LBV. Psychological measures included pain, anxiety, and symptoms; physiological measures included systolic blood pressure (SBP), diastolic blood pressure, heart rate (HR), breathing rate (BR), sympathetic activation (SA), parasympathetic activation (PSA), range of motion (ROM), and isokinetic muscle strength at Weeks 0, 4, and 8. *Results*: Among the psychophysiological variables, pain, anxiety, symptoms, SBP, BR, and SA were significantly reduced in both groups, whereas HR, PSA, isokinetic peak torque (PT) of the knee joint, and ROM were significantly improved only in the LBVG. Comparing both groups, a significant difference appeared in pain, symptom, SA, PSA, isokinetic PT, and ROM at Weeks 4 and 8. *Conclusions*: The results indicate that the LBV intervention mitigated the participants' pain and symptoms and improved their leg strength and ROM, thus highlighting its effectiveness.

Keywords: vibration; pain; symptoms; peak torque; parasympathetic activation; range of motion

1. Introduction

In recent years, various researchers have developed new therapeutic methods using body sounds and have employed techniques such as vibroacoustic sound therapy (VAST) [1]. VAST is a viable form of therapy since bodies are always in motion and the microvibrations that are generated in cells are energy-intensive and involved in an individual's immune response. These microvibrations not only heal damaged cells, but also constantly express energy at the cellular level. These biological phenomena cause immediate vibrations in a human body, which can decrease recovery time from intense stress or fatigue after injury [2]. One study showed that applying vibrations for 30 min with frequency ranges of 10–100 Hz to PC12 cells, which are used to find what prion protein fragments cause neuronal dysfunction, resulted in a significantly higher neurite outgrowth due to the activation of p38 mitogen-activated protein kinases [3]. Another study confirmed the clinical efficacy of VAST when compared to laser and ultrasound therapy [4]. In that study, participants who had a heel spur were classified into two groups to observe differences in pain. One group received VAST, while the other group was treated with ultrasound and laser therapy. The results showed a tentative confirmation of the analgesic effectiveness of VAST in musculoskeletal overload conditions [4]. Another study also observed the effects of VAST among patients with various medical problems by performing a rest program for pain and symptom relief. The authors concluded that the 22-min VAST session had a

53% cumulative reduction in pain and symptoms. Other side effects such as pain, tension, fatigue, headache, and nausea were also reported to have reduced post-treatment [2].

Recently, the development of medical technology has made it easier for people to surgically treat various diseases and injuries. However, rehabilitation often takes a long time because patients feel pain and anxiety post-surgery. This is especially true for patients who have had surgery due to joint disease, and temporarily lose strength and range of motion (ROM). Although an aggressive rehabilitation program including flexibility, strength, and balance training is effective at maintaining or enhancing muscle strength and ROM [5], it may not be easy to apply such measures to patients immediately post-operation.

In general, whole body vibration (WBV) is a rather passive approach to active exercise. It has been suggested that this is similar to common types of exercise that people are accustomed to [6]. There are indications of the positive effects from WBV in immobilized patients. Moreover, VAST waves provide a similar effect to WBV [7]. Additionally, WBV induces improvements in muscular strength and performance and changes in peripheral circulation [8].

Local body vibration (LBV) devices with built-in VAST have been developed in Korea, and they are designed to be hand-operated. Unlike most sonic motors, a new device called Evocell has vibration patterns that are consistent and offer a wide range of sound waves, which change according to the flow of music. Therefore, there is a dual effect in that patients can listen to music while receiving stimuli to injured areas by the synchronized vibrations. Although this technique has been employed in a few hospitals in Korea, its effects have not yet been confirmed. LBV is designed to restore damaged tissue by transmitting vibrations and sound waves in the form of music to specific parts of the body, unlike WBV, where patients must stand on the vibrator to receive stimuli throughout the body. LBV is likely to have an additional psychological effect; however, the mechanisms are not clear.

Therefore, this study hypothesized that LBV penetrates deep into muscle tissues, affects systemic circulation and the autonomic nervous system (ANS), and potentially improves psychological condition. Consequently, such an intervention could lead to decreased pain and anxiety and greater joint flexibility and muscle strength. This study examined a group of patients with an anterior cruciate ligament (ACL) reconstruction in a randomized controlled trial and assessed the psychophysiological effect of a LBV intervention using vibroacoustic sound.

2. Materials and Methods

2.1. Study Design and Participants

This study took place in a research center from 1 December 2017 to 6 February 2018. The first assessment was conducted from 1 to 2 December 2017, the second assessment from 2 to 3 January 2018, and the last assessment from 5 to 6 February 2018. Participants were recruited through the recommendation of a surgeon familiar with LBV. Prior to the study, participants received detailed explanations regarding the study procedures and were then asked to complete questions. The included criteria required that participants underwent an ACL reconstruction no more than seven days before the start of the study. Participants were evaluated by clinical and radiological criteria, level of knee pain during the past month, and pain or difficulty in standing from a sitting position or climbing stairs [9]. All participants were patients who did not exercise regularly for over six months. Additionally, participants were also included if they had not received treatment/medication for weight loss or anything known to affect body composition, and if they did not have any internal metallic materials. The participants' mean (SD) age was 29.25 (14.51) years. After excluding three participants (one had cardiac surgery three years prior and two refused to participate because their homes were too far from the hospital or research center) of fifty-five eligible participants, the remaining fifty-two participants belonged to one of two groups by lot and were randomly allocated to each group as shown in Figure 1. Of the 26 participants in the experimental group who were allocated to the LBV group (LBVG), one did not receive the assessment, two were lost in the follow-up phase, eight underwent arthroscopic surgery for complex injuries to their ACL or posterior cruciate ligament, and four underwent ACL arthroplasty. Therefore, eleven participants of the LBVG who underwent ACL reconstruction were analyzed in our study. Furthermore, of the 26 patients in the control group who were allocated to the non-LBV group (nLBVG), two did not receive the assessment, two were lost in the follow-up phase, and nine underwent arthroscopic surgery with a simple ACL rupture. Therefore, thirteen participants in the nLBVG who underwent ACL reconstruction were analyzed in our study. Exclusion criteria consisted of having a history of impairment of a major organ system or psychiatric disease. Participants with tumors, vascular inflammation, or kidney stones were also excluded. The LBVG received vibroacoustic pulses, whereas the nLBVG received massages by a VAST device without vibroacoustic pulses as a placebo. This study investigated psychological measures such as pain, anxiety, and symptoms; and physiological measures such as systolic blood pressure (SBP), diastolic blood pressure (DBP), heart rate (HR), breathing rate (BR), sympathetic activation (SA), parasympathetic activation (PSA), range of motion (ROM), and isokinetic peak torque (PT) in the quadriceps and hamstrings at Weeks 0, 4, and 8. Finally, twenty-four participants were interviewed and informed about the rehabilitation program they would receive. As shown in Figure 1, the participants were allocated as follows: LBVG (n = 11) and nLBV (n = 13). All participants were assigned using random number tables and assigned identification numbers upon recruitment. Participant characteristics, which indicate homogeneity, are presented in Table 1.

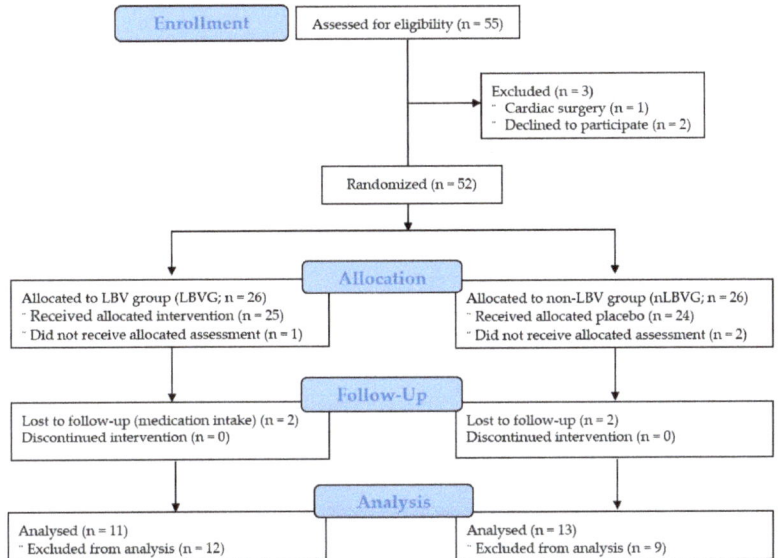

Figure 1. Participant allocation (consolidated standards for reporting of trials flow diagram).

Table 1. Characteristics of the participants.

Items	Groups		Z	p *
	LBVG (n = 11)	nLBVG (n = 13)		
Age, year	26.82 ± 12.08	31.31 ± 16.49	−0.150	0.910
Height, cm	173.00 ± 4.02	174.23 ± 2.35	−0.703	0.494
Weight, kg	74.00 ± 5.37	75.50 ± 6.54	−0.321	0.776
Muscle mass, kg	36.04 ± 5.99	36.94 ± 4.26	−0.933	0.361
Fat mass, kg	14.09 ± 5.38	15.38 ± 3.60	−1.341	0.186
Body mass index, kg/m^2	24.72 ± 1.57	24.85 ± 1.72	−0.349	0.733

All data represent the mean ± standard deviation. LBVG and nLBVG mean local body vibration group and non-local body vibration group, respectively. Symbol * was analyzed by the Mann–Whitney U test.

2.2. Research Ethics

This study was conducted in accordance with the Declaration of Helsinki and was approved by the Institutional Review Board at Sahmyook Univ. (2-7001793-AB-N-012018034HR). All subjects were recruited through advertisements and a written informed consent was obtained before enrollment. First, all of the subjects arrived at the research center to sign an informed consent form and to complete a self-reported questionnaire about their health status. After this procedure, all subjects participated in the experiment conducted by an expert.

2.3. Anthropometric Measurements

To measure body composition, all subjects were weighed while wearing light clothes and without shoes. The bioelectrical impedance analysis method was employed using BMS 330 and InBody 320 Body Composition Analyzer (Biospace Co. Ltd., Seoul, Korea), respectively. The analyzer was a segmental impedance device measuring voltage drops in the upper and lower body. Eight tactile electrodes were placed on the surfaces of the hands and feet. The precision of the repeated measurements expressed as a coefficient of variation was, on average, 0.6% for the percentage of fat mass [7].

2.4. Psychological Condition: Pain, Anxiety, and Symptom

A visual analogue scale (VAS) was used to measure psychological concerns. Each subject was asked to rate how they felt as they received LBV using a bipolar rating scale, which was a 5 × 10 cm bar-shaped box. The pain scale ranged from no pain (close to "0") to severe pain (close to "10"). After participants marked within the box, a transparent paper with a score indicator was placed on top of the boxes to obtain a numerical score. The scales for measuring the levels of anxiety and symptoms were similar to the pain scale. In other words, the anxiety or symptom scale ranged from no anxiety or no symptom (close to "0") to severe anxiety or symptom (close to "10") [10]. Participants were evaluated by a professional psychologist at the beginning and end of the study. The reliabilities of the scales were measured by calculating Cronbach's α, representing internal consistency. The Cronbach's α of pain, anxiety, and symptom were 0.722, 0.816, and 0.799, respectively.

2.5. Physiological Conditions

2.5.1. Blood Pressure and Heart Rate Measurement

The examiner placed an adjustable cuff on each participant's upper arm and electronically pumped air into the cuff by pressing the start button on the digital BP monitor (HEM-741C-C1, Omron Co. Ltd., Seoul, Korea). SBP, DBP, and HR were measured between 1 and 2 min after the air was released automatically once a pressure of 200 mmHg was reached. Thirty minutes before the measurement, participants were not allowed to smoke or consume caffeine. During the measurement, they were placed in a sitting position with their arms raised to their heart height. If a participant's upper arm circumference was more than 33 cm, a larger cuff was used. After two measurements, the mean value was used as data.

2.5.2. Autonomic Nervous System Measurement

ANS was measured by HR variability (HRV). To obtain an accurate measure of HRV, participants were asked to refrain from exercising or consuming alcohol the day before the experiment. Food or caffeine were not consumed for 3 h prior to the measurement. On the day of measurement, HRV was tested twice at 10:00 am and 3:00 pm, and the mean values were recorded. Thirty minutes before the start of the measurement, the participants were asked to sit on a chair and rest. Then, the measurement was taken during the participants' resting HR. HRV was measured for 2.5 min and factors affecting the measurement such as conversation, coughing, and deep breathing were controlled. uBioMacpa (Biosensecreative Co. Ltd., Seoul, Korea) and its embedded software was used for HRV measurements and analyses. HRV is the most commonly used for time domain and frequency domain analyses [11,12]. In the time domain analysis, the interval between normal QRS complexes or the instantaneous HR at a specific point is measured to calculate a normal-to-normal interval (NN interval) between consecutive normal QRS complexes. The standard deviation of NN interval (SDNN) can be determined using the NN interval. SDNN reflects all the cycle elements contributing to HRV. A decrease in SDNN means that the ability to cope with stress is reduced, and the overall health status and ANS control capacity are impaired. The RMSSD (square root of mean squared differences of successive NN intervals) is the square root of the square mean of successive NN interval differences, reflecting the short-term change in HR. This correlates well with the high-frequency index values of the frequency domain analysis and mainly reflects parasympathetic activity. When parasympathetic activity decreases, the RMSSD value also decreases. In general, the larger the RMSSD value, the more physiologically healthy and relaxed one is. Frequency domain analysis of HRV provides information on the HRV spectral components, high frequency, and low frequency range, which reflect the sympathetic and parasympathetic nervous system branches [11,12]. This spectral component is calculated mainly through short-term measurements (i.e., 2–5 min).

2.5.3. Range of Motion Measurement

The ROM of an operated knee joint with an ACL reconstruction was measured using a goniometer in the extended and flexed positions [13]. During the measurement, the ROM of the injured side was measured twice when the participants were actively extended or flexed. Then, the mean values of the two measurements were recorded.

2.5.4. Isokinetic Strength Measurement

Participants were positioned in the isokinetic dynamometer (HUMAC®/NORM™ Testing and Rehabilitation System, CSMi, Stoughton, MA, USA) according to the manufacturer's guidelines for evaluating knee flexion/extension. Each participant sat in an adjustable seat and the tested limb was fixed in place with a Velcro strap on a support over the quadriceps while the knee joint was positioned at their flexed knee angle. The testing apparatus was set up and the participants were positioned and stabilized uniformly while sitting. Testing was performed on the uninjured side first and then performed on the operated side to diminish the possible apprehension of the participants. The designated movement patterns were assessed at a 60°/s concentric protocol. The data were evaluated and analyzed on the operated side. Before each joint measurement, participants were allowed to practice the movement pattern four times as they preferred to become familiar with the movement before performing five maximal test repetitions. All tests were supervised by one trained expert [14].

2.6. Rehabilitation Program and Local Body Vibration Administration

Participants completed a supervised progressive rehabilitation program for eight weeks (Table 2). All participants agreed not to change their daily activity patterns—outside of their participation in this study—or their dietary habits.

Participants performed workout sessions with Evocell (Shinoo Medison, Gangwon-do, Korea; Figure 2). The vibration patterns of Evocell are consistent and have a wide range of sound waves that change frequency according to the flow of music. This device has a maximal impulse of 1658 Hz, which has been developed to reduce pain by delivering stimuli below the skin. To reduce the friction of skin caused by equipment and to relieve pain, an exogenous gel (menthol-based material) was used with a starting impulse intensity at 20% of the maximum impulse for 30 min, similar to protocols from Lundeberg and colleagues [15].

Table 2. Rehabilitation program for the local body vibration group.

Type (Length)	Program Type	Intensity/Time
Warm-up (1 day–8 weeks)	Cycling	RPE 13/15 min
	Upper and lower leg stretching	RPE 13/20 min
1st workout phase (Week 0–2)	Vibroacoustic intervention (331.6 Hz)	20% × 1658 Hz × 30 min
	Q-set	5 s × 10 reps × 3 sets
	Straight leg raise	12 reps × 3 sets
	Ball adduction	6 s × 10 reps × 3 sets
	Half squat	10 reps × 3 sets
	Weight shift	15 reps × 3 sets
	Weight bearing	15 reps × 3 sets
	Calf raise	10 reps × 3 sets
	Balance on floor	2 min × 3 sets
2nd workout phase (Week 3–5)	Vibroacoustic intervention (663.2 Hz)	40% × 1658 Hz × 30 min
	Q-set	10 s × 10 reps × 3 sets
	Straight leg raise	15 reps × 3 sets
	Ball adduction	8 s × 10 reps × 4 sets
	Leg press	10 reps × 3 sets
	Leg extension	15 reps × 3 sets
	Leg curl	15 reps × 3 sets
	Half squat	12 reps × 3 sets
	Calf raise	12 reps × 3 sets
	Balance on pad	4 min × 3 sets
3rd workout phase (Week 6–8)	Vibroacoustic intervention (994.8 Hz)	60% × 1658 Hz × 30 min
	Ball adduction	10 s × 10 reps × 4 sets
	Leg press	12 reps × 3 sets
	Leg extension	15 reps × 3 sets
	Leg curl	15 reps × 3 sets
	Half squat	15 reps × 3 sets
	Calf raise	15 reps × 3 sets
	Balance on air-pad	6 min × 3 sets
Cool-down (1 day–8 weeks)	Upper and lower leg stretching	RPE 13–15/20 min
	Icing	10 min

Note: RPE, ratings of perceived exertion or Borg scale.

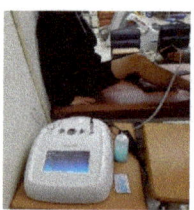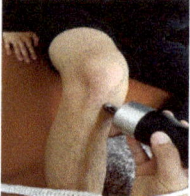

Figure 2. Vibroacoustic intervention applied on an anterior cruciate ligament reconstruction.

The goal of the first stage focused on decreasing pain, tolerating weight bearing, and improving ROM and gait pattern. The goal of the second stage focused on tolerating full weight bearing, increasing passive ROM, and improving neuromuscular control. Finally, the goal of the third stage focused on increasing leg strength, maintaining balance ability, and improving proprioception. The rehabilitation exercises, along with their repetitions and the sets used in this study, were extracted from a study and applied as a method of managing knee problems and preventing reinjury [14].

2.7. Data Analysis

All data were reported as mean (SD). The sample size was determined using G*Power v 3.1.3, considering an a priori effect size $f^2(V) = 0.35$ (medium size effect), α error probability = 0.05, and power (1—β error probability) = 0.95. Although a sample size of 30 was recommended, the current sample included 24 participants. Based on the results of the Kolmogorov–Smirnov test, the non-parametric Mann–Whitney U test and Friedman test were used to examine the differences of variables between groups and to examine the changes of variables among times. Significance was set at $p < 0.05$. SPSS version 18.0 (SPSS Inc., Chicago, IL, USA) was used for all analyses.

3. Results

3.1. Effect of Local Body Vibration on Psychological Condition

The rehabilitation program applied in this study improved the psychological measures of LBVG and nLBVG. As shown in Table 3, although the anxiety was not significantly different between the groups at all times, the pain of the LBVG was significantly lower than that of the nLBVG at Week 8 and the symptoms of the LBVG were significantly lower than those of the nLBVG at Weeks 4 and 8. In other words, a significant effect of the LBV-intervention concerning pain and symptoms was evident.

Table 3. Differences and changes in psychological scales.

Item (Points)	Week	Groups		Z (p) *
		LBVG (n = 11)	nLBVG (n = 13)	
Pain	0	7.56 ± 1.21	7.70 ± 1.58	−0.511 (0.649)
	4	4.10 ± 1.44	4.53 ± 1.20	−0.503 (0.649)
	8	2.13 ± 0.90	4.54 ± 1.33	−3.661 (0.001)
	X^2 (p) **	20.150 (0.001)	17.280 (0.001)	
Anxiety	0	6.39 ± 1.09	6.10 ± 1.24	−1.000 (0.361)
	4	3.72 ± 0.64	4.08 ± 0.95	−1.193 (0.277)
	8	3.01 ± 0.91	3.58 ± 0.95	−1.230 (0.252)
	X^2 (p) **	17.714 (0.001)	17.522 (0.001)	
Symptom	0	7.04 ± 1.46	7.12 ± 1.89	−0.353 (0.733)
	4	3.50 ± 1.16	6.71 ± 1.10	−4.119 (0.001)
	8	2.31 ± 0.90	3.95 ± 1.21	−3.090 (0.002)
	X^2 (p) **	18.558 (0.001)	12.875 (0.002)	

All data represent the mean ± standard deviation. LBVG and nLBVG are the local body vibration group and non-local body vibration group, respectively. Symbols * and ** were analyzed by the Mann–Whitney U test and the Friedman test, respectively.

3.2. Effect of Local Body Vibration on Physiological Condition

3.2.1. Effect of Local Body Vibration on Cardiorespiratory Variables

The rehabilitation program applied in this study somewhat improved the cardiorespiratory measures of the LBVG and nLBVG. As shown in Table 4, SBP, HR, and BR were significantly changed in the LBVG, whereas only SBP and BR were significantly changed in the nLBVG from the baseline to the end of the experiment. However, all of the cardiorespiratory measures were not significantly different between the groups at all times. In other words, a significant effect of the LBV-intervention was not found concerning the cardiorespiratory variables of physiological condition.

Table 4. Differences and changes in cardiorespiratory variables.

Item (Units)	Week	Groups		Z (p) *
		LBVG (n = 11)	nLBVG (n = 13)	
Systolic blood pressure (mmHg)	0	135.09 ± 5.17	134.69 ± 12.59	−0.351 (0.733)
	4	127.09 ± 12.99	126.23 ± 7.17	−0.350 (0.733)
	8	123.45 ± 5.63	124.31 ± 4.85	−0.235 (0.820)
	X^2 (p) **	13.905 (0.001)	7.714 (0.021)	
Diastolic blood pressure (mmHg)	0	80.55 ± 7.15	81.38 ± 12.49	−0.991 (0.331)
	4	79.73 ± 7.73	79.08 ± 11.11	−0.872 (0.392)
	8	79.09 ± 7.11	81.15 ± 11.01	−1.546 (0.134)
	X^2 (p) **	0.800 (0.670)	0.792 (0.673)	
Heart rate (beats/min)	0	77.09 ± 6.47	71.08 ± 8.30	−1.887 (0.063)
	4	73.45 ± 6.22	78.62 ± 9.99	−1.457 (0.150)
	8	69.09 ± 7.71	73.69 ± 7.22	−1.484 (0.150)
	X^2 (p) **	11.538 (0.003)	3.720 (0.156)	
Breathing rate (reps.)	0	29.61 ± 7.16	27.65 ± 5.54	−1.251 (0.228)
	4	19.85 ± 4.19	19.14 ± 3.06	−0.611 (0.569)
	8	19.60 ± 4.34	18.94 ± 3.48	−0.669 (0.531)
	X^2 (p) **	13.818 (0.001)	16.769 (0.001)	

All data represent the mean ± standard deviation. LBVG and nLBVG are the local body vibration group and non-local body vibration group, respectively. Symbols * and ** were analyzed by Mann–Whitney U test and Friedman test, respectively.

3.2.2. Effect of Local Body Vibration on Autonomic Nervous System

The rehabilitation program in this study somewhat improved the measures of autonomic nervous system in the LBVG and nLBVG. As shown in Table 5, SA and PSA were significantly changed in the LBVG, whereas only SA was significantly changed in the nLBVG from the baseline to the end of the experiment. Specifically, the SA measure of LBVG was significantly different when compared with that of the nLBVG at Week 4. The PSA measure of LBVG was significantly higher than that of the nLBVG at Weeks 4 and 8. In other words, a significant effect of the LBV-intervention was found concerning a decreased SA and increased PSA of physiological condition.

Table 5. Differences and changes in autonomic nerve system variables.

Item	Week	Groups		Z (p) *
		LBVG (n = 11)	nLBVG (n = 13)	
Sympathetic activation	0	7.61 ± 0.72	7.23 ± 0.51	−1.352 (0.186)
	4	6.32 ± 0.63	7.69 ± 1.15	−3.023 (0.002)
	8	5.77 ± 0.57	6.46 ± 1.33	−1.257 (0.228)
	X^2 (p) **	14.727 (0.001)	7.882 (0.019)	
Parasympathetic activation	0	3.55 ± 0.40	3.42 ± 0.38	−0.849 (0.424)
	4	4.49 ± 0.36	3.58 ± 0.40	−4.003 (0.001)
	8	4.96 ± 0.28	3.50 ± 0.46	−4.162 (0.001)
	X^2 (p) **	22.000 (0.001)	2.923 (0.232)	

All data represent the mean ± standard deviation. LBVG and nLBVG are the local body vibration group and non-local body vibration group, respectively. Symbols * and ** were analyzed by the Mann–Whitney U test and Friedman test, respectively.

3.2.3. Effect of Local Body Vibration on Strength and Range of Motion

The rehabilitation program in this study improved the measures of isokinetic strength and ROM only in the LBVG. As shown in Table 6, the PTs of the extensor and flexor were significantly changed in the LBVG, but there were no significant changes in the nLBVG from the baseline to the end of the experiment. Specifically, the extensor PT of the LBVG was significantly higher than that of the nLBVG at Week 8. The flexor PTs of the LBVG were also significantly higher than those of the nLBVG at Weeks 4 and 8. The ROM of the LBVG was also significantly higher than those of the nLBVG at Weeks 4 and 8.

In other words, a significant effect of the LBV-intervention was found concerning increased isokinetic strength and improved ROM of the operated knee joint.

Table 6. Differences and changes in strength and range of motion in the knee joint.

Item (Units)	Week	Groups		
		LBVG (n = 11)	nLBVG (n = 13)	Z (p) *
Extensor peak torque (Nm)	0	77.82 ± 12.91	70.00 ± 6.53	−2.311 (0.022)
	4	123.09 ± 35.18	100.15 ± 33.83	−1.574 (0.119)
	8	178.73 ± 27.45	110.23 ± 53.88	−3.229 (0.001)
	X^2 (p) **	13.273 (0.001)	1.385 (0.500)	
Flexor peak torque (Nm)	0	52.36 ± 5.24	47.08 ± 10.47	−1.196 (0.252)
	4	63.91 ± 6.24	43.08 ± 16.27	−3.286 (0.001)
	8	68.00 ± 10.26	50.23 ± 19.43	−2.052 (0.041)
	X^2 (p) **	17.636 (0.001)	3.231 (0.199)	
Range of motion (°)	0	94.55 ± 16.05	86.00 ± 15.35	−1.279 (0.207)
	4	121.73 ± 14.36	89.62 ± 17.47	−3.604 (0.001)
	8	127.82 ± 12.46	92.38 ± 27.65	−2.970 (0.002)
	X^2 (p) **	19.860 (0.001)	1.385 (0.500)	

All data represent the mean ± standard deviation. LBVG and nLBVG are the local body vibration group and non-local body vibration group, respectively. Symbols * and ** were analyzed by Mann-Whitney U test and Friedman test, respectively.

4. Discussion

This study provided evidence that the LBV application on an operated knee joint can improve the patients' psychological condition and physiological capacity including reduced pain and symptoms, improved ANS activity, and increased leg strength and ROM. These positive results may be related to a neurological effect through listening to music and to an improvement in ANS through sound stimuli. Specifically, an increase in vascular circulation during the rehabilitation program played a key role in the healing of the operated knee joint.

Petrofsky and Lee reported that blood circulation plays a vital role in tissue healing and that a richly vascularized area heals faster than a poorly vascularized area [16]. Muscle contractions evoked by imposed vibrations on the body can induce changes in peripheral circulation [13]. In fact, music produces a certain amount of vibration. Objective research has validated the healing effects of combined music and vibrations [17]. In VAST, the relaxing effect of music on the mind is amplified by the relaxing effect that acoustic vibromassage has on the body, producing a deep state of relaxation. VAST converts musical melodies and rhythms into waves that can be felt within a patient's body [17,18]. VAST has long been recognized as a more complex intervention than music alone, and it uses physical stimuli in the form of a pulsed sinusoidal low frequency wave to produce mechanical vibrations that are applied directly to the body [19].

Lane and colleagues reported that the neural correlates of vagal tones developed from the tenth cerebral neuron involve mental stresses that included cognitive and emotional elements such as surgery. The vagal (high frequency) component of HRV predicts survival in patients with post-myocardial infarction, and it reflects the vagal antagonism of sympathetic influences. The results of their research showed the neural correlates of vagal-HRV during various emotional states in real time. They correlated vagal-HRV with measures of regional cerebral blood flow derived from positron emission tomography and 15 O-water in 12 healthy women during diverse emotional states [11]. The heart is dually innervated by the ANS such that relative increases in SA are associated with HR increases and relative increases in PSA are associated with HR decreases; thus, relative sympathetic increases cause the time between heart beats (inter-beat interval) to become shorter and relative parasympathetic increases cause the interval between beats to become longer [11]. One way to index the central control of the heart via the vagal nerve is the use of HRV [20]. Consequently, HRV largely reflects the respiratory gating of the output of the vagal nerve on the sinoatrial node of the heart [21–23].

In this study, psychological problems (i.e., pain, anxiety, and symptoms) from surgery and recovery time improved in the nLBVG and LBVG from the baseline to Week 8. However, the pain and symptoms improved more in the LBVG when compared with the nLBVG at Week 8, highlighting the effects of the rehabilitation program. These results are comparable to those of Lane and colleagues [11]. Moreover, we think that the improvement of psychological problems was affected by ANS, but not by the cardiorespiratory system. As shown in the results of this study, although SBP, HR, and BR were significantly lowered in the LBVG, these cardiorespiratory measures were not significantly different between LBVG and nLBVG from the baseline to the end of the experiment. However, significant effects of the LBV-intervention were found concerning decreased SA and increased PSA of physiological condition in the LBVG. In other words, the positive changes in ANS contributed to improved psychological stability, which may have led to the reduction of pain and symptoms.

Similarly, Lundeberg and colleagues reported that vibrations reduced acute or chronic pain that had a musculoskeletal origin [15]. Moreover, they argued that various modes of electrical stimulation could be used as alternatives to analgesics and surgical procedures. In fact, many authors have suggested that stimulation activates the natural self-healing abilities of the body and its capacity to recover as well as bringing the body and mind into balance, which can reduce inflammation and chronic pain [2,24–26]. Warth and colleagues investigated nine participants with advanced cancer who took part in single-sessions of music therapy, lasting for 30 min [27]. From their results, VAS was feasible; although, a graphical and statistical examination revealed only marginal mean changes between pre- and post-testing. While HRV parameters differed between individuals, mean changes over time remained relatively constant. Examination of individual trajectories revealed that vibroacoustic stimulation may impact the autonomic response. The results above are very similar with the results of our study.

Many patients with osteoarthritis are seeking help with disease management from alternative therapy. When used along with allopathic medicine, these types of therapy may increase a patient's quality of life [28]. The music vibrations harmoniously combine to produce a new type of relaxation for patients. Lundqvist and colleagues reported that vibroacoustic sound waves reduce anxiety and aggression in some patients, thus reducing the need for medical treatment [29]. Koike and colleagues reported that VAST improved the psychological symptoms of 15 nursing home residents with symptoms of depression [30]. Those participants received VAST for 30 min per day for 10 days, and their depression levels were measured using the dementia mood assessment scale (DMAS). Tympanic temperature, pulse, BP, and SpO2 were also measured as physiological indexes of relaxation. Based on DMAS scores, depression was mitigated after participants received VAST. Moreover, significant decreases in tympanic temperature and pulse were observed post-treatment. In their conclusion, VAST provided relaxation effects and reduced depressive symptoms for older patients.

The current study supports and validates the efficacy of VAST, providing additional evidence for the value of these therapies for acute patients who have had ACL reconstruction surgery. The application of LBV improved the patients' muscle strength and ROM as well as fostering psychological stability. Concerning leg strength, extensor and flexor PT were significantly increased only in the LBVG; moreover, the extensor PT of the LBVG was higher than that of the nLBVG at Week 8 and flexor PTs of the LBVG were higher than those of the nLBVG at Weeks 4 and 8. These results were similar for ROM. In other words, the results showed that the vibroacoustic intervention strengthened the quadriceps and hamstrings and expanded the ROM of the operated knee joint. The strength of the tonic vibration reflex tends to increase with increasing muscle length, thus yielding an elastic resistance to slow stretch, similar to the type of resistance encountered in weaker muscles [26,31]. This explanation that the vibration-induced afferent discharge increases with muscle length has been used by many scholars [3,5,6].

In one study, massages using music vibrations were effective in facilitating the release of by-products produced by cells, thereby enabling muscles and organs to improve their function [32]. The development of the muscular vibration provides a means for studying the role played by muscle afferents in motor control, and the technique seems to have therapeutic applications. In this study, not only was LBV highly motivational and relaxing for patients, it also encouraged self-confidence, reduced pain and symptoms, and increased leg strength and ROM. Ultimately, LBV was an effective treatment for pain and symptom management, muscle activation, and ROM expansion in patients who recently underwent an ACL reconstruction operation.

5. Conclusions

This study confirmed that the LBV built-in vibroacoustic sound on an ACL reconstruction could improve patients' psychological condition including pain and symptoms and physiological capacity including ANS activity. These positive changes in psychophysiological conditions may lead to increased leg strength and ROM. Eventually, the results may be related to a neurological effect through listening to music and to an increase in vascular circulation during the rehabilitation program, playing a key role in the healing of the ACL reconstruction of the knee joint.

Author Contributions: Conceptualization, J.-M.P. and Y.-S.J.; Formal Analysis, J.-M.P. and S.P.; Funding Acquisition, Y.-S.J.; Investigation, J.-M.P. and Y.-S.J.; Methodology, J.-M.P., S.P., and Y.-S.J.; Project Administration, Y.-S.J.; Resources, J.-M.P.; Supervision, Y.-S.J.; Visualization, J.-M.P.; Writing—Original Draft Preparation, Y.-S.J.; Writing—Review & Editing, J.-M.P., S.P., and Y.-S.J.

Funding: This research was supported by a grant in 2018 from Hanseo University, Republic of Korea.

Acknowledgments: The authors wish to thank the patients for their participation in this study.

Conflicts of Interest: The authors declare no conflicts of interest.

References

1. Ellis, P. Vibroacoustic sound therapy: Case studies with children with profound and multiple learning difficulties and the elderly in long-term residential care. *Stud. Health Technol. Inf.* **2004**, *103*, 36–42.
2. Patrick, G. The effects of vibroacoustic music on symptom reduction. *IEEE Eng. Med. Biol. Mag.* **1999**, *18*, 97–100. [CrossRef] [PubMed]
3. Koike, Y.; Iwamoto, S.; Kimata, Y.; Nohno, T.; Hiragami, F.; Kawamura, K.; Numata, K.; Murai, H.; Okisima, K.; Iwata, M.; et al. Low frequency vibratory sound induces neurite outgrowth in PC12m3 cells in which nerve growth factor-induced neurite outgrowth is impaired. *Tiss Cult. Res. Commun.* **2004**, *2*, 81–90.
4. Łukasiak, A.; Krystosiak, M.; Widłak, P.; Wołdańska-Okońska, M. Evaluation of the effectiveness of vibroacoustic therapy treatment of patients with so-called "heel spur". A preliminary report. *Ortop. Traumatol. Rehabil.* **2013**, *15*, 77–87. [CrossRef] [PubMed]
5. Bautmans, I.; Van Hees, E.; Lemper, J.C.; Mets, T. The feasibility of whole body vibration in institutionalised elderly persons and its influence on muscle performance, balance and mobility: A randomised controlled trial. *BMC Geriatr.* **2005**, *22*, 17. [CrossRef]
6. Jackson, K.J.; Merriman, H.L.; Vanderburgh, P.M.; Brahler, C.J. Acute effects of whole-body vibration on lower extremity muscle performance in persons with multiple sclerosis. *J. Neurol. Phys. Ther.* **2008**, *32*, 171–176. [CrossRef] [PubMed]
7. Zheng, A.; Sakari, R.; Cheng, S.M.; Hietikko, A.; Moilanen, P.; Timonen, J.; Fagerlund, K.M.; Kärkkäinen, M.; Alèn, M.; Cheng, S. Effects of a low-frequency sound wave therapy programme on functional capacity, blood circulation and bone metabolism in frail old men and women. *Clin. Rehabil.* **2009**, *23*, 897–908. [CrossRef]
8. Kerschan-Schindl, K.; Grampp, S.; Henk, C.; Resch, H.; Preisinger, E.; Fialka-Moser, V.; Imhof, H. Whole-body vibration exercise leads to alterations in muscle blood volume. *Clin. Physiol.* **2001**, *21*, 377–382. [CrossRef]
9. Altman, R.; Asch, E.; Bloch, D.; Bole, G.; Borenstein, D.; Brandt, K.; Christy, W.; Cooke, T.D.; Greenwald, R.; Hochberg, M.; et al. Development of criteria for the classification and reporting of osteoarthritis. Classification of osteoarthritis of the knee. *Arthritis Rheum.* **1986**, *29*, 1039–1049. [CrossRef]
10. Jee, Y.S. The efficacy and safety of whole-body electromyostimulation in applying to human body: Based from graded exercise test. *J. Exerc. Rehabil.* **2018**, *14*, 49–57. [CrossRef]
11. Lane, R.D.; McRae, K.; Reiman, E.M.; Chen, K.; Ahern, G.L.; Thayer, J.F. Neural correlates of heart rate variability during emotion. *Neuroimage* **2009**, *44*, 213–222. [CrossRef]

12. White, D.W.; Raven, P.B. Autonomic neural control of heart rate during dynamic exercise: Revisited. *J. Physiol.* **2014**, *592*, 2491–2500. [CrossRef]
13. Kilinc, B.E.; Kara, A.; Celik, H.; Oc, Y.; Camur, S. Is anterior cruciate ligament surgery technique important in rehabilitation and activity scores? *J. Exerc. Rehabil.* **2016**, *12*, 232–237. [CrossRef] [PubMed]
14. Park, J.S.; Oh, H.W.; Park, E.K.; Ko, I.G.; Kim, S.E.; Kim, J.D.; Jin, J.J.; Jee, Y.S. Effects of rehabilitation program on functional scores and isokinetic torques of knee medial plica-operated patients. *Isokinet. Exerc. Sci.* **2013**, *21*, 19–28. [CrossRef]
15. Lundeberg, T.; Nordemar, R.; Ottoson, D. Pain alleviation by vibratory stimulation. *Pain* **1984**, *20*, 25–44. [CrossRef]
16. Petrofsky, J.S.; Lee, S. The effects of type 2 Diabetes and aging on vascular endothelial and autonomic function. *Med. Sci. Monit.* **2005**, *11*, CR247–CR254.
17. Henry, L.L. Music therapy: A nursing intervention for the control of pain and anxiety in the ICU: A review of the research literature. *Dimens. Crit. Care Nurs.* **1995**, *14*, 295–304. [CrossRef]
18. Boyd-Brewer, C.; McCaffrey, R. Vibroacoustic sound therapy improves pain management and more. *Holist. Nurs. Pract.* **2004**, *18*, 111–118. [CrossRef]
19. Hooper, J. An introduction to vibroacoustic therapy and an examination of its place in music therapy practice. *Br. J. Music Ther.* **2001**, *5*, 69–77. [CrossRef]
20. Thayer, J.; Brosschot, J. Psychosomatics and psychopathology: Looking up and down from the brain. *Psychoneuroendocrinology* **2005**, *30*, 1050–1058. [CrossRef]
21. Saul, J. Beat-to-beat variations of heart rate reflect modulation of cardiac autonomic outflow. *Am. Physiol. Soc.* **1990**, *5*, 32–37. [CrossRef]
22. Grossman, P. Respiratory and cardiac rhythms as windows to central and autonomic biobehavioral regulation: Selection of window frames, keeping the panes clean and viewing the neural topography. *Biol. Psychol.* **1992**, *34*, 131–161. [CrossRef]
23. Zahn, D.; Wenzel, M.; Kubiak, T. Response: Commentary: Heart rate variability and self-control—A meta-analysis. *Front. Psychol.* **2016**, *7*, 1070. [CrossRef] [PubMed]
24. Skille, O.; Wigram, T.; Weeks, L. Vibroacoustic Therapy: The therapeutic effect of low frequency sound on specific physical disorders and disabilities. *Br. J. Music Ther.* **1989**, *3*, 6–10. [CrossRef]
25. Ekhtiari, S.; Horner, N.S.; de Sa, D.; Simunovic, N.; Hirschmann, M.T.; Ogilvie, R.; Berardelli, R.L.; Whelan, D.B.; Ayeni, O.R. Arthrofibrosis after ACL reconstruction is best treated in a step-wise approach with early recognition and intervention: A systematic review. *Knee Surg. Sports Traumatol. Arthrosc.* **2017**, *25*, 3929–3937. [CrossRef] [PubMed]
26. Zhang, X.; Hu, M.; Lou, Z.; Liao, B. Effects of strength and neuromuscular training on functional performance in athletes after partial medial meniscectomy. *J. Exerc. Rehabil.* **2017**, *28*, 110–116. [CrossRef] [PubMed]
27. Warth, M.; Kessler, J.; Kotz, S.; Hillecke, T.K.; Bardenheuer, H.J. Effects of vibroacoustic stimulation in music therapy for palliative care patients: A feasibility study. *BMC Complement. Altern. Med.* **2015**, *15*, 436. [CrossRef] [PubMed]
28. Dottie, R. Alternative therapies for arthritis treatment: Part 2. *Holist. Nurs. Pract.* **2004**, *3*, 167–174.
29. Lundqvist, L.O.; Andersson, J.; Viding, J. Effects of vibroacoustic music on challenging behaviors in individuals with autism and developmental disabilities. *Res. Autism Spectr. Disord.* **2009**, *3*, 390–400. [CrossRef]
30. Koike, Y.; Hoshitani, M.; Tabata, Y.; Seki, K.; Nishimura, R.; Kano, Y. Effects of vibroacoustic therapy on elderly nursing home residents with depression. *J. Phys. Ther. Sci.* **2012**, *24*, 291–294. [CrossRef]
31. Imai, R.; Osumi, M.; Ishigaki, T.; Kodama, T.; Shimada, S.; Morioka, S. Effects of illusory kinesthesia by tendon vibratory stimulation on the postoperative neural activities of distal radius fracture patients. *Neuroreport* **2017**, *28*, 1144–1149. [CrossRef] [PubMed]
32. Skille, O.; Wigram, T. The effect of music, vocalization and vibration on brain and muscle tissue: Studies in vibroacoustic therapy. In *The Art and Science of Music Therapy: A Handbook*; Wigram, T., Saperston, B., West, R., Eds.; Harwood Academic Press: London, UK, 1995.

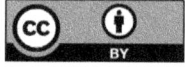

© 2019 by the authors. Licensee MDPI, Basel, Switzerland. This article is an open access article distributed under the terms and conditions of the Creative Commons Attribution (CC BY) license (http://creativecommons.org/licenses/by/4.0/).

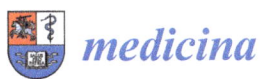

Case Report

Pain and Function in the Runner a Ten (din) uous Link

Peter Francis [1,2,*], Isobel Thornley [2], Ashley Jones [2] and Mark I. Johnson [2,3]

1 Department of Science and Health, Institute of Technology Carlow, Carlow, Ireland
2 Musculoskeletal Health Research Group, Leeds Beckett University, Leeds LS13HE, UK; i.thornley@leedsbeckett.ac.uk (I.T.); Ashley.D.Jones@leedsbeckett.ac.uk (A.J.); m.johnson@leedsbeckett.ac.uk (M.I.J.)
3 Centre for Pain for Research, Leeds Beckett University, Leeds LS13HE, UK
* Correspondence: peter.francis@itcarlow.ie; Tel.: +353-59917-5000

Received: 28 November 2019; Accepted: 27 December 2019; Published: 7 January 2020

Abstract: A male runner (30 years old; 10-km time: 33 min, 46 s) had been running with suspected insertional Achilles tendinopathy (AT) for ~2 years when the pain reached a threshold that prevented running. Diagnostic ultrasound (US), prior to a high-volume stripping injection, confirmed right-sided medial insertional AT. The athlete failed to respond to injection therapy and ceased running for a period of 5 weeks. At the beginning of this period, the runner completed the Victoria institute of sports assessment–Achilles questionnaire (VISA-A), the foot and ankle disability index (FADI), and FADI sport prior to undergoing an assessment of bi-lateral gastrocnemius medialis (GM) muscle architecture (muscle thickness (MT) and pennation angle (PA); US), muscle contractile properties (maximal muscle displacement (Dm) and contraction time (Tc); Tensiomyography (TMG)) and calf endurance (40 raises/min). VISA-A and FADI scores were 59%/100% and 102/136 respectively. Compared to the left leg, the right GM had a lower MT (1.60 cm vs. 1.74 cm), a similar PA (22.0° vs. 21.0°), a lower Dm (1.2 mm vs. 2.0 mm) and Tc (16.5 ms vs. 17.7 ms). Calf endurance was higher in the right leg compared to the left (48 vs. 43 raises). The athlete began a metronome-guided (15 BPM), 12-week progressive eccentric training protocol using a weighted vest (1.5 kg increments per week), while receiving six sessions of shockwave therapy concurrently (within 5 weeks). On returning to running, the athlete kept daily pain (Numeric Rating Scale; NRS) and running scores (miles*rate of perceived exertion (RPE)). Foot and ankle function improved according to scores recorded on the VISA-A (59% vs. 97%) and FADI (102 vs. 127/136). Improvements in MT (1.60 cm vs. 1.76 cm) and PA (22.0° vs. 24.8°) were recorded via US. Improvements in Dm (1.15 mm vs. 1.69 mm) and Tc (16.5 ms vs. 15.4 ms) were recorded via TMG. Calf endurance was lower in both legs and the asymmetry between legs remained (L: 31, R: 34). Pain intensity (mean weekly NRS scores) decreased between week 1 and week 12 (6.6 vs. 2.9), while running scores increased (20 vs. 38) during the same period. The program was maintained up to week 16 at which point mean weekly NRS was 2.2 and running score was 47.

Keywords: chronic pain; pain management; Achilles; tendon; running

---

1. Introduction

Achilles tendinopathy (AT) is the 2nd most common running injury [1,2]. It is primarily located in the mid-portion of the tendon or at the insertion with the calcaneus (insertional tendinopathy) [3]. The stages of tendinopathy have been characterized as reactive (a non-inflammatory cellular response to acute loading that results in tendon thickening), dysrepair (failed healing that demonstrates greater matrix breakdown and the separation of collagen) and degenerative (increased cell death, matrix breakdown, neuronal and capillary in growth) [4]. Pain can be present or absent at any stage of the tendon pathology continuum. Furthermore, tendons can have discrete regions at different stages of the pathology-continuum at the same time [4,5]. Pathological findings as a result of imaging the tendon do not always correlate with patient symptoms [6].

The majority of running injuries are characterized by repetitive overuse and are usually to tissues ill-equipped for load absorption (i.e., non-contractile) [1]. The insidious onset of pain at a threshold (e.g., <5/10 on a Numeric Rating Scale; NRS) [7] below that experienced during traumatic insults often allows the runner to continue to run. In other words, there is a dissociation between pain and function in chronic injuries [8]. There are several pharmacological (e.g., NSAID's, injection therapy) and non-pharmacological (e.g., heavy isometric loading, shock-wave therapy, cross-training) aids that produce short-term analgesic effects in tendinopathy [9–13]. However, chronic pain can reach a threshold whereby it is more akin to that experienced in traumatic pain (>5/10 on an NRS). This can force the athlete to stop running and seek longer-term resolutions.

The strongest evidence for the long-term resolution for Achilles tendon pain comes from exercise protocols [14]. Variations of the Alfredsson protocol (straight and bent knee eccentric exercise on the edge of a step) [15,16] appear to be most effective in patients with mid-portion tendinopathy. Excessive dorsi-flexion on the edge of a step is thought to increase the compressive load at the tendon insertion and therefore, straight leg exercises on a flat surface appear to be more effective for those with insertional tendinopathy [17]. These protocols have been further enhanced by a greater understanding of the other neuromuscular deficits that occur as a result of Achilles tendon injury. For example, externally paced eccentric exercise using a metronome standardizes the time the muscle is under tension and enhances neural plasticity [18].

The reasons pain and function respond positively to this form of training are multi-factorial [19]. To the best of the authors' knowledge, there are no scientific reports which capture self-reported function (Victoria institute of sports assessment–Achilles questionnaire; VISA-A, the foot and ankle disability index FADI, and FADI Sport) [20–22], muscle architecture (Ultrasonography; US), muscle contractile properties (Tensiomyography; TMG), muscle endurance (Calf Endurance Test) and pain (Numeric Rating Scale; NRS) pre and post conservative Achilles tendon management.

2. Case Report

2.1. Case History

The patient provided written informed consent for the publication of this case report. A male runner (30 years, 10-km time: 33 min 46 s) had been running with suspected insertional AT for 110 weeks (~2 years) having had the symptoms for the previous 5 years. The average miles per week for the 2-year period was 30. The average miles per week during phases of race preparation was ~40 and the maximum miles per week was 50. During this period, pain (~≤5/10; NRS) and or stiffness was present every morning during the first steps on walking. Pain usually subsided as running progressed and returned after periods of prolonged rest. The runner used a 4-day-per-week running schedule and a 3-day-per-week cross-training schedule to manage running loads applied to the tendon and to lower the risk of other injury. Occasionally, pain increased (≥5/10; NRS) and was relieved using heavy double-legged isometric exercise (~85 kg) and reducing running from four days to three. No structured Achilles tendon rehabilitation was undertaken other than calf raise exercises on days the runner attended the gym (maximum 2*per week). The above summarises the training and pain status of the runner for much of the 2 years prior to cessation. This period included personal bests over 5 km (16:10), 10 km (33:46) and half-marathon (78:00).

Nine weeks before cessation (week 101/110), the runner began to increase the volume and sometimes intensity of one weekly run in an attempt to train for a marathon. This elevated daily pain to 7/10 and to a point where conservative self-management (as above) was no longer effective. The runner attended a sports medicine physician for an ultrasound guided high-volume stripping injection as prescribed in Humphreys et al. [10]. The diagnosis of right-sided medial insertional AT was made by a qualified medical doctor using ultrasonography. The doctor had ~20-years' experience in the diagnosis of musculoskeletal conditions, diagnostic ultrasound and steroid injection therapy. The doctor was a member of the British Association of Sports and Exercise Medicine. Diagnosis was obtained by palpating the painful site on the medial calcaneus and using ultrasonography to image the same area (Figure 1). Over the course of 1 week (no running), the runner failed to respond to injection therapy and ceased running.

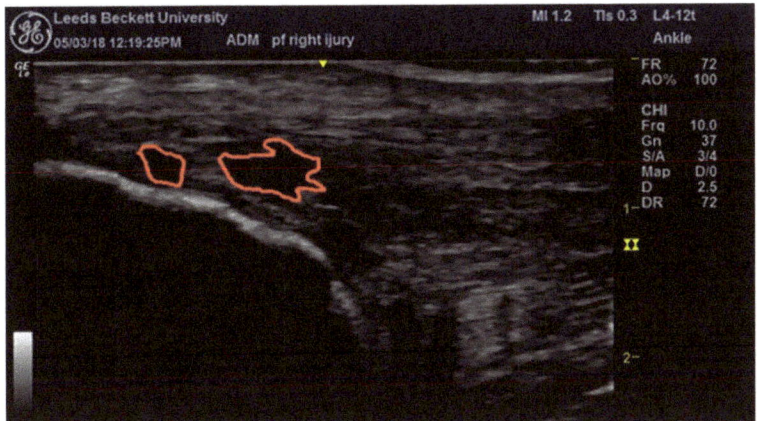

Figure 1. Identification of right-sided medial insertional tendinopathy.

2.2. Assessment

The runner reported to the laboratory (Figure 2) at Leeds Beckett University and completed the Victoria institute of sports assessment-Achilles questionnaire (Victoria institute of sports assessment-Achilles questionnaire; VISA-A), the foot and ankle disability index (FADI and FADI Sport), prior to undergoing an assessment of bi-lateral gastrocnemius medialis (GM) muscle architecture (muscle thickness (MT) and pennation angle (PA); US), muscle contractile properties (maximal muscle displacement (Dm) and contraction time (Tc); Tensiomyography (TMG)) and calf endurance (40 raises/min).

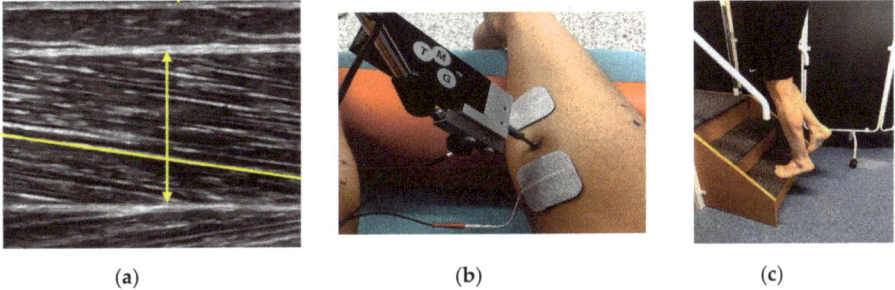

Figure 2. The use of ultrasonography (US), tensiomyography (TMG) and the calf endurance test in the assessment of (**a**) muscle architecture, (**b**) contractile properties, and (**c**) endurance.

VISA-A and FADI scores were 59%/100% and 102/136, respectively. Compared to the left leg, the right GM had a lower MT (1.60 cm vs. 1.74 cm), a similar PA (22.0° vs. 21.0°), a lower Dm (1.2 mm vs. 2.0 mm) and Tc (16.5 ms vs. 17.7 ms). Calf endurance was higher in the injured leg (right) compared to the left (48 vs. 43 raises).

2.3. Intervention

The athlete ceased running for 5 weeks and began a metronome guided (15-BPM), 12-week progressive eccentric training protocol (3 sets, 12 reps, 2*day) on a flat surface, using a weighted-vest (1.5 kg increments per week). The exercise was performed by bilaterally plantar flexing both legs and lowering unilaterally on the affected leg to a count of 4 s (15 BPM). The athlete also received six sessions of shockwave therapy (2000 shocks per session at a pressure and frequency of 1.8–2.2 bar and 10 Hz, respectively) concurrently within the first 5 weeks. The athlete recorded daily pain scores (NRS) [23] throughout the intervention (Figure 3). On return to running (after 5 weeks), the athlete also recorded a score composed of miles * rate of perceived exertion (RPE) [24]. Running miles* rate of perceived exertion (RPE) was recorded in order to provide a crude estimate of running load. Running began with a 2.5-mile jog, barefoot and on a hard grass surface (British Summer Time). This was progressed (week 6–13) until the athlete could run 8 miles, three times per week at an RPE of 11 (light). The laboratory measures were re-assessed at the 12-week point. The athlete continued to perform the eccentric training protocol and record pain and running load data up to week 16 (Figure 3). Between week 13 and 16, the three 8-mile runs were replaced with an 8-mile run over an undulating surface (shod; RPE: 13), a track session that began with 4 × 400 m and progressed to 16 × 400 m (shod; RPE 15) and a long run that progressed to 12 miles (barefoot and occasionally shod; RPE 11).

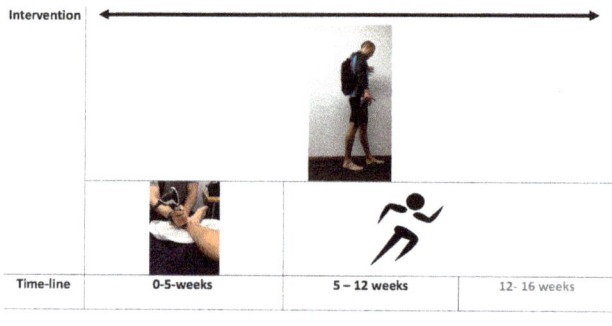

Figure 3. The intervention for the management of medial insertional Achilles tendinopathy.

2.4. Outcomes

The athlete had a compliance of 80.4% (135/168 possible sessions) to the 12-week eccentric training protocol. At the 12-week point, foot and ankle function improved according to scores recorded on the VISA-A (59% vs. 97%) and FADI (102 vs. 127/136). Figure 4 displays pre and post left–right differences in gastrocnemius muscle architecture and contractile properties.

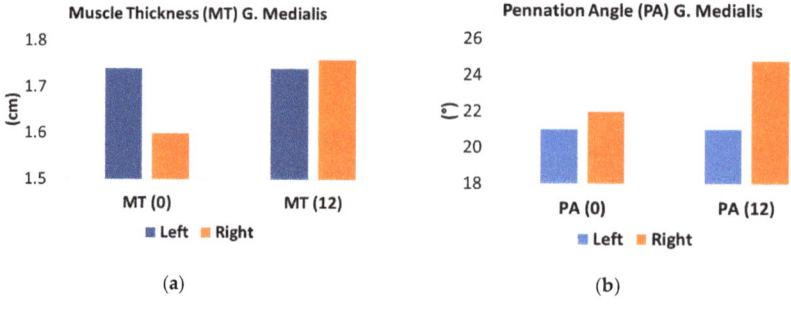

Figure 4. Cont.

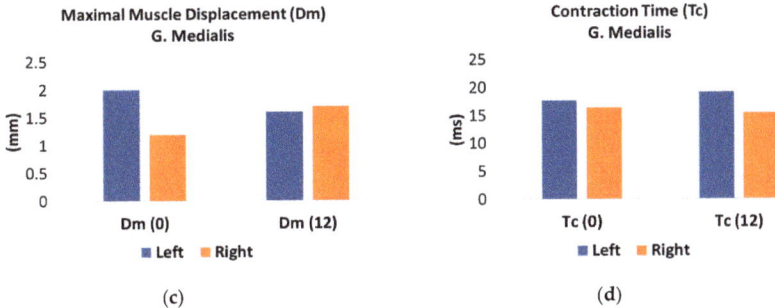

(c)   (d)

Figure 4. Changes in gastrocnemius muscle architecture ((**a**) muscle thickness and (**b**) pennation angle) and contractile properties ((**c**) muscle displacement and (**d**) contraction time) pre and post intervention.

In the injured leg, improvements in MT (1.60 cm vs. 1.76 cm) and PA (22.0° vs. 24.8°) were recorded via US. Improvements in Dm (1.15 mm vs. 1.69 mm) and Tc (16.5 ms vs. 15.4 ms) were recorded via TMG. Calf endurance was lower in both legs and the asymmetry between legs remained (L: 31, R: 34). Pain intensity (mean weekly NRS scores) decreased between week 1 and week 12 (6.6 vs. 2.9), while running scores increased (20 vs. 38) during the same period. The program was maintained up to week 16 at which point mean weekly NRS was 2.2 and running score was 47 (Figure 5).

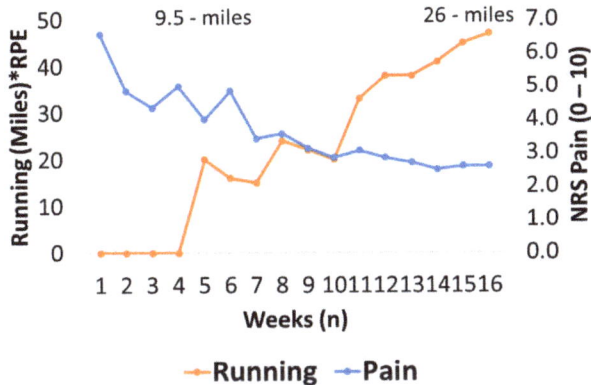

Figure 5. Weekly pain (numeric rating scale; NRS) and function (miles*rate of perceived exertion; RPE) response to intervention. Weekly mileage totals began with 9.5 on week 5 and ended with 26 on week 16.

3. Discussion

The runner in this case report ran for ~2 years with persistent pain and achieved several personal bests. This demonstrates, in this athlete at least, that pain can be managed in a way that allows a high level of athletic function. This underscores the title of this paper which suggests that pain and function are not as closely linked in chronic pain as they may be in pain resulting from traumatic insult. In fact, baseline results of the calf endurance test appear to demonstrate a compensatory mechanism whereby calf endurance in the injured leg was higher than that of the non-injured [25]. Calf endurance, and to a lesser extent PA, may have helped to compensate for the asymmetry in MT and Dm reported.

This athlete did not respond to a high-volume stripping injection, which may suggest that this type of intervention is not as effective in insertional tendinopathy as it appeared to be for mid-portion tendinopathy [10]. It may also reflect intra-individual responses to injection therapy. Overall, pain and function appeared to respond positively as a result of the combined shockwave therapy and eccentric loading protocol administered over the 16-week period. It is difficult to know from a case report whether the effects demonstrated were due to one or both interventions. It should be noted that pain did not begin to lower on a consistent basis until week 7, and all shockwave therapy had been administered by week 5. These findings, combined with the rise in function and fall in pain from ~week 10, suggest that the eccentric loading protocol was the dominant factor in recovery. This suggestion is underpinned by the substantial improvements in neuromuscular function reported.

In the injured leg (right), there were improvements in gastrocnemius medialis MT (~10%) and PA (~12.7%), as measured by US, which appeared to be reflected by the relative improvement in Dm (~47%) and, to a lesser extent, Tc (~6.7%). These findings were expected, as they mirror improvements in muscle size and function in response to resistance exercise [25]. Strength increases prior to changes in muscle size and is usually proportionally greater, i.e., modest gains in muscle size are usually associated with 3–4 times the relative strength gains [26,27]. In the early stages of resistance training, this is suggested to be as a result of an increase in the neural drive to muscle [28]. Häkkinen and colleagues reported the largest motor units to be recruited within the first 7 weeks of resistance training [29]. The force output of a muscle increases in response to the number of sarcomeres in parallel. An increase in PA facilitates more sarcomeres in parallel, i.e., an increase in physiological cross-sectional area (CSA) without a change in anatomical CSA [30]. It is likely that the increase in PA and the overall increase in contractile mass (MT) contributed to the increase in Dm reported in this athlete. However, Dm is not a measure of force but of stiffness and therefore, it is likely to be heavily influenced by the tendon aponeurosis complex and intramuscular connective tissue. These are the structures which transfer muscle force to the bone. Increases in musculotendinous stiffness have previously been reported in response to resistance training [31,32] and likely contribute to changes reported in Dm. These changes in connective tissue stiffness are thought to be primarily driven by an increase in type I collagen synthesis [33].

This interpretation of an increase in Dm representing an increase in stiffness is somewhat at odds with researchers in the field who suggest a lower Dm to be associated with a greater muscle stiffness [34]. These interpretations are based primarily on cross-sectional studies comparing power and endurance athletes [35] and founded on what remains a limited understanding of the physiology that underpins measures obtained from Tensiomyography. In our laboratory, we are still optimizing the standard operating procedures [36,37] in order to obtain stable measurements prior to a more in-depth interpretation of what the data might indicate physiologically. Our experience from this case report and on-going investigations in our laboratory suggest that differences in Dm are dependent on the context in which they are reported. We suggest that in the case of cross-sectional comparisons, as mentioned above, lower Dm is indeed indicative of higher muscle stiffness. However, in the case of training or detraining we suggest that the increase or decrease in contractile mass and PA can lead to an increase in or decrease in Dm. We advise caution in the interpretation of these findings and others, as interpretation of the data obtained from Tensiomyography remains in its infancy.

The modest reduction in Tc might be expected from an intervention that did not challenge the speed of muscle contraction. The improvements reported are likely due to an increase in the number of sarcomeres in series [38] and the increase in PA, which would allow sarcomeres to operate closer to their optimum length [25]. Calf endurance appeared to decline during the 12-week period, which we suggest is due to the initial 5 weeks without running and the gradual buildup of running up to week 12. It is likely that the removal of a stimulus that had been there for ~2 years led to this reduction. The asymmetry between legs remained, suggesting that some of the adaptations which occurred in the painful leg over time remained.

There are several limitations we would like to acknowledge related to the interpretation of this case report. Firstly, although tendon structural abnormalities are present on ultrasound, this cannot be inferred to represent pathology [39]. In fact, the link between findings on imaging and pain in runners is weak for several musculoskeletal conditions [40–42]. That being said, the presence of loading specific pain and pain on palpation suggest an accurate diagnosis was received. Secondly, although we suggest the eccentric exercise protocol was the primary driver behind improvements demonstrated in this case, the influence of the injection and the shockwave therapy cannot be ruled out. Recent evidence suggests that high-volume image-guided injections, as used in this case, demonstrate improvements in pain and function with or without steroid in mid-portion AT [43]. This did not appear to be the case in this report. Although pain did not decrease on a consistent basis until week 7, a significant dose of shockwave therapy was administered during the first 5 weeks. Furthermore, there are promising results in terms of medium and long-term follow-up in mid-portion AT following shockwave therapy [44]. There are several mechanisms by which shockwave is speculated to have an effect on pain and tissue healing. The short-term effects on pain are thought to occur due to hyper stimulation analgesia [45]. In the medium term, it has been suggested that a sharp rise in substance P release and a subsequent long decrease may lead to longer lasting relief from pain [46]. Tendon repair is speculated to be promoted post shockwave therapy via an increase in tenocyte proliferation and an induction of growth factors [47]. Finally, tendinopathy is a condition associated with chronic pain. Disability levels associated with chronic musculoskeletal pain are more closely associated with cognitive and behavioral aspects of pain than sensory and biomedical ones. Positive outcomes are associated with changes in psychological distress, fear avoidance beliefs, self-efficacy in controlling pain and coping strategies [48]. Therefore, in this case, the break from running, and the knowledge of a combined shockwave therapy and exercise intervention coupled with an expected timeline of improvement may have had just as big an impact as the intervention itself.

4. Conclusions

This athlete ran at a high level for 2 years with persistent Achilles pain. Even after an evidence-based rehabilitation programme and a gradual return to running, this athlete was never entirely pain-free. The findings in this runner appear to underscore the need for greater awareness among clinicians about the dissociation between pain and function in Achilles tendinopathy. Pain education and limiting fear avoidance may be as important as physical rehabilitation. The neuromuscular adaptations in this study were substantial and the physiology which underpins them is multifactorial. To what extent these neuromuscular adaptations contribute to the reduction in pain and increase in running specific function is unknown and it will perhaps always be an almost impossible research question to answer. However, it is likely that the combination of neuromuscular adaptations and structural adaptations within the tendon itself help to better balance stress on biological tissue preventing overload of a specific portion of tendon.

Author Contributions: Conceptualization, P.F.; methodology, I.T. and A.J.; formal analysis, I.T. and A.J.; writing—original draft preparation, P.F.; writing—review and editing, M.I.J. All authors have read and agreed to the published version of the manuscript.

Funding: This research received no external funding.

Acknowledgments: The authors would like to acknowledge the institutions of Leeds Beckett University and Institute of Technology Carlow for providing the facilities and support in writing the full manuscript respectively.

Conflicts of Interest: The authors declare no conflict of interest. The funders had no role in the design of the study; in the collection, analyses, or interpretation of data; in the writing of the manuscript, or in the decision to publish the results.

References

1. Francis, P.; Whatman, C.; Sheerin, K.; Hume, P.; Johnson, M.I. The proportion of lower limb running injuries by gender, anatomical location and specific pathology: A systematic review. *J. Sports Sci. Med.* **2019**, *18*, 21–31. [PubMed]
2. Lopes, A.D.; Hespanhol Junior, L.C.; Yeung, S.S.; Costa, L.O. What are the main running-related musculoskeletal injuries? A Systematic Review. *Sports Med.* **2012**, *42*, 891–905. [CrossRef] [PubMed]

3. Cook, J.L.; Stasinopoulos, D.; Brismee, J.M. Insertional and mid-substance Achilles tendinopathies: Eccentric training is not for everyone-updated evidence of non-surgical management. *J. Man. Manip. Ther.* **2018**, *26*, 119–122. [CrossRef] [PubMed]
4. Cook, J.L.; Purdam, C.R. Is tendon pathology a continuum? A pathology model to explain the clinical presentation of load-induced tendinopathy. *Br. J. Sports Med.* **2009**, *43*, 409–416. [CrossRef] [PubMed]
5. Cook, J.L.; Rio, E.; Purdam, C.R.; Docking, S.I. Revisiting the continuum model of tendon pathology: What is its merit in clinical practice and research? *Br. J. Sports Med.* **2016**, *50*, 1187–1191. [CrossRef] [PubMed]
6. Khan, K.M.; Forster, B.B.; Robinson, J.; Cheong, Y.; Louis, L.; Maclean, L.; Taunton, J.E. Are ultrasound and magnetic resonance imaging of value in assessment of Achilles tendon disorders? A two year prospective study. *Br. J. Sports Med.* **2003**, *37*, 149–153. [CrossRef]
7. Silbernagel, K.G.; Thomee, R.; Eriksson, B.I.; Karlsson, J. Continued sports activity, using a pain-monitoring model, during rehabilitation in patients with Achilles tendinopathy: A randomized controlled study. *Am. J. Sports Med.* **2007**, *35*, 897–906. [CrossRef]
8. Moseley, G.L.; Butler, D.S. Fifteen years of explaining pain: The past, present, and future. *J. Pain* **2015**, *16*, 807–813. [CrossRef]
9. Bussin, E.R.; Cairns, B.; Bovard, J.; Scott, A. Randomised controlled trial evaluating the short-term analgesic effect of topical diclofenac on chronic Achilles tendon pain: A pilot study. *BMJ Open* **2017**, *7*, e015126. [CrossRef]
10. Humphrey, J.; Chan, O.; Crisp, T.; Padhiar, N.; Morrissey, D.; Twycross-Lewis, R.; King, J.; Maffulli, N. The short-term effects of high volume image guided injections in resistant non-insertional Achilles tendinopathy. *J. Sci. Med. Sport* **2010**, *13*, 295–298. [CrossRef]
11. Rio, E.; Kidgell, D.; Purdam, C.; Gaida, J.; Moseley, G.L.; Pearce, A.J.; Cook, J. Isometric exercise induces analgesia and reduces inhibition in patellar tendinopathy. *Br. J. Sports Med.* **2015**, *49*, 1277–1283. [CrossRef] [PubMed]
12. Wiegerinck, J.I.; Kerkhoffs, G.M.; van Sterkenburg, M.N.; Sierevelt, I.N.; van Dijk, C.N. Treatment for insertional Achilles tendinopathy: A systematic review. *Knee Surg. Sports Traumatol. Arthrosc.* **2013**, *21*, 1345–1355. [CrossRef] [PubMed]
13. Paquette, M.R.; Peel, S.A.; Smith, R.E.; Temme, M.; Dwyer, J.N. The impact of different cross-training modalities on performance and injury-related variables in high school cross country runners. *J. Strength Cond. Res.* **2018**, *32*, 1745–1753. [CrossRef] [PubMed]
14. Beyer, R.; Kongsgaard, M.; Hougs Kjaer, B.; Ohlenschlaeger, T.; Kjaer, M.; Magnusson, S.P. Heavy slow resistance versus eccentric training as treatment for achilles tendinopathy: A randomized controlled trial. *Am. J. Sports Med.* **2015**, *43*, 1704–1711. [CrossRef]
15. Alfredson, H.; Pietila, T.; Jonsson, P.; Lorentzon, R. Heavy-load eccentric calf muscle training for the treatment of chronic Achilles tendinosis. *Am. J. Sports Med.* **1998**, *26*, 360–366. [CrossRef]
16. Woodley, B.L.; Newsham-West, R.J.; Baxter, G.D. Chronic tendinopathy: Effectiveness of eccentric exercise. *Br. J. Sports Med.* **2007**, *41*, 188–198. [CrossRef]
17. Jonsson, P.; Alfredson, H.; Sunding, K.; Fahlstrom, M.; Cook, J. New regimen for eccentric calf-muscle training in patients with chronic insertional Achilles tendinopathy: Results of a pilot study. *Br. J. Sports Med.* **2008**, *42*, 746–749. [CrossRef]
18. Rio, E.; Kidgell, D.; Moseley, G.L.; Gaida, J.; Docking, S.; Purdam, C.; Cook, J. Tendon neuroplastic training: Changing the way we think about tendon rehabilitation: A narrative review. *Br. J. Sports Med.* **2016**, *50*, 209–215. [CrossRef]
19. O'Neill, S.; Watson, P.J.; Barry, S. Why are eccentric exercises effective for achilles tendinopathy? *Int. J. Sports Phys. Ther.* **2015**, *10*, 552–562.
20. Robinson, J.M.; Cook, J.L.; Purdam, C.; Visentini, P.J.; Ross, J.; Maffulli, N.; Taunton, J.E.; Khan, K.M. The VISA-A questionnaire: A valid and reliable index of the clinical severity of Achilles tendinopathy. *Br. J. Sports Med.* **2001**, *35*, 335–341. [CrossRef]
21. Martin, R.; Burdett, R.; Irrgang, J. Development of the foot and ankle disability index (FADI). *J. Orthop. Sports Phys. Ther.* **1999**, *29*, A32–A33.
22. Hale, S.A.; Hertel, J. Reliability and sensitivity of the Foot and Ankle Disability Index in subjects with chronic ankle instability. *J. Athl. Train.* **2005**, *40*, 35–40.

23. Hawker, G.A.; Mian, S.; Kendzerska, T.; French, M. Measures of adult pain: Visual Analog Scale for Pain (VAS Pain), Numeric Rating Scale for Pain (NRS Pain), McGill Pain Questionnaire (MPQ), Short-Form McGill Pain Questionnaire (SF-MPQ), Chronic Pain Grade Scale (CPGS), Short Form-36 Bodily Pain Scale (SF-36 BPS), and Measure of Intermittent and Constant Osteoarthritis Pain (ICOAP). *Arthritis Care Res.* **2011**, *63* (Suppl. S11), S240–S252.
24. Borg, G.; Exertion, B.P.; Scales, P. *Champaign*; Human Kinetics: Champaign, IL, USA, 1998; pp. 1–104.
25. Blazevich, A.J. Effects of physical training and detraining, immobilisation, growth and aging on human fascicle geometry. *Sports Med.* **2006**, *36*, 1003–1017. [CrossRef] [PubMed]
26. Francis, P.; Mc Cormack, W.; Toomey, C.; Norton, C.; Saunders, J.; Kerin, E.; Lyons, M.; Jakeman, P. Twelve weeks' progressive resistance training combined with protein supplementation beyond habitual intakes increases upper leg lean tissue mass, muscle strength and extended gait speed in healthy older women. *Biogerontology* **2016**, *18*, 881–891. [CrossRef] [PubMed]
27. Seynnes, O.R.; de Boer, M.; Narici, M.V. Early skeletal muscle hypertrophy and architectural changes in response to high-intensity resistance training. *J. Appl. Physiol.* **2007**, *102*, 368–373. [CrossRef] [PubMed]
28. Gabriel, D.A.; Kamen, G.; Frost, G. Neural adaptations to resistive exercise: Mechanisms and recommendations for training practices. *Sports Med.* **2006**, *36*, 133–149. [CrossRef]
29. Hakkinen, K.; Pakarinen, A.; Kraemer, W.J.; Hakkinen, A.; Valkeinen, H.; Alen, M. Selective muscle hypertrophy, changes in EMG and force, and serum hormones during strength training in older women. *J. Appl. Physiol.* **2001**, *91*, 569–580. [CrossRef]
30. Aagaard, P.; Andersen, J.L.; Dyhre-Poulsen, P.; Leffers, A.M.; Wagner, A.; Magnusson, S.P.; Halkjaer-Kristensen, J.; Simonsen, E.B. A mechanism for increased contractile strength of human pennate muscle in response to strength training: Changes in muscle architecture. *J. Physiol.* **2001**, *534*, 613–623. [CrossRef]
31. Geremia, J.M.; Baroni, B.M.; Bobbert, M.F.; Bini, R.R.; Lanferdini, F.J.; Vaz, M.A. Effects of high loading by eccentric triceps surae training on Achilles tendon properties in humans. *Eur. J. Appl. Physiol.* **2018**, *118*, 1725–1736. [CrossRef]
32. Kubo, K.; Kanehisa, H.; Ito, M.; Fukunaga, T. Effects of isometric training on the elasticity of human tendon structures in vivo. *J. Appl. Physiol.* **2001**, *91*, 26–32. [CrossRef]
33. Langberg, H.; Ellingsgaard, H.; Madsen, T.; Jansson, J.; Magnusson, S.P.; Aagaard, P.; Kjaer, M. Eccentric rehabilitation exercise increases peritendinous type I collagen synthesis in humans with Achilles tendinosis. *Scand. J. Med. Sci. Sports* **2007**, *17*, 61–66. [CrossRef]
34. Macgregor, L.J.; Hunter, A.M.; Orizio, C.; Fairweather, M.M.; Ditroilo, M. Assessment of Skeletal Muscle Contractile Properties by Radial Displacement: The Case for Tensiomyography. *Sports Med.* **2018**, *48*, 1607–1620. [CrossRef]
35. Valenzuela, P.L.; Sanchez-Martinez, G.; Torrontegi, E.; Vazquez-Carrion, J.; Montalvo, Z.; Lucia, A. Comment on: Assessment of skeletal muscle contractile properties by radial displacement: The case for tensiomyography. *Sports Med.* **2019**, *49*, 973–975. [CrossRef]
36. Wilson, H.V.; Johnson, M.I.; Francis, P. Repeated stimulation, inter-stimulus interval and inter-electrode distance alters muscle contractile properties as measured by Tensiomyography. *PLoS ONE* **2018**, *13*, e0191965. [CrossRef] [PubMed]
37. Wilson, H.V.; Jones, A.D.; Johnson, M.I.; Francis, P. The effect of inter-electrode distance on radial muscle displacement and contraction time of the biceps femoris, gastrocnemius medialis and biceps brachii, using Tensiomyography in healthy participants. *Physiol. Meas.* **2019**, *40*. [CrossRef]
38. Franchi, M.V.; Atherton, P.J.; Reeves, N.D.; Fluck, M.; Williams, J.; Mitchell, W.K.; Selby, A.; Beltran Valls, R.M.; Narici, M.V. Architectural, functional and molecular responses to concentric and eccentric loading in human skeletal muscle. *Acta Physiol.* **2014**, *210*, 642–654. [CrossRef]
39. Docking, S.I.; Ooi, C.C.; Connell, D. Tendinopathy: Is imaging telling us the entire story? *J. Orthop. Sports Phys. Ther.* **2015**, *45*, 842–852. [CrossRef]
40. Kornaat, P.R.; Van de Velde, S.K. Bone marrow edema lesions in the professional runner. *Am. J. Sports Med.* **2014**, *42*, 1242–1246. [CrossRef]

41. Stahl, R.; Luke, A.; Ma, C.B.; Krug, R.; Steinbach, L.; Majumdar, S.; Link, T.M. Prevalence of pathologic findings in asymptomatic knees of marathon runners before and after a competition in comparison with physically active subjects—A 3.0 T magnetic resonance imaging study. *Skelet. Radiol.* **2008**, *37*, 627–638. [CrossRef]
42. Shaikh, Z.; Perry, M.; Morrissey, D.; Ahmad, M.; Del Buono, A.; Maffulli, N. Achilles tendinopathy in club runners. *Int. J. Sports Med.* **2012**, *33*, 390–394.
43. Abdulhussein, H.; Chan, O.; Morton, S.; Kelly, S.; Padhiar, N.; Valle, X.; King, J.; Williams, S.; Morrissey, D. High Volume Image Guided Injections with or without steroid for mid-portion Achilles Tendinopathy: A Pilot Study. *Clin. Res. Foot Ankle* **2017**, *5*, 249. [CrossRef]
44. Vulpiani, M.C.; Trischitta, D.; Trovato, P.; Vetrano, M.; Ferretti, A. Extracorporeal shockwave therapy (ESWT) in Achilles tendinopathy. A long-term follow-up observational study. *J. Sports Med. Phys. Fit.* **2009**, *49*, 171–176.
45. Hausdorf, J.; Schmitz, C.; Averbeck, B.; Maier, M. Molecular basis for pain mediating properties of extracorporeal shock waves. *Schmerz* **2004**, *18*, 492–497. [CrossRef] [PubMed]
46. Maier, M.; Averbeck, B.; Milz, S.; Refior, H.J.; Schmitz, C. Substance P and prostaglandin E2 release after shock wave application to the rabbit femur. *Clin. Orthop. Relat. Res.* **2003**, *406*, 237–245. [CrossRef]
47. Notarnicola, A.; Moretti, B. The biological effects of extracorporeal shock wave therapy (eswt) on tendon tissue. *Muscles Ligaments Tendons J.* **2012**, *2*, 33–37.
48. O'Sullivan, P. It's time for change with the management of non-specific chronic low back pain. *Br. J. Sports Med.* **2012**, *46*, 224–227. [CrossRef]

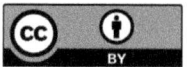

© 2020 by the authors. Licensee MDPI, Basel, Switzerland. This article is an open access article distributed under the terms and conditions of the Creative Commons Attribution (CC BY) license (http://creativecommons.org/licenses/by/4.0/).

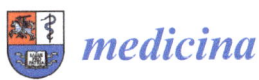

Article

The Beliefs and Attitudes of Cypriot Physical Therapists Regarding the Use of Deep Friction Massage

Alexios Pitsillides [1] and Dimitrios Stasinopoulos [1,2,*]

[1] Department of Health Sciences, School of Sciences, European University Cyprus, Nicosia 1516, Cyprus
[2] Cyprus Musculoskeletal and Sports Trauma Research Centre (CYMUSTREC), Nicosia 1516, Cyprus
* Correspondence: d.stasinopoulos@euc.ac.cy; Tel.: +357-22713044

Received: 13 June 2019; Accepted: 7 August 2019; Published: 12 August 2019

Abstract: *Background*: Deep friction massage (DFM) is a widely used technique by physical therapists worldwide for chronic pain management. According to Dr. James Cyriax, compliance with the proposed guidelines is vital to obtain the desired therapeutic results. *Objectives*: This study explored the beliefs and attitudes of Cypriot physical therapists to DFM and their compliance with the suggested guidelines to identify any empirical-based application patterns and compare them to the suggestions of Cyriax. In addition, the prevalence of DFM use in clinical practice in Cyprus was investigated. *Methods*: Questionnaires, consisting of 18 multiple choice questions and a table of six sub-questions, were distributed to 90 local physical therapists. *Results*: A total of 70% of respondents declared that they perform DFM in their daily practice. The respondents answered 11 out of the 19 technical questions in compliance with the guidelines. *Conclusion*: The study revealed the DFM application pattern of Cypriot physical therapists. The compliance percentage of this pattern to Cyriax guidelines was 58% in general and 62.5% for patients with chronic conditions.

Keywords: Cyriax method; transverse frictions; deep friction massage; deep transverse massage; friction massage; chronic pain; chronic musculoskeletal pain

1. Introduction

Physical therapists worldwide treat chronic pain on a daily basis. A widely known technique for treating chronic musculoskeletal pain is deep friction massage (DFM) [1]. Although Mennell proposed a special massage technique called "frictions" in 1982 [2], DFM was officially introduced to and popularized in the clinical world by Dr. James Cyriax in 1984. According to Cyriax, DFM can be distinguished from general massage as it reaches the deep structures of the body, such as the ligaments, tendons, and muscles [1]. DFM has four key aims: (1) To induce pain relief, (2) to produce therapeutic movement, (3) to produce traumatic hyperemia in chronic lesions, and (4) to improve function [3–5]. The technique can be found in the literature under several names. However, incorrect terminology may negatively affect the results of the technique through differences in execution [1,6]. In the authors' opinion, the general term should be transverse friction massage (TFM) with individual terms used according to the chronicity of the injury. Specifically, the terms gently transverse massage (GTM) for acute injuries and deep transverse friction (DTF) for chronic injuries are apt descriptions of the procedure that must be followed in each case [7].

However, the effectiveness of DFM has not been clearly documented [4,5]. A considerable number of reviews concluded that sample sizes and methodological limitations were the main limiting factors. One such limitation is the lack of standardization of the DFM protocol [3–6].

In 2017, Chaves et al. conducted a cross-sectional study of 478 respondents to determine the prevalence of DFM in clinical practice in Portugal. Further, they aimed to characterize the application parameters used by local physical therapists and identify empirical model-based patterns of DFM application in degenerative tendinopathy. The study concluded that Portuguese physical therapist application patterns were in conflict with the rules of Cyriax. As alluded to above, the aim of their study [8] was not to identify the effectiveness of DFM, but to measure their subjects' compliance to Cyriax guidelines, as according to the proposed guidelines, absolute compliance is vital for successful therapeutic results.

Taking the above-mentioned study into consideration, we designed and conducted the present study on the Cypriot therapeutic community. The purpose of the study was to explore the beliefs and attitudes of Cypriot physical therapists on DFM. The results will be beneficial on a local level, as they could help to highlight whether there is a need to improve application patterns locally. Furthermore, helpful conclusions may be deducted through comparisons with similar studies conducted in other countries. As an example, non-compliance to Cyriax's protocol in clinical practice may translate into a need for revised, more comprehensive guidelines or into a need for improvement and modernization of the current guidelines [7]. Furthermore, the results of the study will add to the existing body of evidence on DFM. The present study is innovative as no other work in the literature has explored this particular issue in Cyprus.

2. Materials and Methods

2.1. Aims of the Study

The aims of this study were firstly, to determine the prevalence of DFM used in clinical practice in Cyprus, secondly, to explore the application of parameters used by local physical therapists, and more specifically, to check if the guidelines proposed by Cyriax were being applied by Cypriot physical therapists, and finally, to identify any empirical model-based patterns.

2.2. Questionnaire Design

The questionnaire was designed as part of a postgraduate degree research project based on the relevant literature. Following corrections from the student's advisor, the questionnaire was finalized. It was then distributed to five physical therapists to confirm that the questions were easily comprehensible; subsequently, some amendments were made. The questionnaire used closed-ended questions with an open comments section at the end of each question.

2.3. Questionnaire Sharing

The questionnaire was distributed to 90 of the 943 registered Cypriot physical therapists. The process started on 28 November 2018 and ended on 28 January 2019. Some of the questionnaires were completed by local physical therapists who were present at the annual meeting of the Cyprus Physical Therapists' Association. The rest were distributed by the author to private physical therapy clinics.

In order to be considered eligible to take part in the study, one had to be a registered physical therapist. Physical therapy students or physical therapy assistants were not eligible to participate. Once the questionnaire was distributed, no further verbal communication between the participants and the author was allowed. The questionnaire was completed in the presence of the author to minimize the likelihood of the results being altered by copying or searching for the correct answer using the internet.

2.4. Ethics

All questionnaires were completed anonymously. Precautions were taken to ensure that all participating physical therapists were fully informed of the purpose and parameters of the questionnaire and consented to the completion of the questionnaire. Relevant information concerning the exact purpose of the study, information on the authors, and the fact that the results might be published were provided on the first page of the questionnaire. Any participant could decline to take part in the survey after consenting, if they so wished.

2.5. Questionnaire Content

The first page of the questionnaire described the purpose and subject of the survey. It further clarified the anonymity of the answers. The first column of Table 1 below lists the 18 multiple-choice questions and a table of 6 sub-questions related to Question 7 contained in the questionnaire.

Table 1. Professional characteristics of the sample ($n = 90$). DFM: Deep friction massage.

Question	Final Sample	
Academic qualifications	n	%
BSc	62	69
Master	26	29
PhD	2	2
Other	0	0
Total	90	100
Years of experience		
1–3	16	18
3–5	16	18
5–10	21	23
Other	37	41
Total	90	100
Field of specification		
Cardiorespiratory	9	7.5
Musculoskeletal	74	61.6
Neurological	25	20.9
Other	12	10
Total	120	100
Use of DFM in daily practice		
Yes	63	70
No	27	30
Total	90	100
Learned the technique from:		
Book	14	16
University	51	59
Seminar	17	20
Other	4	5
Total	86	100

2.6. Data Management and Analysis

The data were tallied by simple counting of the responses for every possible answer in each question. Due to the fact that the respondents were allowed to choose more than one answer or even skip a question, the total number of given answers was also counted for every question individually. The percentage of every answer was calculated in relation to the total number of collected answers to that specific question. The number of each answer was multiplied by one hundred and then divided by the sample size of that question.

3. Results

Table 1 summarizes the participants' professional characteristics. Table 2 displays the answers to all the questions answered by respondents. Table 3 consists of three columns, which display (1) the questions, (2) the most frequent answer, and (3) a comparison of this study's results with the guidelines proposed by Cyriax (shown in the following column). The majority of participants were graduate physical therapists (BSc) with more than 10 years of experience who claimed to specialize in musculoskeletal rehabilitation. Most participants (63 out of 90, 70%) also declared that they used DFM in their daily practice. A total of 59% (51 out of 81) of the sample were taught the technique in their pre-graduate education.

Table 2. Questions and answers given by participants ($n = 90$).

Question	Final Sample	
	n	%
6. Do you use the technique as ... ?		
A single treatment	3	5
In combination with another technique (which one)	43	52
In combination with physical modalities	33	40
Other	2	3
Total	81	100
7a. Acute phase (friction intensity)		
Gentle	48	77.4
Deep	2	3.3
Other	12	19.3
Total	62	100
7b. Acute phase (frequency)		
Daily	8	11.4
Every 48 h	33	47
Once per week	9	12.8
Other	9	12.8
Total	69	100
7c. Acute phase (duration)		
Until analgesia plus 10 maneuvers more	23	38.2
10 min after analgesia	17	28.8
Other	19	32
Total	59	100
7d. Chronic phase (friction intensity)		
Gentle	3	4.8
Deep	57	90.4
Other	3	4.8
Total	63	100
7e. Chronic phase (frequency)		
Daily	15	23.4
Every 48 h	36	56.3
Once per week	9	14
Other	4	6.3
Total	64	100
7f. Chronic phase (duration)		
Until analgesia plus 10 maneuvers more	27	43.5
10 min after analgesia	26	42
Other	9	14.5
Total	62	100

Table 2. Cont.

Question	Final Sample n	Final Sample %
8. Where do you apply DFM?		
Around the point of pain	27	32
On the exact point of pain	54	64
Other	3	4
Total	84	100
9. What is the direction of the applied force?		
Transverse	51	74
Parallel	12	17
Other	6	9
Total	69	100
10. What is the ideal depth?		
Enough to ensure the compression and friction of the target tissue	40	60
Until pain reaches 3/10 on a Visual Analog Scale (VAS)	21	31
Other	6	9
Total	67	100
11. What criteria do you use to choose the applied depth?		
Injury phase	35	37
Pain scale	39	41
Experience	19	20
Other	2	2
Total	92	100
12. Speed of application		
Slow, gradually increase	46	72
Fast	8	12
Other	10	16
Total	64	100
13. Patient positioning		
Comfortable position	46	67
With the area of application stretched	18	26
Other	5	7
Total	69	100
14. If the target tissue is a muscle, it should be positioned		
Stretched	27	37
Accessible	39	53
Shortened	4	5
Other	3	5
Total	73	100
15. If the target tissue is a ligament, it should be positioned		
Stretched	24	35
Accessible	37	54
Shortened	7	10
Other	1	1
Total	69	100

Table 2. Cont.

Question	Final Sample	
	n	%
16. If the target tissue is a tendon, it should be positioned		
Stretched	27	38
Accessible	35	49
Shortened	7	10
Other	2	3
Total	71	100
17. If the target tissue is a tendon with sheath, it should be positioned		
Stretched	31	49
Accessible	26	41
Shortened	5	8
Other	1	2
Total	63	100
18. What grip do you use?		
With the edge of the last phalanx and the last interphalangeal joint bent	24	28.5
With the edge of the last phalanx and the last interphalangeal joint in flexion	31	37
With tools	24	28.5
Other	5	6
Total	84	100
19. Intermediate material		
Oil	24	28
Gel	10	12
Anti-inflammatory cream	22	25
Other	30	35
Total	86	100

Table 3. Questions, answers, and guidelines.

Question	Respondents	n	%	Cyriax
6. Application of DFM in combination with any other technique/single therapy/physical modalities.	In combination with another technique	43	52	Combined with manual therapy
7a. Acute injury, friction intensity	Gently	48	77.4	Gently
7b. Acute injury, frequency	Every 48 h	33	47	Daily
7c. Acute injury, friction duration	Until analgesia plus 10 maneuvers more	23	38.2	Until analgesia plus 10 maneuvers more
7d. Chronic injury, friction intensity	Deep	57	90.4	Deep
7e. Chronic injury, frequency	Every 48 h	36	56.3	Every 48 h minimum
7f. Chronic injury, friction duration	Until analgesia plus 10 maneuvers more	27	43.5	Until analgesia plus 10 min more
8. Spot of application	Exact spot of pain	54	64	Exact spot of pain
9. Applied force direction	Transverse	51	74	Transverse
10. Ideal depth of friction	That ensures tissue compression	40	60	That ensures tissue compression
11. Criteria for ideal depth	Injury chronicity and patient pain.	39	41	Injury chronicity and patient pain.
12. Application speed	Slow, gradually increasing	46	72	Slow

Table 3. Cont.

Question	Respondents	n	%	Cyriax
13. Patient position	Comfortable	46	67	Comfortable
14. Muscle position while applying DFM	Accessible	39	53	Shortened
15. Ligament position while applying DFM	Accessible	37	54	Accessible
16. Tendon position while applying DFM	Accessible	35	49	Accessible
17. Tendon with sheath position while applying DFM	Stretched	31	49	Stretched
18. Preferred hand grip	2 out of 6 suggested by Cyriax	31	37	Cyriax suggested 6 hand grips
19. Intermediate material	Anti-inflammatory gel	22	25	No intermediate material

4. Discussion

4.1. General Discussion

Out of the 90 questionnaires distributed, 27 were not completed beyond Question 4. This most likely suggests that 30% of the sample did not perform DFM in their daily practice or they did not specialize in musculoskeletal injuries. However, is not possible to say that all of those who did not proceed beyond Question 4 did not use the technique, as they may have chosen to stop for other reasons, such as lack of motivation. We believe that asking our subjects if they wished to participate before we shared the questionnaire minimized this possibility.

Seventy percent of our sample declared that they performed the technique and specialized in musculoskeletal injuries. The remaining 63 questionnaires were analyzed in order to investigate the beliefs of Cypriot physical therapists on DFM.

The majority of respondents were graduate physical therapists who mainly specialized in musculoskeletal treatments and applied DFM in their daily practice. Respondents were mainly taught the technique during their university studies.

One of the aims of the study was to identify the presence of any empirical model-based patterns. The questionnaire results revealed that DFM was applied by local physical therapists in a different way to the technique proposed by Cyriax. This empirical model-based pattern is described in the "Respondents" column in Table 3.

The local application pattern differed as compared with the guidelines for seven parameters. Firstly, local physical therapists combined DFM with a variety of other techniques, not only manual therapy, as proposed. Secondly, Cypriot physical therapists applied the technique every 48 h in cases of acute injury, rather than daily. In addition, a stricter interval (every 48 h) than that suggested by Cyriax (48 h minimum) was preferred for chronic conditions. With regard to the speed of application, Cypriot physical therapists claimed to use a slow but gradually increasing speed, whereas Cyriax suggests a slow speed and clarifies that a faster speed mostly affects the superficial tissues [1,3]. When a muscle is the target, local physical therapists preferred to apply DFM with the tissue in an accessible rather than a shortened position. Attention must be given to the therapist's hand position to avoid fatigue. Out of the six hand positions proposed by Cyriax, only two were used by Cypriot physical therapists. The last difference identified concerned the intermediate material used. The respondents stated that they preferred to use an anti-inflammatory gel instead of not using anything, as suggested by Cyriax.

Apart from Questions 7a–c, the survey could be analyzed as an independent questionnaire for chronic pain treatment. In such a case, sixteen technical questions concerned the beliefs and attitudes of local physical therapists regarding chronic pain management. The results of a questionnaire in this scenario would lead us to the same conclusions as the original questionnaire used in the study. In more detail, 10 out of the 16 questions would be in compliance with the suggested guidelines. Even if chronic pain management was investigated in isolation, a substantial percentage of physical therapists in Cyprus did not comply with the suggested guidelines.

Similar to a study published [8] in Portugal, our results demonstrate that the daily application of DFM in Cyprus is not in complete compliance with the proposed instructions of Cyriax. This could be interpreted in different ways. Firstly, it could be that the guidelines need to be revised and improved. The second reason could be that better instructions are needed with regard to this particular technique. Alternatively, the technique proposed by Cyriax may not provide clinicians with adequate therapeutic results, leading to modifications to the technique during daily practice.

The observed non-compliance with the instructions suggested by Cyriax is not only observed among Cypriot physical therapists. As mentioned previously, Portuguese physical therapists were also found to apply DFM in their own ways [8]. In addition, a lack of awareness or differentiation between some technical details of DFM can be observed in the literature. For example, in chronic conditions, the technique must be applied for 10 min after analgesia [1]. However, this proposed duration was neither used by the subjects of this study nor by the authors of previous studies related to DFM [6,9–18].

To date, the effectiveness of this technique has not been documented sufficiently [4,5]. Combined with the observed tendencies of clinicians from different countries, the question of whether the suggested guidelines need to be modified or whether this technique should be used at all has been raised. It is the authors' opinion that DFM should undergo important modifications and a thorough investigation on its effectiveness should be made before it can be recommended to the clinical world [7].

DFM is an old technique, thus, its characteristics are strongly challenged by the better understanding of certain pathologies [7]. For example, the currently suggested technique for tendinopathy is considerably different from that suggested by Cyriax. The use of DFM in such a condition would only result in the breakage of any adhesions, thereby producing traumatic hyperemia. This approach, in cases of tendinopathy, does not target the ability of tendons to store and release energy [19] or their neuroplasticity [20], both of which are vital in tendon rehabilitation.

Our study adds to the body of evidence on DFM. It is the second study to reveal non-compliance of physical therapists to the guidelines. Further, in addition to the observed lack of awareness or the differentiation of some technical details of DFM in the literature, we conclude that physical therapy professionals may have to move on from this traditional technique.

Bearing in mind the insufficiently documented effectiveness of DFM and having observed that physical therapists in different countries tend to change the proposed guidelines—possibly in an effort to improve their therapeutic results—the authors conclude that DFM should, at present, not be included as a first-line treatment.

4.2. Study Limitations

This study is not free of limitations. It concerns the beliefs of Cypriot physical therapists and, therefore, the results cannot be generalized to other countries. Another limitation is that there was no randomization. A third limitation might be the fact that respondents were allowed to choose more than one answer in some questions or even skip one. Despite the use of an equation to calculate the percentage of each answer in relation with the sample size of each question individually, this might have introduced bias associated with double-counting responses.

5. Conclusions

In the current study, 58% of respondents were found to apply DFM in compliance with the suggestions of Cyriax. However, when treating chronic pain, 62.5% complied with the suggested guidelines.

The study revealed the application pattern of DFM followed by Cypriot physical therapists. This pattern differs from the suggestions of Cyriax for seven of the measured parameters.

Author Contributions: Supervision, D.S.; writing—review and editing, A.P.

Funding: This research received no external funding.

Acknowledgments: We would like to thank all the participants for kindly taking the time to answer our questionnaire.

Conflicts of Interest: The authors declare no conflict of interest.

Appendix A

Questionnaire translated to English.

(1) Academic qualifications?

   1. BSc
   2. MSc
   3. PhD
   4. Other … … … … … … … … … …

(2) Years of experience?

   1. 1–3
   2. 3–5
   3. 5–10
   4. Other … … … … … … … … … …

(3) Field of specificity?

   1. Cardiorespiratory
   2. Musculoskeletal
   3. Neurological
   4. Other … … … … … … … … … …

(4) Do you use DFM in your daily practice?

   YES/NO

If in question 3 your answer was NOT «Musculoskeletal» or/and in question 4 your answer was NO, please do not complete the questionnaire further.

(5) How did you learn the technique?

   1. From a book
   2. University
   3. Seminar
   4. Other … … … … … … … … … …

(6) Do you use the technique as

   1. A single treatment
   2. In combination with another technique (which one)
   3. In combination with physical modalities
   4. Other … … … … … … … … … …

(7) Choose an answer in each section of the table (√).

Choose what is correct in every question (√). There may be more than one correct answer. In case you chose other, please clarify.

Injury Phase	Friction Intensity	Frequency	Duration
Acute	☐ Gentle ☐ Deep ☐ Other … … … … … …	☐ Daily ☐ Every 48 h ☐ Once per week ☐ Other … … … … … … .	☐ Until analgesia plus 10 maneuvers more ☐ 10 min after analgesia ☐ Other … … … … … … … .
Chronic	☐ Gentle ☐ Deep ☐ Other … … … … … …	☐ Daily ☐ Every 48 h ☐ Once per week ☐ Other … … … … … … .	☐ Until analgesia plus 10 maneuvers more ☐ 10 min after analgesia ☐ Other … … … … … … … .

(8) Where do you apply DFM?

 1. Around the point of pain
 2. At the exact point of pain
 3. Other … … … … … … … … … …

(9) What is the direction of the applied force?

 1. Transverse
 2. Parallel
 3. Other … … … … … … … … … …

(10) What is the ideal depth?

 1. Enough to ensure the compression and friction of target tissue
 2. Until pain reaches 3/10 on the VAS scale
 3. Other … … … … … … … … … …

(11) What criteria you use to choose the applied depth?

 1. Injury phase
 2. Pain scale
 3. Experience
 4. Other … … … … … … … … … …

(12) Speed of application?

 1. Slow but gradually increasing
 2. Fast
 3. Other … … … … … … … … … …

(13) Patient positioning?

 1. Comfortable position
 2. With the area of application stretched
 3. Other … … … … … … … … … …

(14) If the target tissue is a muscle, where should it be positioned?

 1. Stretched
 2. Accessible
 3. Shortened

4. Other ... ...

(15) If the target tissue is a ligament, where should it be positioned?

1. Stretched
2. Accessible
3. Shortened
4. Other ... ...

(16) If the target tissue is a tendon, where should it be positioned?

1. Stretched
2. Accessible
3. Shortened
4. Other ... ...

(17) If the target tissue is a tendon with sheath, where should it be positioned?

1. Stretched
2. Accessible
3. Shortened
4. Other ... ...

(18) What grip do you use?

1. With the edge of the last phalanx and the last interphalangeal joint bent
2. With the edge of the last phalanx and the last interphalangeal joint in flexion
3. With tools
4. Other ... ...

(19) Intermediate material?

1. Oil
2. Gel
3. Anti-inflammatory cream
4. Other ... ...

References

1. Atkins, E.; Kerr, J.; Goodlad, E. A Practical Approach to Musculoskeletal Medicine. *Phys. Ther. Sport* **2016**, *19*, 49.
2. Chamberlain, G.J. Cyriax's Friction Massage: A Review. *J. Orthop. Sports Phys. Ther.* **1982**, *4*, 16–22. [CrossRef] [PubMed]
3. Chaves, P. Is There a Role for Deep Friction Massage in the Management of Patellar Tendinopathy? Technique Characterization and Short-Term Clinical Outcomes. Ph.D. Thesis, University of Porto, Porto, Portugal, 2018.
4. Joseph, M.F.; Taft, K.; Moskwa, M.; Denegar, C.R. Deep Friction Massage to Treat Tendinopathy: A Systematic Review of a Classic Treatment in the Face of a New Paradigm of Understanding. *J. Sport Rehabil.* **2012**, *21*, 343–353. [CrossRef] [PubMed]
5. Loew, L.M.; Brosseau, L.; Tugwell, P.; Wells, G.A.; Welch, V.; Shea, B.; Poitras, S.; De Angelis, G.; Rahman, P. Deep transverse friction massage for treating lateral elbow or lateral knee tendinitis. *Cochrane Database Syst. Rev.* **2014**, *11*. [CrossRef] [PubMed]
6. Stasinopoulos, D. Cyriax physiotherapy for tennis elbow/lateral epicondylitis. *Br. J. Sports Med.* **2004**, *38*, 675–677. [CrossRef] [PubMed]

7. Pitsillides, A.; Stasinopoulos, D. Cyriax friction massage, opinion for improvements. *Medicina* **2019**, *55*, 185. [CrossRef] [PubMed]
8. Chaves, P.; Simões, D.; Paço, M.; Pinho, F.; Duarte, J.A.; Ribeiro, F. Cyriax's deep friction massage application parameters: Evidence from a cross-sectional study with physical therapists. *Musculoskelet. Sci. Pract.* **2017**, *32*, 92–97. [CrossRef] [PubMed]
9. Blackwood, J.; Ghazi, F. Can the addition of transverse friction massage to an exercise programme in treatment of infrapatellar tendinopathy reduce pain and improve function? A pilot study. *Int. Musculoskelet. Med.* **2012**, *34*, 108–114. [CrossRef]
10. Cooil, R.; Gahzi, F. A pilot study to compare the outcome measures in patients with supraspinatus tendinopathy when treated with either transverse frictions or transverse frictions combined with ultrasound. *Int. Musculoskelet. Med.* **2010**, *32*, 124–128. [CrossRef]
11. Lee, H.M.; Wu, S.K.; You, J.Y. Quantitative application of transverse friction massage and its neurological effects on flexor carpi radialis. *Man. Ther.* **2009**, *14*, 501–507. [CrossRef] [PubMed]
12. Nagrale, A.V.; Herd, C.R.; Ganvir, S.; Ramteke, G. Cyriax Physiotherapy Versus Phonophoresis with Supervised Exercise in Subjects with Lateral Epicondylalgia: A Randomized Clinical Trial. *J. Man. Manip. Ther.* **2009**, *17*, 171–178. [CrossRef] [PubMed]
13. Olaussen, M.; Holmedal, Ø.; Mdala, I.; Brage, S.; Lindbæk, M. Corticosteroid or placebo injection combined with deep transverse friction massage, Mills manipulation, stretching and eccentric exercise for acute lateral epicondylitis: A randomised, controlled trial. *BMC Musculoskelet. Disord.* **2015**, *16*, 122. [CrossRef] [PubMed]
14. Senbursa, G.; Baltaci, G.; Atay, Ö.A. The effectiveness of manual therapy in Supraspinatus Tendinopathy. *Acta Orthop. Traumatol. Turc.* **2011**, *45*, 162–167. [CrossRef] [PubMed]
15. Senbursa, G.; Baltacı, G.; Atay, A. Comparison of conservative treatment with and without manual physical therapy for patients with shoulder impingement syndrome: A prospective, randomized clinical trial. *Knee Surg. Sports Traumatol. Arthrosc.* **2007**, *15*, 915–921. [CrossRef] [PubMed]
16. Stasinopoulos, D.; Stasinopoulos, I. Comparison of effects of Cyriax physiotherapy, a supervised exercise programme and polarized polychromatic non-coherent light (Bioptron light) for the treatment of lateral epicondylitis. *Clin. Rehabil.* **2006**, *20*, 12–23. [CrossRef] [PubMed]
17. Yi, R.; Bratchenko, W.W.; Tan, V. Deep Friction Massage Versus Steroid Injection in the Treatment of Lateral Epicondylitis. *Hand* **2018**, *13*, 56–59. [CrossRef] [PubMed]
18. Stasinopoulos, D.; Stasinopoulos, I. Comparison of effects of exercise programme, pulsed ultrasound and transverse friction in the treatment of chronic patellar tendinopathy. *Clin. Rehabil.* **2004**, *18*, 347–352. [CrossRef] [PubMed]
19. Malliaras, P.; Cook, J.; Purdam, C.; Rio, E. Patellar Tendinopathy: Clinical Diagnosis, Load Management, and Advice for Challenging Case Presentations. *J. Orthop. Sports Phys. Ther.* **2015**, *45*, 887–898. [CrossRef] [PubMed]
20. Rio, E.; Kidgell, D.; Lorimer Moseley, G.; Gaida, J.; Docking, S.; Purdam, C.; Cook, J. Tendon neuroplastic training: Changing the way we think about tendon rehabilitation: A narrative review. *Br. J. Sports Med.* **2016**, *50*, 209–215. [CrossRef] [PubMed]

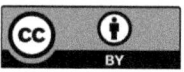

© 2019 by the authors. Licensee MDPI, Basel, Switzerland. This article is an open access article distributed under the terms and conditions of the Creative Commons Attribution (CC BY) license (http://creativecommons.org/licenses/by/4.0/).

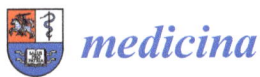

Opinion

Cyriax Friction Massage—Suggestions for Improvements

Alexios Pitsillides [1] and Dimitrios Stasinopoulos [1,2,*]

[1] Department of Health Sciences, School of Sciences, European University Cyprus, Nicosia 1516, Cyprus; alexpitsillides@gmail.com
[2] Director of Cyprus Musculoskeletal and Sports Trauma Research Centre (CYMUSTREC), Nicosia 1516, Cyprus
[*] Correspondence: D.stasinopoulos@euc.ac.cy; Tel.: +357-22713044

Received: 30 March 2019; Accepted: 17 May 2019; Published: 21 May 2019

Abstract: *Background and objectives:* Cyriax friction massage is a widely known and used technique in the field of chronic pain management. Despite its frequent use in daily clinical practice, the technique lacks evidence to support its therapeutic value. While this might be due to various factors, the authors of this paper suggest that the technique might need to be improved and/or modernized according to the recent literature. The purpose of this letter is to further analyze our point of view. *Materials and Methods:* Using the most relevant methods to the subject literature, the authors intended to point out a few technical details that might need reconsideration and/or modernization. *Results:* An appropriate terminology is suggested in the text. Further, suggestions are made regarding the technique's interval time, a possible addition of self-treatment, a discussion of the combination with Mill's manipulation, tendon positioning and other parameters. *Conclusions:* As a therapeutic value has not yet been clearly documented, and since the modernization and/or improvement of the technique might be needed, we suggest that this technique should not be used as a first-line treatment for the management of chronic pain.

Keywords: Cyriax method; transverse frictions; deep friction massage; deep transverse massage; friction massage

1. Introduction

Deep friction massage (DFM) has been promoted and popularized by Cyriax to the clinical world, even though Mennell first suggested the use of specific massage movements called frictions [1,2]. To date, the efficiency of the technique has not been documented, despite the fact that DFM is a widely known technique. Relevant reviews have been hampered by deterrent factors such as sample sizes as well as several methodological limitations of the included studies, such as the lack of standardization of the DFM protocol [3–5]. We believe that is indeed a possibility that the therapeutic results of the method have not been documented yet due to the factors found by the authors of the previously mentioned reviews. On the other hand, we suspect that the inability to record the therapeutic results of DFM might be due to technical faults of the instructions proposed by Cyriax.

2. Terminology

Incorrect terminology may have negative effects on the results of the technique, as it appears to affect how it is executed [6]. This observation has been made by other researchers as well [7], but a proposal for an appropriate terminology cannot be found in the published literature as far as we know. The only discrimination we could find is the one between an acute and a chronic injury in the latest edition of Cyriax's book, but this only describes the grade of the technique that has to be applied [6].

Considering firstly that the correct application depends on proper friction intensity, duration and frequency, and secondly that nonspecific terms might be a deterrent factor, we believe that setting specific terms might influence clinical results.

In our opinion, the general term of the technique should be transverse friction massage (TFM). We believe that previously suggested terms are not completely correct. Any term that includes the word "deep" should not be used. We believe that any term with this characteristic cannot include the application that has to be done for an acute injury, since it will have to be mostly superficial to the tissue, and only six sweeps should be performed on the target tissue [6]. The word "friction" should be included in our opinion. Even though, in an acute stage, the friction on the target tissue is limited to six sweeps, we suggest that the word "friction" should be part of the general terminology of the technique. Our suggestion comes from the fact that friction on the target tissue is the aim of the technique, and thus this has to be clear in the general terminology. The term "massage" has to be included as well. In this way, a new reader will understand that that technique does not only involve friction. Thus, in an acute phase, transverse massage is applied until analgesia and from that point, once target tissue is reached, six sweeps (frictions) more. Additionally, as in chronic injuries transverse massage is applied until analgesia, and from that point 10 minutes of friction is applied to the target tissue, we suggest as a general term the one mentioned above, transverse friction massage (TFM).

In an acute injury, we suggest the term gentle transverse massage (GTM). The differentiation from the term suggested in Cyriax's book is the word "massage" instead of "friction". We believe massage is a better term to describe the procedure performed at an acute stage, which is a gentle transverse massage of the area until analgesia and then six sweeps more.

On the other hand, we are in agreement with the suggestion made in the book for chronic injuries. We support the term deep transverse friction (DTF) since it is what is mostly performed in this situation.

3. Interval between Sessions

We believe that the instructions concerning the interval between interventions in a chronic stage are incorrectly left to the discretion of the therapist. While a comparison of different intervals between TFM sessions does not exist, the instruction of a minimum 48 h [6] is not enough in our opinion. We believe that basic biological differences between the tissues that the technique could be applied to are ignored.

Specifically, oxygen consumption by tendons and ligaments is 7.5 times lower than skeletal muscles. Given their low metabolic rate and well-developed anaerobic energy generation capacity, tendons are able to carry loads and maintain tension for long periods while avoiding the risk of ischemia and subsequent necrosis. However, a low metabolic rate results in slow healing after injury [8]. Thus, we believe that guidelines should be suggested according to the target tissue. We suggest that tendons and ligaments are treated every third day, securing a balance between collagen synthesis and degradation [9]. Another reason that leads to this suggestion is the slower healing after micro injuries due to the technique, due to the aforementioned biological differences. We believe tendons and ligaments should be treated every third day due to the fact that type I collagen's response to high load in a normal tendon peaks at around 3 days after intense loading [10–12]. This response to load appears to be greater in pathological tendons than normal tendons, with a lower resting level and elevated response to loading [10]. We believe that, during the interval time, the tendon should still be somehow loaded to favor the healing process. A possible way to follow this is suggested and further analyzed in the following paragraph. It is also important to mention that the biological tendon response to TFM on humans has not been reported yet, and our suggestions come as a result of studies investigating changes induced by exercise [9,11,12].

4. Self-Treatment

We believe that the technique as proposed by Cyriax does not include the element of self-treatment. It is in our opinion impossible to compare a method that loads the affected tissue for a minimum of

10 min every 48 h (current Cyriax suggestion) to any other technique that loads the same tissue in a more logically structured way [13]. In such a comparison, the results might not support TFM. This might be due to the loading frequency and not the efficiency of the technique itself, since the healing process will be favored by light loading in the interval between sessions. By concluding our thinking, we believe that educating the patient to self-execute GTM between sessions may improve TFM results and offer more equality in the comparison of the technique with others. Training the patient to execute GTM might be beneficial in an acute injury. Since the analgesic effect of TFM can last from 0.3 min to 48 h [14], the patient will be given a way to control their pain, at least for those in which the analgesic duration would have been below the mean (24 h). Unfortunately, only one previous study [14] has examined the duration of the TFM analgesic effect. Due to this lack of evidence, we are unable to recommend a possible dosage of GTM to control pain.

With all this in mind, we suggest that the patient should be taught to control their pain by gently massaging the affected area only until analgesia. In this way, in the case of an acute injury, better pain control will be offered. In the case of a chronic injury, a moderated load will be applied on the tissue in the interval between sessions, positively affecting the new tissue produced by the caused micro injuries during the physiotherapy session, aiding the healing process.

5. Mill's Manipulation for Lateral Elbow Tendinopathy (LET)

In our opinion, Cyriax's suggestion that TFM should always be followed by Mill's manipulation when faced with lateral elbow tendinopathy (LET) is wrong and restrictive for the results of the method. The only reason that the technique is followed by this specific manipulation in the case of LET is because of Cyriax's suggestion [15]. With no evidence supporting the idea that the combination of the technique with Mill's manipulation is superior to a combination with another manipulation or TFM alone [15], we believe that such a restriction is anecdotal.

It is our belief that LET should be either treated similarly to other tendinopathies, or that specific manipulations should be combined in every tendinopathy treatment. To answer this, well-designed RCTs should be designed.

6. Tendon Position

Another point that we believe needs modernization is the position of the tendon during the application of the technique. In our opinion, tendons should be placed in a stretched position, which should be determined by the perception of discomfort and not pain. It has been shown that when the muscle–tendon unit is stretched, most of the stretching occurs in the muscle [16]. A percentage of the force exerted on the tendon during the TFM is possibly absorbed by the muscle. A greater stretch, in our opinion, might be translated into better therapeutic results, as it would correspond to a higher probability of the alignment of the tendon fibers.

7. Other Parameters

As described by Cyriax [6], the guidelines are largely based on clinical opinion. In terms of application duration and sessions, we believe as much as necessary should be used to produce the required therapeutic results. In order to suggest a proper treatment time and number of sessions, we believe that relative RCTs should be designed.

It is widely known and supported by evidence that treating a musculoskeletal disorder is not simply about breaking adhesions and promoting collagen alignment (if this effect is indeed produced by TFM). A good rehabilitation should also address specific tissue characteristics. In the example of tendons, energy storage and release are essential and vital [7]. TFM does not affect this parameter, and so we disagree with Cyriax that TFM combined with manual therapy can efficiently rehabilitate a tendon. Another tissue-specific parameter that is not addressed by TFM is tendon neuroplasticity [17].

We believe that, at the moment, TFM is not supported by sufficient evidence, which creates difficulties for proper parameters to be suggested. This might be a reason that the technique's efficacy has not yet been shown [1,2]. It is also a possibility this is the origin of the non-compliance with Cyriax's protocol in clinical practice, where physiotherapists undertake their clinical reasoning based on the patient's specific needs, adjusting the recommended dose to their interpretation of the clinical condition [1,2].

We believe that there is a reasonable theoretical background behind the theory of TFM, but that it needs modernization and further investigation. A better application of the technique will be translated not only to a better management of pain, but also to a better rehabilitation of musculoskeletal injuries.

8. Conclusions

While there is not sufficient evidence regarding the efficacy of TFM, it is our personal opinion that it should not be in the first line of musculoskeletal treatments.

Author Contributions: The letter was conducted for the needs of a postgraduate degree by one of the authors (A.P.) and supervised by the other (D.S.).

Funding: This letter received no external funding.

Conflicts of Interest: The authors declare no conflict of interest.

References

1. Chaves, P.; Simões, D.; Paço, M.; Pinho, F.; Duarte, J.A.; Ribeiro, F. Cyriax's deep friction massage application parameters: Evidence from a cross-sectional study with physiotherapists. *Musculoskelet. Sci. Pract.* **2017**, *32*, 92–97. [CrossRef]
2. Chamberlain, G.J. Cyriax's friction massage: A review. *J. Orthop. Sports Phys. Ther.* **1982**, *4*, 16–22. [CrossRef] [PubMed]
3. Chaves, P. Is There a Role for Deep Friction Massage in the Management of Patellar Tendinopathy? Technique Characterization and Short-Term Clinical Outcomes. Ph.D. Thesis, Faculty of Sport, University of Porto, Porto, Portugal, 2018.
4. Joseph, M.F.; Taft, K.; Moskwa, M.; Denegar, C.R. Deep friction massage to treat tendinopathy: A systematic review of a classic treatment in the face of a new paradigm of understanding. *J. Sport Rehabil.* **2016**, *21*, 343–353. [CrossRef]
5. Loew, L.M.; Brosseau, L.; Tugwell, P.; Wells, G.A.; Welch, V.; Shea, B.; Poitras, S.; De Angelis, G.; Rahman, P. Deep transverse friction massage for treating lateral elbow or lateral knee tendinitis. *Cochrane Database Syst. Rev.* **2014**. [CrossRef] [PubMed]
6. Atkins, E.; Kerr, J.; Goodlad, E. A practical approach to musculoskeletal medicine. *Phys. Ther. Sport* **2016**, *19*, 49. [CrossRef]
7. Stasinopoulos, D.; Johnson, M.I. Cyriax physiotherapy for tennis elbow/lateral epicondylitis. *Br. J. Sports Med.* **2004**, *38*, 675–677. [CrossRef] [PubMed]
8. Sharma, P.; Maffulli, N. Biology of tendon injury: Healing, modeling and remodeling. *J. Musculoskelet. Neuronal Interact.* **2006**, *6*, 181–190. [PubMed]
9. Magnusson, S.P.; Langberg, H.; Kjaer, M. The pathogenesis of tendinopathy: Balancing the response to loading. *Nat. Rev. Rheumatol.* **2010**, *6*, 262–268. [CrossRef] [PubMed]
10. Cook, J.L.; Purdam, C.R. The challenge of managing tendinopathy in competing athletes. *Br. J. Sports Med.* **2014**, *48*, 506–509. [CrossRef] [PubMed]
11. Langberg, H.; Skovgaard, D.; Asp, S.; Kjær, M. Time pattern of exercise-induced changes in type I collagen turnover after prolonged endurance exercise in humans. *Calcif. Tissue Int.* **2000**, *67*, 41–44. [CrossRef] [PubMed]
12. Langberg, H.; Skovgaard, D.; Petersen, L.J.; Bülow, J.; Kjær, M. Type I collagen synthesis and degradation in peritendinous tissue after exercise determined by microdialysis in humans. *J. Physiol.* **1999**, *521*, 299–306. [CrossRef] [PubMed]
13. Malliaras, P.; Cook, J.; Purdam, C.; Rio, E. Patellar tendinopathy: Clinical diagnosis, load management, and advice for challenging case presentations. *J. Orthop. Sport. Phys. Ther.* **2015**, *45*, 887–898. [CrossRef] [PubMed]

14. de Bruijn, R. Deep transverse friction; its analgesic effect. *Int. J. Sports Med.* **1984**, *5*, 35–36. [CrossRef]
15. Stasinopoulos, D.; Johnson, M.I. It may be time to modify the Cyriax treatment of lateral epicondylitis. *J. Bodyw. Mov. Ther.* **2007**, *11*, 64–67. [CrossRef]
16. Wilhelm, M.; Matthijs, O.; Browne, K.; Seeber, G.; Matthijs, A.; Sizer, P.S.; Brismée, J.-M.; James, C.R.; Gilbert, K.K. Deformation response of the iliotobia band-tensor fasia lata complex to clinical-grade longitudinal tension loading in-vitro. *Int. J. Sports Phys. Ther.* **2017**, *12*, 16–24. [PubMed]
17. Rio, E.; Kidgell, D.; Lorimer Moseley, G.; Gaida, J.; Docking, S.; Purdam, C.; Cook, J. Tendon neuroplastic training: Changing the way we think about tendon rehabilitation: A narrative review. *Br. J. Sports Med.* **2016**, *50*, 209–215. [CrossRef] [PubMed]

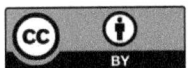

© 2019 by the authors. Licensee MDPI, Basel, Switzerland. This article is an open access article distributed under the terms and conditions of the Creative Commons Attribution (CC BY) license (http://creativecommons.org/licenses/by/4.0/).

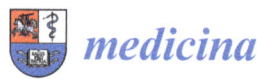

Article

Factors Affecting Psychological Stress in Healthcare Workers with and without Chronic Pain: A Cross-Sectional Study Using Multiple Regression Analysis

Yuta Sakamoto [1,*], Takeru Oka [2], Takashi Amari [3] and Satoshi Shimo [4]

1. Department of Physical Therapy, Health Science University, Fujikawaguchiko-machi 401-0380, Japan
2. Department of Rehabilitation Technique, Fuefuki Central Hospital, Fuefuki 406-0032, Japan; okakaookakao16@yahoo.co.jp
3. Department of Rehabilitation Technique, Ageo Central General Hospital, Ageo 362-8588, Japan; amaritaka@gmail.com
4. Department of Occupational Therapy, Health Science University; Fujikawaguchiko-machi 401-0380, Japan; sshimo@kenkoudai.ac.jp
* Correspondence: y.sakamoto@kenkoudai.ac.jp; Tel.: +81-555-83-5200

Received: 27 June 2019; Accepted: 23 September 2019; Published: 27 September 2019

Abstract: *Background and Objectives:* Pain affects psychological stress and general health in the working population. However, the factors affecting psychological job stress related to chronic pain are unclear. This study aimed to clarify the structural differences among factors affecting psychological job stress in workers with chronic pain and those without pain. *Materials and Methods:* A stepwise multiple regression analysis revealed the differences in structure between the psychological stress of workers with chronic pain and those with no pain. Psychological job stress by the Brief Job Stress Questionnaire was used as the dependent variable, with psychological state (depression and anxiety), specifically that characteristic of chronic pain (pain catastrophizing); information on the nature of the pain (intensity and duration); and number of years of service as independent variables. Selected independent variables were evaluated for collinearity. *Results:* In the model with psychological stress as a dependent variable (chronic pain: $r^2 = 0.57$, $F = 41.7$, $p < 0.0001$; no-pain: $r^2 = 0.63$, $F = 26.3$, $p < 0.0001$), the difference between the experiences of workers with chronic pain and those with no pain was that chronic pain was associated with depression (Beta = 0.43, $p < 0.0001$) and no pain with anxiety (Beta = 0.34, $p < 0.0001$). In the model with chronic pain-related depression as a dependent variable ($r^2 = 0.62$, $F = 41.7$, $p < 0.0001$), job-life satisfaction (Beta = −0.18, $p = 0.0017$) and magnification (a dimension of pain catastrophizing; Beta = 0.16, $p < 0.0001$) were significant. *Conclusions:* The results of this study suggest that the psychological characteristics of chronic pain, such as depression and magnification, should be considered when evaluating and intervening in the job stress of workers with chronic pain.

Keywords: mental health; psychological stress; chronic pain; job stress; medical staff

1. Introduction

A focus on the practical implications of an aging population, driven mainly by an increase in average life expectancy and a decline in birthrate, has become a conspicuous feature of the 21st century. While the focus is usually on increases in this population, the situation affects a number of societal aspects, including the decline of the workforce and its downstream effects [1]. The Japanese population started its decline following the recording of its largest population in 2015; however, the country's workforce has been on the decline, from 53% in 1995—the country's largest workforce on record—to

48% in 2015 [2]. The 5% drop in workforce means that the population supporting social security is declining while the number of elderly people receiving social security is increasing, and the burden on workers is increasing. The continued decline in the size of the working population demonstrates the lack of effective interventions to address this issue, even though it has been recognized for more than 20 years. Furthermore, psychosocial and work environments can contribute to health damage caused by mental stress and physical burden, which highlights the socio-economic importance of healthy work conditions [3–5]. Thus, it has been shown that improving the health of workers is an important issue not only for individuals but also for society.

Work-related stress is an occupational health challenge and has been identified as a significant contributing factor to burnout syndrome [6], high staff turnover [7], absenteeism [8], and low labor productivity [9]. To counter this, the Japanese government increased its focus on workers' mental health by launching an occupational health policy, the Stress Check Program, in 2015 [10]. However, since job stress and related psychological states are affected by a number of factors, its uniform evaluation is difficult.

Pain is one of the factors affecting psychological stress in workers, and the cost of pain-related lost productivity ranged from $299 to $335 billion in a large-scale survey using 2008 data on economic loss from pain in the United States; the annual cost of pain is greater than lifestyle-related diseases (heart disease, cancer, diabetes), which are considered to drive large economic losses [11]. Current pain measures often fail to take into account deterioration caused by various factors, including psychological and cognitive aspects, in addition to the sensory experience of noxious stimuli. Since the characteristics of chronic pain are intensified, its assessment should take into account psychological state, such as the presence of anxiety and depression, and level of pain catastrophizing, as evidenced through rumination, helplessness, and magnification of symptoms [12]. Work in the field of chronic pain has shown that psychological states affect pain experience; for example, low social support in the workplace and low job satisfaction are risk factors for back pain [13], while work stress is an independent predictor of chronic neck and shoulder pain [14]. Work-related psychosocial factors are critical in the assessment of health-related quality of life for chronic pain patients [15]. However, thus far the investigation of mental health as it relates to pain is inadequate. We reported on psychological job stress and depression related to chronic pain, as well as psychological stress and anxiety related to the absence of pain, in a previous study on rehabilitation workers [16]. However, a detailed structural explanation for this difference has not yet been provided. The purpose of this cross-sectional study, therefore, was to clarify differences between the factors affecting psychological job stress in hospital workers with chronic pain and in those without pain, using a structural model and multiple regression analysis.

2. Materials and Methods

2.1. Study Design

This study utilized a cross-sectional design. The sample was recruited from medical staff at a core hospital, and data was collected in February 2018 using questionnaires. The questionnaire survey was distributed to medical staff in all departments who had worked at least 6 months, with the exception of the department in charge of all physicians, which did not provide consent for their staff to participate. Valid questionnaire responses were used to divide the sample into two groups based on duration of pain: a chronic pain group (CPG) and no pain group (NPG). The CPG was defined by continuing or intermittent pain lasting ≥6 months, while the NPG was defined by no pain at the time of the survey and no repetitive pain in the past month. Although previous studies have defined chronic pain as pain lasting longer than 3, or in some cases, 6 months and of at least moderate intensity [17–19], our study builds on the notion that chronic pain cannot be evaluated uniformly. We therefore adopted a pain duration of over 6 months as characteristic of chronic pain.

The procedures were fully explained to participants, in accordance with the Declaration of Helsinki, before the survey, and informed consent was obtained from all subjects prior to participation. The participants were identified by a randomly assigned identifier. This study was conducted with the approval of the Research Ethics Committee of Fuefuki Central Hospital on the 15 August 2017 (Fuefuki, Japan; approval number, 17-4).

2.2. Outcome Measure

Job stress was evaluated with the Brief Job Stress Questionnaire (BJSQ), which is used as part of Japanese policy [10]. The BJSQ evaluates job stressors (nine subscales, namely quantity of work, quality of work, physical burden, interpersonal factors, work environment, job control, use of skills, job fit, and job value); psychological stress (five subscales: vigor, irritability, fatigue, feelings of anxiety, and depressed mood); physical stress, based on an evaluation of somatic symptoms; support (three subscales: support from superiors, from colleagues, and from family and friends); and job-life satisfaction. The main outcome was used to evaluate psychological stress [20]. Scores were calculated by summing the outcome scores of the four-point Likert scale (1 = low stress to 4 = high stress); some items were reverse-scored.

One of the chronic pain models [21] suggests pain catastrophizing, anxiety, and depression worsen pain symptoms; additional measures were therefore used to evaluate psychological state and pain-related psychological factors. With this in mind, we used the Hospital Anxiety Depression Scale (HADS), which includes 14 items rated according to a four-point Likert scale and is used to measure anxiety and depression. Physical symptoms are not assessed by HADS, positioning it as a useful measure of chronic pain-related anxiety or depression independent of insomnia or deep symptoms caused by chronic pain. The Pain Catastrophizing Scale (PCS) [22] was used to evaluate pain catastrophizing—a psychological state characteristic of chronic pain. The scale contains 13 items scored on a five-point Likert scale. A subscale assessing rumination, magnification, and helplessness was developed based on the Japanese version of the PCS [23]. Pain characteristics were evaluated as follows: pain intensity was measured using a visual analog scale (VAS) for pain—a subjective evaluation of pain on a scale of 0–100, indicated on a 100 mm line; pain-related disability was measured using the Brief Pain Inventory (BPI), specifically related to the impact of pain on the participant's life and job; pain duration, measured in number of weeks; and site of pain.

2.3. Statistical Analysis

First, the differences between the two groups in terms of basic characteristics, performance on the five scales of the BJSQ, and psychological state were measured and compared using Mann–Whitney U and chi-square tests. Second, the structural model was verified. Structural model analysis can usually be done using path analysis or structural equation modeling. There are two ways to analyze path models; one of them uses multiple regression analysis. The multiple regression strategy for computing a path analysis employs the ordinary least squares method to calculate the path coefficients [24]. In this approach, the path coefficient is the beta weight of the independent variable, and usually, several multiple regression analyses are used. In this way, an analysis that models multiple independent variables and multiple dependent variable relationships is expressed as multivariate multiple regression [25]. Based on this analysis method, multiple regression analyses were performed twice for each group. A first multiple regression analysis was conducted using psychological stress as dependent variable; analyses were conducted in a stepwise manner according to p-value and Bayesian information criterion instead of Akaike's information criterion, as the emphasis was on model fitness rather than predictive accuracy. Number of years of service, job stress subscales (except that of psychological stress), depression, and anxiety were introduced as independent variables to test for collinearity. The results of the VAS, BPI, and PCS subscales, along with pain duration, were also included into chronic pain as independent variable. Third, another iteration of the multiple regression analysis was performed with the extracted independent variables from the second analysis as dependent variables. The independent variables introduced in the third round were set to the same conditions as for the second analysis, with the exception of the subscale for psychological stress. Furthermore, the validity of model structure in each group was verified through a comparison with the alternative model (AM), which used multiple regression analysis with psychological stress as the independent variable and the dependent variable in a second multiple regression (intragroup-AM). Moreover, the validity of the independent variable in the first multiple regression analysis was verified by comparing the AM, which swapped independent variables between groups (intergroup-AM).

Unless otherwise specified, variables were expressed according to median (lower quartile (LQ) to higher quartile (HQ)). JMP software (version 11.2; SAS Institute, Inc., Cary, NC, USA) was used to conduct the statistical analyses. The indices of multiple regression analysis results were r^2, F-value, and standardized coefficients (Beta). Beta was used as a value representing the degree of influence of the relevant structure. The critical value for significance was set at p value < 0.05.

3. Results

The number of participants is depicted in Figure 1. Out of 284 medical staff members initially contacted, 205 responded with valid answers, resulting in a response rate of 72%. A total of 97 respondents (47%) were included in the CPG, 68 (33%) in the NPG, and 40 participants (20%) could not be included in either group (sub-chronic and acute pain). This division occurred per the criteria discussed previously. The characteristics of the two groups and comparisons between them are shown in Table 1. Mean age in the CPG was 34 years (range: 29.5–41 years). NPG mean age was 34 years (range: 27–37 years; $p = 0.11$). There was no significant difference in gender between the two groups ($p = 0.083$), although the number of females in the CPG was 13% more than in the NPG. The number of years of service showed a similar trend to age, with both the CPG and NPG at 6 years (with ranges of 3–11 and 3–9 years, respectively). There was no difference between office position ($p = 1$) and type of labor contract ($p = 1$). In terms of professional registration or licensing, most participants were nurses (CPG: 47%; NPG: 37%), followed by respondents with no professional registration (CPG: 12%; NPG: 17%). Differences between the two groups were observed for professional registration; however, it was difficult to verify the significance of this difference due to the sample size and research design.

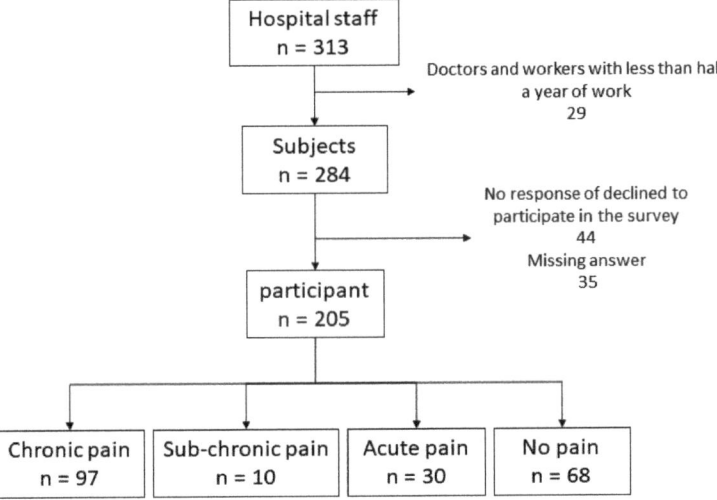

Figure 1. Classification of participants by pain duration. We classified participants according to pain duration. Those included in the no pain group were not experiencing pain at the time of the survey and had not experienced repeated pain in the same site within one month. Acute pain was classified as pain experienced for less than three months, sub-chronic pain was experienced for three to six months, and chronic pain was experienced for over six months. The incidence of chronic pain was the highest, at 47%.

Table 1. Comparison between groups.

		Chronic Pain Group n = 97		No Pain Group n = 68		p-Value
Age	Median (LQ–HQ) years	34	(29.5–41)	34	(27–37)	0.11
Gender	Female (%)	74	(76)	43	(63)	0.083
Years of service	Median (LQ–HQ) years	6	(3–11)	6	(3–9)	0.26
Office Position	None (%)	81	(84)	57	(84)	1
Labor contract	Regular workers (%)	87	(89)	61	(90)	1
License	Nurse (%)	46	(47)	25	(37)	
	None (%)	12	(12)	12	(17)	
	Physical therapist (%)	9	(9)	4	(6)	
	Medical Social worker (%)	6	(6)	2	(3)	
	Pharmacist (%)	5	(5)	5	(7)	
	Occupational therapist (%)	4	(4)	8	(12)	
	Radiologist (%)	4	(4)	1	(6)	
	Other (%)	12	(13)	11	(12)	

LQ: lower quartile. HQ: higher quartile.

The pain characteristics of the CPG are contained in Table 2. Pain intensity (according to VAS scores) was 48 mm (Interquartile range: 30.5–63.5 mm); BPI-life and BPI-job were 3 (range: 1–5); PCS was 20 (range: 8.5–27); and duration of pain was 208 weeks (range: 91–520). The median for pain persistence experienced as "always" was 22%; 58% of respondents reported that pain affected their work performance; and 13% reported absenteeism. Approximately half had a history of consultation with healthcare providers, and 5% had undergone surgery. The majority of pain sites were reported as, in order, lower back (61%), shoulder (55%), and neck (30%); where multiple pain sites were reported, all were recorded.

Table 2. Pain characteristics of the chronic pain group (CPG).

Evaluation Item		Measured Value
Visual analog scale	median (LQ–HQ) mm	48 (30.5–63.5)
Brief pain inventory-life	median (LQ–HQ)	3 (1–5)
Brief pain inventory-job	median (LQ–HQ)	3 (1–5)
Pain catastrophizing scale	median (LQ–HQ)	20 (8.5–27)
Rumination	median (LQ–HQ)	10 (6–13)
Helplessness	median (LQ–HQ)	5 (2–9)
Magnification	median (LQ–HQ)	4 (1–6)
Duration of pain	median (LQ–HQ) week	208 (91–520)
Recalled trigger [A]	not reported (%)	51 (55)
Pain persistence [B]	always (%)	21 (22)
	often (%)	44 (47)
	sometimes (%)	21 (22)
Consultation history	reported (%)	51 (53)
Surgical history	not reported (%)	92 (95)
Influence at work	reported (%)	41 (58)
Absenteeism	not reported (%)	84 (87)
Pain site [C]	low back (%)	59 (61)
	shoulder (%)	53 (55)
	neck (%)	29 (30)
	head (%)	11 (11)
	knee (%)	10 (10)
	groin (%)	9 (9)
	other (%)	18 (19)

[A] Missing value was five. [B] Missing value was three. [C] The site of pain was added respectively. LQ: lower quartile. HQ: higher quartile.

The result of the comparison between group outcomes is shown in Table 3. In terms of BJSQ scores, significant differences were found for psychological stress [CPG: 40 (34–47); NPG: 38 (32–42); p = 0.039]; physical stress [CPG: 22 (18–25); NPG: 16 (13–19.8); $p < 0.0001$]; and job-life satisfaction [CPG: 6 (5–6); NPG: 6 (5–7); $p = 0.043$]. Differences between job stressors and support were not significant. A significant difference on the scale of psychological states was found for depression [CPG: 6 (3.5–9); NPG: 4.5 (2–8); $p = 0.037$]. Anxiety tended to be higher in the CPG [CPG: 7 (4–9); NPG: 5 (3–8); $p = 0.054$].

Table 3. Comparison between the chronic pain and no pain groups.

	Chronic Pain Group		No Pain Group		p-Value
	Median	(LQ–HQ)	Median	(LQ–HQ)	
BJSQ					
Psychological stress	40	(34–47)	38	(32–42)	0.039 [A]
Physical stress	22	(18–25)	16	(13–19.8)	$p < 0.0001$
Job stressors	64	(56–68)	63	(57–67)	0.83
Support	26	(23–30)	26	(23–28)	0.39
Job-life satisfaction	6	(5–6)	6	(5–7)	0.043 [A]
HADS					
Anxiety	7	(4–9)	5	(3–8)	0.054
Depression	6	(3.5–9)	4.5	(2–8)	0.037 [A]

LQ: lower quartile. HQ: higher quartile. BJSQ: Brief Job Stress Questionnaire. HADS: Hospital Anxiety Depression Scale. [A]: $p < 0.05$.

The factors affecting psychological stress in the CPG, as determined by multiple regression analysis, are shown in Table 4. In the model with psychological stress as a dependent variable ($r^2 = 0.57$, F = 41.7, $p < 0.0001$), depression (Beta = 0.43, $p < 0.0001$), physical stress (Beta = 0.37, $p < 0.0001$), and interpersonal factors (Beta = 0.25, $p = 0.0005$) were independent variables. The result of a multiple regression analysis with these independent variables as dependent variables showed that depression as dependent variable ($r^2 = 0.62$, F = 41.7, $p < 0.0001$) affected anxiety (Beta = 0.41, $p < 0.0001$), vigor (Beta = −0.35, $p < 0.0001$), job-life satisfaction (Beta = −0.18, $p = 0.0017$), and magnification (a dimension of pain catastrophizing; Beta = 0.16, $p < 0.0001$). Physical stress as dependent variable ($r^2 = 0.40$, F = 20.3, $p < 0.0001$) had an impact on depressed mood (Beta = 0.35, $p = 0.0003$), fatigue (Beta = 0.30, $p = 0.0016$), and VAS (Beta = 0.26, $p = 0.002$). Interpersonal factors as dependent variable ($r^2 = 0.28$, F = 12.0, $p < 0.0001$) was linked to depressed mood (Beta = 0.35, $p = 0.0003$), job control (Beta = −0.22, $p = 0.020$), and number of years of service (Beta = −0.20, $p = 0.028$). The structure created by multiple regression analysis of CPG data is shown in Figure 2.

Table 4. Factors contributing to psychological stress in the chronic pain group.

Dependent Variable	Independent Variable	r²	Adj-r²	RMSE	F-Value	B	SE	95% CI Lower	95% CI Upper	β	T Value	p-Value
Psychological stress		0.57	0.56	6.78	41.7							p < 0.0001
	1 Depression					1.24	0.22	0.81	1.68	0.43	5.64	p < 0.0001
	2 Physical stress					0.74	0.15	0.45	1.04	0.37	5.01	p < 0.0001
	3 Interpersonal					1.34	0.37	0.60	2.08	0.25	3.58	0.0005
1 Depression		0.62	0.61	2.20	38.3							p < 0.0001
	Anxiety					0.39	0.081	0.25	0.54	0.41	5.26	p < 0.0001
	Vigor					−0.56	0.11	−0.78	−0.34	−0.35	−4.97	p < 0.0001
	Job-life satisfaction					−0.50	0.20	−0.90	−0.01	−0.18	−2.42	0.017
	Magnification					0.17	0.08	0.01	0.34	0.16	2.14	0.035
2 Physical stress		0.40	0.38	4.00	20.3							p < 0.0001
	Depressed mood					0.43	0.11	0.20	0.65	0.35	3.76	0.0003
	Fatigue					0.59	0.18	0.23	0.96	0.30	3.25	0.0016
	Pain intensity (VAS)					0.06	0.02	0.02	0.10	0.26	3.17	0.002
3 Interpersonal		0.28	0.26	1.65	12.0							p < 0.0001
	Depressed mood					0.16	0.04	0.08	0.25	0.35	3.77	0.0003
	Job control					−0.28	0.12	−0.52	−0.04	−0.22	−2.36	0.020
	Years of service					−0.06	0.03	−0.11	−0.01	−0.20	−2.23	0.028

Adj-r²: adjusted r-square. RMSE: root mean square error. SE: standard error. CI: confidence interval. β: standardized coefficients. VAS: visual analog scale. Note: The analysis' first step was confirmed by the method of matching factors to variable increase with the Bayesian information criterion and the method of variable increase/decrease with the p-value. The second step utilized the least squares method.

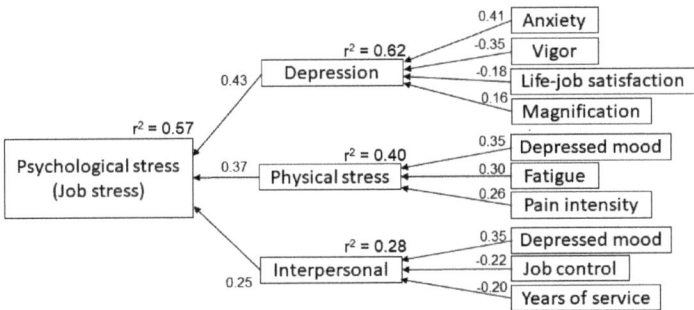

Figure 2. The factor effect model for psychological job stress related to chronic pain. The factor effect model was developed using the results of the stepwise multiple regression analysis using the Bayesian information criterion and *p*-values. The arrow direction moves from the independent variable to the dependent variable, and its numerical value indicates the standardized estimated value. The psychological stress related to chronic pain was most affected by depression, with satisfaction and pain catastrophizing associated through depression.

In the intragroup-AM of the CPG, the AM with an independent variable of depression ($r^2 = 0.55$, $F = 28.1$, $p < 0.0001$) showed that anxiety (Beta = 0.42, $p < 0.0001$) and vigor (Beta = −0.46, $p < 0.0001$) were higher than Beta in the original model; moreover, job-life satisfaction (Beta = −0.08, $p = 0.31$) and magnification (Beta = −0.012, $p = 0.88$) were lower than Beta in the original model, with no significant difference in *p*-value. The AM with an independent variable of physical stress ($r^2 = 0.89$, $F = 245.5$, $p < 0.0001$) showed that depressed mood (Beta = 0.70, $p < 0.0001$) and fatigue (Beta = 0.39, $p < 0.0001$) were higher than Beta in the original model; moreover, pain intensity (Beta = 0.01, $p = 0.69$) was lower than Beta in the original model, with no significant difference in *p*-value. The AM with an independent variable of interpersonal ($r^2 = 0.77$, $F = 105.7$, $p < 0.0001$) showed that depressed mood (Beta = 0.86, $p < 0.0001$) was higher than Beta in the original model; moreover, years of service (Beta = 0.03, $p = 0.51$) and job control (Beta = −0.072, $p = 0.17$) were lower than Beta in the original model, with no significant difference in *p*-value. This result of intragroup p-AM was compared to the original model fit (r^2) and to the independent variable Beta to determine the appropriate model. The r^2 of some intragroup-AMs showed a higher increase than in the original model because the intragroup-AM included a subscale of psychological stress as an independent variable. This model was not appropriate because the sum of the subscales was psychological stress. Furthermore, Beta of job-life satisfaction and magnification (a dimension of pain catastrophizing) reduced further than in the original model. This showed that the original model of the CPG was a better model to explain the influential factors than intragroup-AM.

The effect factors of psychological stress in the NPG, as determined by multiple regression analysis, are shown Table 5. In the model with psychological stress as a dependent variable ($r^2 = 0.63$, $F = 26.3$, $p < 0.0001$), physical stress (Beta = 0.45, $p < 0.0001$), anxiety (Beta = 0.34, $p < 0.0001$), quality of work (Beta = 0.25, $p = 0.0002$), and job fit (Beta = −0.21, $p < 0.0001$) were independent variables. The result of multiple regression analysis with physical stress as dependent variable ($r^2 = 0.41$, $F = 26.3$, $p < 0.0001$) had depressed mood (Beta = 0.43, $p < 0.0001$), irritability (Beta = 0.28, $p = 0.0085$), and support from coworkers (Beta = −0.21, $p = 0.036$) as independent variables. Where anxiety was the dependent variable ($r^2 = 0.63$, $F = 26.5$, $p < 0.0001$), depression (Beta = 0.37, $p = 0.0003$), feelings of anxiety (Beta = 0.33, $p = 0.0004$), vigor (Beta = −0.14, $p = 0.0041$), and work environment (Beta = 0.19, $p = 0.015$) were affected. Quality of work as dependent variable ($r^2 = 0.51$, $F = 16.1$, $p < 0.0001$) was associated with quantity of work (Beta = 0.34, $p = 0.0022$), feelings of anxiety (Beta = 0.30, $p = 0.0036$), physical burden (Beta = 0.28, $p = 0.0063$), and support from family and friends (Beta = 0.19, $p = 0.044$). Job fit as dependent variable ($r^2 = 0.51$, $F = 16.1$, $p < 0.0001$) was linked to job value (Beta = 0.62, $p < 0.0001$) and job-life satisfaction (Beta = 0.29, $p = 0.0012$). The structure created by multiple regression analysis of the NPG is shown in Figure 3.

Table 5. Impact factors for psychological stress in the no pain group.

Dependent Variable	Independent Variable	r^2	Adj-r^2	RMSE	F-Value	B	SE	95% CI Lower	95% CI Upper	β	T Value	p-Value
Psychological stress		0.63	0.60	5.90	26.3							p < 0.0001
	1 Physical stress					0.75	0.14	0.48	1.03	0.45	5.45	p < 0.0001
	2 Anxiety					0.94	0.24	0.46	1.43	0.34	3.90	0.0002
	3 Quality of work					1.26	0.24	0.45	2.07	0.25	3.10	0.0029
	4 Job fit					−3.19	1.21	−5.61	−0.77	−0.21	−2.64	0.0104
1 Physical stress		0.41	0.38	4.41	15.0							p < 0.0001
	Depressed mood					0.59	0.14	0.31	0.86	0.43	4.24	p < 0.0001
	Irritability					0.78	0.29	0.21	1.36	0.28	2.72	0.0085
	Support from coworkers					−0.65	0.30	−1.25	−0.04	−0.21	−2.14	0.036
2 Anxiety		0.63	0.60	2.09	26.5							p < 0.0001
	Depression					0.31	0.08	0.16	0.46	0.37	4.18	p < 0.0001
	Feelings of anxiety					0.53	0.14	0.25	0.82	0.33	3.75	0.0004
	Vigor					−0.43	0.14	−0.72	−0.14	−0.28	−2.98	0.0041
	Work environment					0.92	0.37	0.19	1.65	0.19	2.51	0.015
3 Quality of work		0.51	0.47	1.36	16.1							p < 0.0001
	Quantity of work					0.32	0.10	0.12	0.52	0.34	3.20	0.0022
	Feelings of anxiety					0.27	0.09	0.09	0.44	0.30	3.02	0.0036
	Physical burden					0.59	0.21	0.17	1.00	0.28	2.83	0.0063
	Support from family and friends					0.18	0.09	0.004	0.36	0.19	2.05	0.044
4 Job fit		0.52	0.50	0.43	35.1							p < 0.0001
	Job value					0.71	0.10	0.51	0.91	0.62	7.15	p < 0.0001
	Job-life satisfaction					0.17	0.05	0.07	0.26	0.29	3.38	0.0012

Adj-r^2: adjusted r-square. RMSE: root mean square error. SE: standard error. CI: confidence interval. B: standardized coefficients. VAS: visual analog scale. Note: The first step of the analysis was confirmation of matching factors through the variable increase method, using the Bayesian information criterion and variable increase/decrease method by p-value. The secondary step used the least squares method.

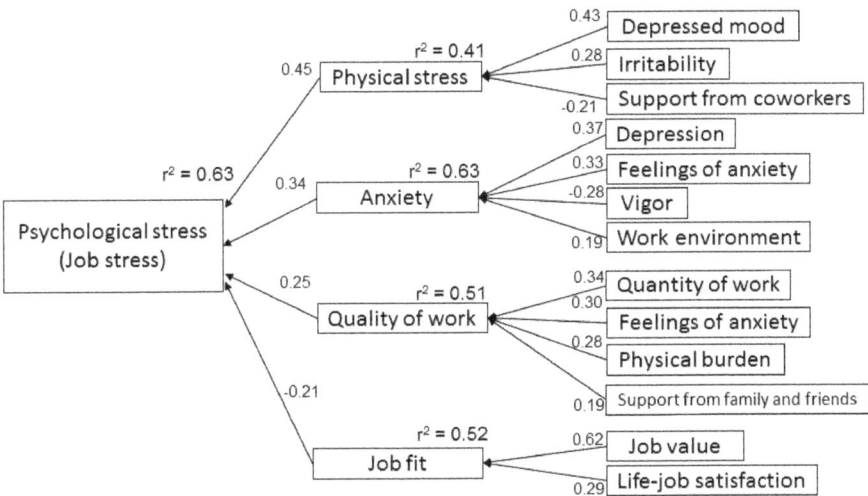

Figure 3. The effect factor model for psychological job stress with no pain. The effect factor model was created through stepwise multiple regression analysis with the Bayesian information criterion and *p*-value. The arrow direction flows from the independent variable to the dependent variable, and its numerical value indicates the standardized estimated value.

In the intragroup-AM of the NPG, the AM with an independent variable of physical stress ($r^2 = 0.89$, F = 165.8, $p < 0.0001$) showed that depressed mood (Beta = 0.82, $p < 0.0001$) and irritability (Beta = 0.26, $p < 0.0001$) were higher than Beta in the original model; moreover, support from coworkers (Beta = −0.037, $p = 0.39$) was lower than Beta in the original model, with no significant difference in *p*-value. The AM with an independent variable of anxiety ($r^2 = 0.83$, F = 75.4, $p < 0.0001$) showed that feelings of anxiety (Beta = 0.71, $p < 0.0001$) and vigor (Beta = −0.29, $p < 0.0001$) were higher than Beta in the original model; moreover, depression (Beta = 0.036, $p = 0.55$) and work environment (Beta = −0.063, $p = 0.23$) were lower than Beta in the original model, with no significant difference in *p*-value. The AM with an independent variable of quality of work ($r^2 = 0.75$, F = 48.4, $p < 0.0001$) showed that feelings of anxiety (Beta = 0.84, $p < 0.0001$) was higher than Beta in the original model; moreover, quantity of work (Beta = 0.032, $p = 0.47$), support from family and friends (Beta = −0.040, $p = 0.55$), and physical burden (Beta = −0.032, $p = 0.65$) were lower than Beta in the original model, with no significant difference in *p*-value. The AM with an independent variable of job fit ($r^2 = 0.11$, F = 4.1, $p = 0.007$) showed job-life satisfaction (Beta = −0.33, $p = 0.007$) to be slightly higher than Beta in the original model; moreover, job value (Beta = −0.025, $p = 0.84$) was lower than Beta in the original model, with no significant difference in *p*-value. A comparison of this result with the original model fit (r^2) and independent variable Beta showed a similarity with the results of the CPG. The r^2 of some intragroup-AMs of the NPG showed a higher increase than the original model because the intragroup-AM included a subscale of psychological stress as an independent variable. This model was not appropriate because the sum of the subscales was psychological stress. Furthermore, the r^2 of job fit was reduced further than in the original model. This showed that the original model for the NPG was also a better model to explain the affecting factors than the intragroup-AM.

In the intergroup-AM, the model fit for the CPG was lower than in the first multiple regression model of the CPG ($r^2 = 0.47$, F = 20.6, $p < 0.0001$), and this model showed physical stress (Beta = 0.36, $p < 0.0001$), anxiety (Beta = 0.40, $p < 0.0001$), quality of work (Beta = 0.068, $p = 0.46$), and job fit (Beta = −0.13, $p = 0.10$). Moreover, the model fit for the NPG was lower than in the first multiple regression model of the NPG ($r^2 = 0.50$, F = 21.2, $p < 0.0001$), and this model showed depression (Beta = 0.35, $p < 0.0001$), physical stress (Beta = 0.56, $p < 0.0001$), interpersonal (Beta = 0.079, $p = 0.38$), and job fit (Beta

= −0.13, $p = 0.10$). This result differed from the original model in that the most influential independent variable of the intergroup-AM for the CPG was anxiety, not physical stress, and the main independent variable of the intergroup-AM for the NPG was physical stress, not depression.

4. Discussion

4.1. Participant Characteristics

This cross-sectional study investigated the factors affecting psychological stress in hospital workers with and without chronic pain. The study had a high response rate (72%) and groups, classified based on the presence or absence of chronic pain, had a median age of 34 years, in line with trends among the labor population. Focusing on the feature of pain in the CPG, 75% of respondents experienced moderate or higher pain, based on the LQ of pain intensity at 30.5 mm on the VAS [26]. However, studies have shown that VAS scores do not coincide with verbal ratings of intensity of chronic pain, and VAS evaluation alone is considered inadequate in the later stages of chronic pain [27]. The median pain duration for CPG participants was 208 weeks—meeting the criteria for chronic pain. Site of pain in the CPG was consistent with the findings of an epidemiological survey in Japan, which also found that the lower back was the most frequent site of chronic pain, followed by the neck and shoulders, respectively [28]. However, the degree of pain-related interference in life and work assessed by two BPI scales had a score of five in the HQ, and more than moderate interference was 25% [29,30]. Based on our results, we can assume that chronic pain affects younger medical staff. Moreover, disability due to chronic pain was not that prevalent.

4.2. Validation of Outcome Comparison between Two Groups

The outcome was nonparametric in that there were many mild cases and few severe cases in this study design, and comparison of both groups needed a suitable statistical test. Thus, outcome comparisons were considered along with medians and quartiles. In the comparison of job stress, psychological stress and physical stress were significantly high in the CPG. The difference between psychological stress in the two groups was five points for the HQ and two points for the LQ, suggesting that chronic pain is linked to higher levels of psychological stress. It was considered that the difference of 6 points in the median score for physical stress was caused by the inclusion of pain-related items in the scale. We considered it unlikely that the work-related environment differed among the groups because there was no significant difference in job stressors and support structures. Job-life satisfaction was significantly lower in the CPG, but the degree of difference was small: the HQ in the NPG was only one point higher. In terms of psychological state, the depression levels of the CPG were significantly higher, confirming findings linking high depression to chronic pain in previous studies [31,32]. However, at least approximately 25% of participants in both groups had symptomatic depression, based on their high HADS scores [33]. This suggests that chronic pain is a significant contributor to job stress, in particular psychological and physical stress, regardless of the presence of job stressors or support.

4.3. Validation of Structure Model by Multiple Regression Analysis

The multiple regression analysis showed that each group had different factors affecting psychological stress. Our findings positioned depression as an independent variable in the CPG and anxiety as an independent variable in the NPG. In addition, in the multiple regression analysis, CPG-depression had anxiety as an independent variable, and NPG-anxiety had depression as an independent variable. This finding emphasizes earlier findings that depression is important to consider in cases of chronic pain, while anxiety is an important consideration in the absence of pain [16]. However, this finding may also simply involve the effects of participants' differential abilities to deal with high stress, as CPG scores were significantly higher in the comparison of the two groups.

In the second multiple regression analysis, CPG-depression had job-life satisfaction and magnification (a dimension of pain catastrophizing) as independent variables. There was a difference in job-life satisfaction between the CPG and NPG, and NPG satisfaction had the independent variable of job fit, which is a subscale of job stressors. We interpreted the satisfaction effects of job fit to be appropriate, as the biggest determinant of job satisfaction in epidemiological studies has been found to be an "interesting" job [34]. Furthermore, a job satisfaction and health meta-analysis reported stronger relationships with psychological stress than physical distress [35]. Accordingly, the results of the present study contribute to the understanding of differences in job-life satisfaction affecting job-related psychological stress between people with chronic pain and those with no pain. Our interpretation that magnification increases depression is appropriate; while the differences regarding the PCS subscales were slight, several studies have reported the importance of magnification as a psychological factor [16,36]. Furthermore, pain catastrophizing and depression have additive and adverse effects on the impact of pain, hence both are important assessment measures for chronic pain [31].

The validation process of intragroup-AM reflected that the original model by repeated regression analysis was valid because Beta in the intragroup-AM decreased more than in the original model, except in the independent variable of the psychological stress subscale in both groups. Thus, depression in the CPG and physical stress in the NPG, extracted by the first multiple regression analysis, were the most influential independent variables for each group. This finding was also emphasized in the comparison results between intergroup-AM and the original model. Consequently, our findings are reasonable and suggest that pain catastrophizing, which is a psychological condition that exacerbates chronic pain, can also aggravate psychological job stress by mediating depression.

4.4. Highlight of This Study

A highlight of our findings is that workers with chronic pain who had low satisfaction and a high rate of pain catastrophizing show an increase in psychological stress through depression. This is very different to the group with no pain and implies that mental health interventions for medical workers with chronic pain need to consider the psychological conditions characteristic of chronic pain.

The epidemiological investigation of chronic pain in Japan showed that professional workers had the highest chronic pain prevalence of several occupation types [28]. Participants in this study included many professional hospital workers, about half of whom had chronic pain. Thus, hospital workers are responsible for the patient's health, but they may also themselves be suffering from pain. The health and working environment of hospital workers may be important considerations for ensuring proper quality of medical care. If a mental health improvement program, as a worker health policy, is verified without considering chronic pain, the effect on psychological stress may be overestimated or underestimated. Therefore, the assessment and treatment of chronic pain may also be effective in patients who face high levels of psychological stress.

4.5. Limitations

There were some limitations that should be considered in the interpretation of this study. Participants were workers at the medical center but doctors were not included, thus the study cannot explain the situation with doctors. Moreover, the study did not consider the severity of chronic pain or physical and joint function, and the index of satisfaction was one scale for both groups. Furthermore, it is possible that insufficient evaluations contributed to the low r^2 for physical stress in both groups and in the interspersion of NPG scores (e.g., physical functions that are the origin of physical stress, and pain-related interpersonal factors such as role clarity and recognition) [37]. In addition, it is possible that more specific models could be developed by examining the factors affecting pain and job stress, such as the effort—reward imbalance [38], demand and control [39], and job characteristics [40]. In addition, model verification to burnout, absence, retirement, and chronic pain requires research utilizing different designs, including longitudinal and intervention research. However, the findings of the present study show that the factors affecting job psychological stress differ between workers who experience chronic pain and those who are pain-free, and we consider our findings to be important for future studies of workers' mental health and chronic pain.

5. Conclusions

This cross-sectional study investigated the effect of various factors on psychological stress in hospital workers with chronic pain and those without. Chronic pain is associated with high psychological job stress and physical stress, regardless of the absence or presence of job stressors or support. Furthermore, depression was found to affect psychological job stress in those with chronic pain, while anxiety affected psychological job stress of those with no pain. Moreover, workers with chronic pain, through the effects of job satisfaction and pain catastrophizing, showed increased psychological job stress related to depression. Additionally, the structural model developed for the CPG differed from that developed for the NPG.

Chronic pain is multifaceted in terms of its socio-psychological effects, and this should be considered when evaluating the issue. Based on the results of the present study, it is important to consider the psychological conditions characteristic of chronic pain in order to evaluate and improve the job stress of workers with chronic pain.

Author Contributions: Conceptualization, Y.S. and S.S.; methodology, Y.S., T.O., and T.A.; software, Y.S.; validation, Y.S., T.O., and T.A.; formal analysis, Y.S.; data curation, Y.S. and T.O.; writing—original draft preparation, Y.S.; writing—review and editing, T.O., T.A., and S.S.; visualization, Y.S.; supervision, Y.S. and S.S.; project administration, Y.S.

Funding: This research received no external funding.

Acknowledgments: We would like to thank Editage (www.editage.com) for English language editing.

Conflicts of Interest: The authors declare no conflict of interest.

References

1. Meltem, I.Y. Economic and Social Consequences of Population Aging the Dilemmas and Opportunities in the Twenty-First Century. *Appl. Res. Qual. Life* **2015**, *10*, 735–752.
2. Statistics Bureau Portal Site of Official Statistics of Japan, 2015 Population Census. Available online: http://www.stat.go.jp/english/data/kokusei/index.html (accessed on 11 June 2019).
3. Stansfeld, S.; Candy, B. Psychosocial work environment and mental health–a meta-analytic review. *Scand. J. Work. Environ. Health* **2006**, *32*, 443–462. [CrossRef] [PubMed]
4. Grimani, A.; Bergström, G.; Casallas, M.I.R.; Aboagye, E.; Jensen, I.; Lohela-Karlsson, M. Economic Evaluation of Occupational Safety and Health Interventions from the Employer Perspective: A Systematic Review. *J. Occup. Environ. Med.* **2018**, *60*, 147–166. [CrossRef] [PubMed]
5. Ravesteijn, B.; van Kippersluis, H.; van Doorslaer, E. The wear and tear on health: What is the role of occupation? *Health Econ.* **2018**, *27*, e69–e86. [CrossRef] [PubMed]
6. Seidler, A.; Thinschmidt, M.; Deckert, S.; Then, F.; Hegewald, J.; Nieuwenhuijsen, K.; Riedel-Heller, S.G. The role of psychosocial working conditions on burnout and its core component emotional exhaustion—A systematic review. *J. Occup. Med. Toxicol.* **2014**, *9*, 10. [CrossRef] [PubMed]
7. Avey, J.B.; Luthans, F.; Jensen, S.M. Psychological capital: A positive resource for combating employee stress and turnover. *Hum. Resour. Manag.* **2009**, *48*, 677–693. [CrossRef]
8. Darr, W.; Johns, G. Work strain, health, and absenteeism: A meta-analysis. *J. Occup. Health Psychol.* **2008**, *13*, 293–318. [CrossRef]
9. Bubonya, M.; Cobb-Clark, D.A.; Wooden, M. Mental Health and Productivity at Work: Does What You Do Matter? *Labour Econ.* **2017**, *46*, 150–165. [CrossRef]
10. Kawakami, N.; Tsutsumi, A. The Stress Check Program: A new national policy for monitoring and screening psychosocial stress in the workplace in Japan. *J. Occup. Health* **2016**, *58*, 1–6. [CrossRef]
11. Gaskin, D.J.; Richard, P. The Economic Costs of Pain in the United States. *J. Pain* **2012**, *13*, 715–724. [CrossRef]

12. Wideman, T.H.; Asmundson, G.G.; Smeets, R.J.; Zautra, A.J.; Simmonds, M.J.; Sullivan, M.J.; Haythornthwaite, J.A.; Edwards, R.R. Re-Thinking the Fear Avoidance Model: Toward a Multi-Dimensional Framework of Pain-Related Disability. *Pain* **2013**, *154*, 2262–2265. [CrossRef] [PubMed]
13. Hoogendoorn, W.E.; Van Poppel, M.N.M.; Bongers, P.M.; Koes, B.W.; Bouter, L.M. Systematic Review of Psychosocial Factors at Work and Private Life as Risk Factors for Back Pain. *Spine* **2000**, *25*, 2114–2125. [CrossRef] [PubMed]
14. Fanavoll, R.; Nilsen, T.I.; Holtermann, A.; Mork, P.J. Psychosocial work stress, leisure time physical exercise and the risk of chronic pain in the neck/shoulders: Longitudinal data from the Norwegian HUNT Study. *Int. J. Occup. Med. Environ. Health* **2016**, *29*, 585–595. [CrossRef] [PubMed]
15. Yamada, K.; Matsudaira, K.; Imano, H.; Kitamura, A.; Iso, H. Influence of work-related psychosocial factors on the prevalence of chronic pain and quality of life in patients with chronic pain. *BMJ Open* **2016**, *6*, 010356. [CrossRef] [PubMed]
16. Sakamoto, Y.; Amari, T.; Shimo, S. The relationship between pain psychological factors and job stress in rehabilitation workers with or without chronic pain. *Work* **2018**, *61*, 357–365. [CrossRef] [PubMed]
17. Andersen, C.H.; Andersen, L.L.; Gram, B.; Pedersen, M.T.; Mortensen, O.S.; Zebis, M.K.; Sjøgaard, G. Influence of frequency and duration of strength training for effective management of neck and shoulder pain: A randomised controlled trial. *Br. J. Sports Med.* **2012**, *46*, 1004–1010. [CrossRef]
18. Treede, R.-D.; Rief, W.; Barke, A.; Aziz, Q.; Bennett, M.I.; Benoliel, R.; Cohen, M.; Evers, S.; Finnerup, N.B.; First, M.B.; et al. A classification of chronic pain for ICD-11. *Pain* **2015**, *156*, 1003–1007. [CrossRef]
19. Fillingim, R.B.; Loeser, J.D.; Baron, R.; Edwards, R.R. Assessment of Chronic Pain: Domains, Methods, and Mechanisms. *J. Pain* **2016**, *17*, T10–T20. [CrossRef]
20. Tsutsumi, A.; Shimazu, A.; Eguchi, H.; Inoue, A.; Kawakami, N. A Japanese Stress Check Program screening tool predicts employee long-term sickness absence: A prospective study. *J. Occup. Health* **2018**, *60*, 55–63. [CrossRef]
21. Hirsh, A.T.; George, S.Z.; Bialosky, J.E.; Robinson, M.E. Fear of pain, pain catastrophizing, and acute pain perception: Relative prediction and timing of assessment. *J. Pain* **2008**, *9*, 806–812. [CrossRef]
22. Sullivan, M.J.L.; Bishop, S.R.; Pivik, J. The Pain Catastrophizing Scale: Development and validation. *Psychol. Assess.* **1995**, *7*, 524–532. [CrossRef]
23. Matsuoka, H.; Sakano, Y. Assessment of cognitive aspect of pain: Development, reliability, and validation of Japanese version of pain catastrophizing scale. *Jpn. J. Psychosom. Med.* **2007**, *47*, 95–102. (In Japanese)
24. Meyers, L.S.; Gamst, G.; Guarino, A. *Applied Multivariate Research: Design and Interpretation*; SAGE Publishing: Thousand Oaks, CA, USA, 2006; pp. 594–595.
25. Patrick, D. *Analysis of Multiple Dependent Variables*; Oxford Scholarship Online, Oxford University Press: Oxford, UK, 2013. [CrossRef]
26. Collins, S.L.; Moore, R.A.; McQuay, H.J. The visual analogue pain intensity scale: What is moderate pain in millimeters? *Pain* **1997**, *72*, 95–97. [CrossRef]
27. Kliger, M.; Stahl, S.; Haddad, M.; Suzan, E.; Adler, R.; Eisenberg, E. Measuring the Intensity of Chronic Pain: Are the Visual Analogue Scale and the Verbal Rating Scale Interchangeable? *Pain Pract.* **2015**, *15*, 538–547. [CrossRef] [PubMed]
28. Nakamura, M.; Nishiwaki, Y.; Ushida, T.; Toyama, Y. Prevalence and characteristics of chronic musculoskeletal pain in Japan. *J. Orthop. Sci.* **2011**, *16*, 424–432. [CrossRef] [PubMed]
29. Li, K.K.; Harris, K.; Hadi, S.; Chow, E. What Should be the Optimal Cut Points for Mild, Moderate, and Severe Pain? *J. Palliat. Med.* **2007**, *10*, 1338–1346. [CrossRef] [PubMed]
30. Kapstad, H.; Hanestad, B.R.; Langeland, N.; Rustøen, T.; Stavem, K. Cutpoints for mild, moderate and severe pain in patients with osteoarthritis of the hip or knee ready for joint replacement surgery. *BMC Musculoskelet. Disord.* **2008**, *9*, 55. [CrossRef] [PubMed]
31. Linton, S.J.; Nicholas, M.K.; MacDonald, S.; Boersma, K.; Bergbom, S.; Maher, C.; Refshauge, K. The role of depression and catastrophizing in musculoskeletal pain. *Eur. J. Pain* **2011**, *15*, 416–422. [CrossRef] [PubMed]
32. Lerman, S.F.; Rudich, Z.; Brill, S.; Shalev, H.; Shahar, G. Longitudinal Associations Between Depression, Anxiety, Pain, and Pain-Related Disability in Chronic Pain Patients. *Psychosom. Med.* **2015**, *77*, 333–341. [CrossRef] [PubMed]
33. Stern, A.F. The Hospital Anxiety and Depression Scale. *Occup. Med.* **2014**, *64*, 393–394. [CrossRef] [PubMed]

34. Alfonso, S.P.; Andres Avelino, S.P. Well-Being at Work: A Cross-National Analysis of the Levels and Determinants of Job Satisfaction. *J. Socio-Econ.* **2000**, *29*, 517–538. [CrossRef]
35. Faragher, E.B.; Cass, M.; Cooper, C.L. The relationship between job satisfaction and health: A meta-analysis. *Occup. Environ. Med.* **2005**, *62*, 105–112. [CrossRef] [PubMed]
36. Masselin-Dubois, A.; Attal, N.; Fletcher, D.; Jayr, C.; Albi, A.; Fermanian, J.; Bouhassira, D.; Baudic, S. Are Psychological Predictors of Chronic Postsurgical Pain Dependent on the Surgical Model? A Comparison of Total Knee Arthroplasty and Breast Surgery for Cancer. *J. Pain* **2013**, *14*, 854–864. [CrossRef] [PubMed]
37. Bergsten, E.L.; Mathiassen, S.E.; Vingård, E. Psychosocial Work Factors and Musculoskeletal Pain: A Cross-Sectional Study among Swedish Flight Baggage Handlers. *BioMed Res. Int.* **2015**, *2015*, 1–11. [CrossRef] [PubMed]
38. Halonen, J.I.; Virtanen, M.; Leineweber, C.; Rod, N.H.; Westerlund, H.; Magnusson Hanson, L.L. Associations between onset of effort-reward imbalance at work and onset of musculoskeletal pain: Analyzing observational longitudinal data as pseudo-trials. *Pain* **2018**, *159*, 1477–1483. [CrossRef] [PubMed]
39. Foppa, I.; Noack, R.H. The relation of self-reported back pain to psychosocial, behavioral, and health-related factors in a working population in Switzerland. *Soc. Sci. Med.* **1996**, *43*, 1119–1126. [CrossRef]
40. Barro, D.; Olinto, M.T.A.; Macagnan, J.B.A.; Henn, R.L.; Pattussi, M.P.; Faoro, M.W.; Garcez, A.D.S.; Paniz, V.M.V. Job characteristics and musculoskeletal pain among shift workers of a poultry processing plant in Southern Brazil. *J. Occup. Health* **2015**, *57*, 448–456. [CrossRef]

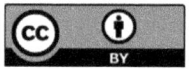

© 2019 by the authors. Licensee MDPI, Basel, Switzerland. This article is an open access article distributed under the terms and conditions of the Creative Commons Attribution (CC BY) license (http://creativecommons.org/licenses/by/4.0/).

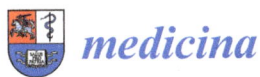

Erratum

Factors Affecting Psychological Stress in Healthcare Workers with and without Chronic Pain: A Cross-Sectional Study Using Multiple Regression Analysis

Yuta Sakamoto [1],*, Takeru Oka [2], Takashi Amari [3] and Satoshi Shimo [4]

1. Department of Physical Therapy, Health Science University, Fujikawaguchiko-machi 401-0380, Japan
2. Department of Rehabilitation Technique, Fuefuki Central Hospital, Fuefuki 406-0032, Japan; okakaookakao16@yahoo.co.jp
3. Department of Rehabilitation Technique, Ageo Central General Hospital, Ageo 362-8588, Japan; amaritaka@gmail.com
4. Department of Occupational Therapy, Health Science University, Fujikawaguchiko-machi 401-0380, Japan; sshimo@kenkoudai.ac.jp
* Correspondence: y.sakamoto@kenkoudai.ac.jp; Tel.: +81-555-83-5200

Received: 19 December 2019; Accepted: 20 December 2019; Published: 24 December 2019

The authors did not realize the error made in the front matter in the proofreading phase. The authors wish to make the following correction to this paper [1]:

An author's name was originally stated as **Satoshi Simo**, but should be changed to **Satoshi Shimo**.

The authors would like to apologize for any inconvenience caused to the readers by these changes. The manuscript will be updated, and the original copy will remain online on the article webpage.

References

1. Sakamoto, Y.; Oka, T.; Amari, T.; Simo, S. Factors Affecting Psychological Stress in Healthcare Workers with and without Chronic Pain: A Cross-Sectional Study Using Multiple Regression Analysis. *Medicina* **2019**, *55*, 652. [CrossRef] [PubMed]

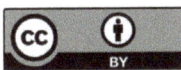

© 2019 by the authors. Licensee MDPI, Basel, Switzerland. This article is an open access article distributed under the terms and conditions of the Creative Commons Attribution (CC BY) license (http://creativecommons.org/licenses/by/4.0/).

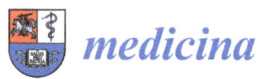

Article

Chronic Pain Patients' Gaze Patterns toward Pain-Related Information: Comparison between Pictorial and Linguistic Stimuli

Jieun Lee [1], Jaewon Beom [2], Seoyun Choi [1], Seulgi Lee Amy Wachholtz [1,3] and Jang-Han Lee [1,*]

[1] Department of Psychology, Chung-Ang University, Seoul 06974, Korea
[2] Department of Physical Medicine and Rehabilitation, Chung-Ang University Hospital, Chung-Ang University College of Medicine, Seoul 06973, Korea
[3] Department of Psychology, University of Colorado-Denver, Denver, CO 80204, USA
* Correspondence: clipsy@cau.ac.kr; Tel.: +82-2-820-5751

Received: 28 June 2019; Accepted: 21 August 2019; Published: 27 August 2019

Abstract: *Background and Objectives:* The attentional bias and information processing model explained that individuals who interpret pain stimuli as threatening may increase their attention toward pain-related information. Previous eye tracking studies found pain attentional bias among individuals with chronic pain; however, those studies investigated this phenomenon by using only one stimulus modality. Therefore, the present study investigated attentional engagement to pain-related information and the role of pain catastrophizing on pain attentional engagement to pain-related stimuli among chronic pain patients by utilizing both linguistic and visual stimulus. *Materials and Methods:* Forty chronic pain patients were recruited from the rehabilitation center, the back pain clinic, and the rheumatology department of Chung-Ang University Hospital in Seoul, Korea. Patients observed pictures of faces and words displaying pain, presented simultaneously with neutral expressions, while their eye movements were measured using the eye tracking system. A *t*-test and ANOVA were conducted to compare stimulus pairs for the total gaze duration. *Results:* Results revealed that chronic pain patients demonstrated attentional preference toward pain words but not for pain faces. An ANOVA with bias scores was conducted to investigate the role of pain catastrophizing on attentional patterns. Results indicated that chronic pain patients with high pain catastrophizing scores gazed significantly longer at pain- and anger-related words than neutral words compared to those with low pain catastrophizing scores. The same patterns were not observed for the facial expression stimulus pairs. *Conclusions:* The results of the present study revealed attentional preference toward pain-related words and the significant role of pain catastrophizing on pain attentional engagement to pain-related words. However, different patterns were observed between linguistic and visual stimuli. Clinical implications related to use in pain treatment and future research suggestions are discussed.

Keywords: attentional preference; linguistic; visual stimuli; chronic pain

1. Introduction

Attentional bias toward pain-related information is well established [1]. However, the evidence for attentional bias toward pain stimuli has not always been supported and authors argued that the inconsistency in results is due to differences in the methodologies [1,2]. These meta-analytic studies found consistent evidence for attentional engagement toward pain-related information for maintained attention at the supraliminal level (i.e., presentation time longer than 1250 ms) but inconsistent results at the subliminal level (i.e., presentation time shorter than 500 ms). These results indicated a need for researchers to consider a stimulus presentation time that is longer than 1250 ms in order to examine maintained attention to pain-related stimuli. Furthermore, to address limitations associated with the visual-probe task (i.e., attentional bias to specific stimuli can only be observed at certain specified time points), an eye tracker was used to observe attentional patterns toward pain-related stimuli continuously across time in recent attentional bias studies.

Previous studies utilizing eye tracking methods [3–5] found that individuals with chronic pain have a tendency to gravitate toward pain stimuli in their attentional process. However, literature indicated that attentional bias is "a complex process", which includes not only attentional engagement toward threatening stimuli but also attentional avoidance from threatening stimuli [6]. Previous studies [6,7] found attentional avoidance from threat-related information when facing real threatening and painful conditions (e.g., operation, dental treatment). This result indicates that when the degree of threat is high (i.e., situations where individuals anticipate high levels of acute pain), individuals may turn their attention away from threatening stimuli in order to manage anxiety. When a threat becomes chronic, chronic pain patients demonstrated difficulty in disengaging their attention from pain stimuli [3–5].

Maintaining attention toward pain-related information shown in chronic pain patients [3–5] may be an attentional process similar to the rumination process observed in depressed individuals. This implies that repetitive negative thoughts related to pain increase and maintain the attention of pain suffers to pain-related information [1]. Pain catastrophizing is defined as cognitive and emotional responses (i.e., rumination, exaggeration, and helplessness) to actual or anticipated pain. Pain catastrophizing is known to be one of the important psychological factors associated with frequency and severity of chronic pain [8–10]. Previous eye tracking studies [3,4] implied attentional engagement toward pain-related information could be influenced by pain catastrophizing, however, those studies were conducted with a non-clinical population. The current study investigated the role of pain catastrophizing on maintained attention toward pain-related information in a clinical population in order to confirm previous results obtained from non-clinical sample studies.

Meta-analytic studies mentioned above suggested that one of the reasons why attentional bias studies demonstrated inconsistent results was due to different stimulus types [1,2]. People may respond to visual and linguistic stimuli differently. According to the dual-coding theory, visual and linguistic information are processed through distinct channels in the human brain [11]. The results of previous studies [12–14] support the notion suggested by the dual-coding theory (i.e., differences in the processing between visual and verbal information). Those studies found not only functional differences but also anatomical differences in processing visual and linguistic stimuli in human brain. Although previous studies found evidence for attentional engagement toward pain-related linguistic stimuli [1,2] and attentional engagement toward pain-expression pictures [3–5] among chronic pain individuals, similarities and differences in the attentional engagement of chronic pain individuals toward different pain stimulus modalities have rarely been compared using eye tracking methodology. Studies, such as ours, that directly compare different pain stimulus modalities as part of investigating the pain attentional bias of chronic pain patients will provide valuable information to develop the most effective psychological intervention for chronic pain patients.

In summary, the present study examined how the attentional engagement toward pain-related information differs depending on different stimulus modalities (word vs. facial expression) and a psychological factor, particularly pain catastrophizing levels. Moreover, to investigate pain-specific attentional patterns, anger-related information pairs (anger vs. neutral stimuli) were included and compared with pain-related stimuli pairs. Inconsistent results in previous attentional bias studies among individuals with chronic pain might have occurred due to a diversity of chronic pain conditions, therefore the current study only recruited patients who were diagnosed with musculoskeletal disorders. Based on previous studies, the present study proposed that (1) chronic pain patients would demonstrate attentional engagement toward pain-related information regardless of types of stimuli presented (i.e., word and pictorial stimuli); (2) attentional engagement toward pain-related information would be maintained across 3000 ms for both pain-related word and pictorial stimuli; and (3) attentional engagement toward pain-related information would be influenced by pain catastrophizing levels for both pain-related word and pictorial stimuli.

2. Materials and Methods

2.1. Participants

We conducted the power analysis of repeated measure ANOVA with within-subjects using G*Power 3.1 program and 28 participants (effect size = 0.25, type I error = 0.05, power of test = 0.80) were the minimum sample size. To account for a possibility of a minimum 10% dropout rate, we increased the sample size to 40. Forty patients with chronic pain that was diagnosed by medical doctors were recruited from the rehabilitation center, the back pain clinic, and the department of rheumatology in Chung-Ang University Hospital in Seoul, Korea. Inclusion criteria were: (1) aged 18 years or older; (2) having no cognitive disability; (3) having no difficulty in understanding and completing the survey; (4) having no eye diseases such as glaucoma and cataract; (5) experiencing chronic pain for more than 3 months; and (6) experiencing musculoskeletal pain as a major source of pain. After medical doctors referred patients to research assistants, the aims and design of the study were explained to patients and informed consent obtained from those who agreed to participate in the present study. This study was approved by the Institutional Review Board of Chung-Ang University Hospital and conforms to the Ethical Guidelines of the 1975 Declaration of Helsinki (approval number IRB#: 1813-002-313, approved on 28 November 2018).

2.2. Measures

Participants completed a questionnaire that contained demographic questions (i.e., age, gender, smoking and drinking) and pain-related questions (i.e., current pain level, levels of pain in the past month, and levels of pain in past 3 months). Regarding pain-related questions, the participants rated their pain on an 11-point numeric rating scale (NRS). In addition to the brief survey regarding demographic and pain-related questions, the following measures were administered.

A Korean-language version of the pain catastrophizing scale (PCS) has been translated and standardized in Korean population [15]. The original PCS was developed by Sullivan et al. [16]. The PCS has 13 items that assess three components of pain catastrophizing: rumination (e.g., "I can't seem to keep it out of my mind"), magnification (e.g., "I wonder whether something serious may happen"), and helplessness (e.g., "There is nothing I can do to reduce the intensity of pain"). Participants were asked to rate their responses on a five-point Likert scale ranging from 0 (not at all) to 4 (always). Cronbach's alpha of K-PCS was 0.93 [15] and internal consistency of this study was 0.91.

The pain disability index (PDI) that was originally developed by Pollard [17] and the present study utilized the Korean-language version of the PDI which was translated by Hong [18]. PDI is a questionnaire that measures the degree of subjective disruption experienced due to chronic pain in seven different domains of life (e.g., home, social, recreational, occupational, sexual life, self-management, and life-support). For each life domain, participants were asked to provide disability ratings on 11-point scales from 0 (no disability) to 10 (total disability). The higher score represents pain interfering more with life. Cronbach's alpha was 0.87 [18] and internal consistency of this study was 0.91.

2.3. Stimulus Materials

2.3.1. Photo Stimulus

As an experimental stimulus, photos displaying facial expressions were obtained by the Korea University Collection (KUFEC) [19] that contained different facial expressions such as anger, happiness, and neutral. Since facial expressions displaying pain were not included in the KUFEC, 32 photos displaying pained expressions were obtained from the previous study [3]. Two pilot studies were conducted to validate photos displaying pained expressions. In pilot studies, 15 participants (five male graduate students, 10 female graduate students) rated the extent manufactured photos are related to pain expression and valence of each photo on a 7-point scale. Based on the results of pilot studies, eight photos (four male, four female) were selected. The mean of rating for pained facial expression was M = 5.67, SD = 0.51 and the mean of rating for valence of pained facial expressions was M = 4.79, SD = 0.30.

Regarding photos displaying anger-related and neutral expression, pictures from the KUFEC corresponding to the selected painful faces were selected. A total of 24 pictures were used in this study (eight pain, eight anger, eight neutral).

2.3.2. Word Stimulus

As another visual experimental stimulus, words describing different emotions including the state of experiencing pain (8 sensory pain words, 8 anger-related words, and 8 neutral words) were utilized in the present study. Total 24 sensory pain words were extracted from the previous studies [20,21]. The present study only included sensory pain words because previous studies including a meta-analysis study indicated that attentional bias was reliably established only to sensory pain words [2,22]. Two pilot studies (9 pain patients, 30 undergraduate and graduate students) were performed to select and validate sensory pain words. Participants rated the degree each word is related to sensory pain expression and rated valence for each word on a 7-point scale. As a result, 8 sensory pain words were selected (Degree each word is related to pain expression: M = 5.26, SD = 0.25; valence of pain words: M = 5.11, SD = 0.33).

Eight anger-related and neutral words were selected from the National Korean Language Institute and anger-related and neutral words were comparable in terms of their word lengths with pain words. All word stimuli were noun forms.

2.3.3. Experimental Design

The paradigm of the experiment in the present study was based on previous studies [3,23–25]. Pairs of photos and words displaying different emotions were presented side by side on the gray background. The eye movements during viewing the stimuli were measured by the Tobii TX300 eye tracker system, which included an LCD 22-inch monitor screen and a camera attached to the bottom of the screen. The word and the picture stimuli were presented in the following order: a central fixation point (1000 ms), picture and word stimuli (3000 ms), and the blank screen (1000 ms). After sitting on a chair, the participants were asked to hold their head still to minimize head movement and view the stimuli through a monitor which was located 60 cm away from the chair. All words and photos were presented with a resolution of 1920 × 1080 pixels and the viewing angle was 38°.

In terms of stimuli, in total 32 picture pairs and word pairs (i.e., 16 pairs of 'pain–neutral', 16 pairs of 'anger–neutral') were shown. Each photo and word appeared equally on the left and right side to control the position bias (i.e., the habit of reading from the left to the right) [3]. To prevent the effect of learning influencing the gaze behaviors of the participants, the presentation sequence of picture and word stimuli was randomized for each participant. The Tobii TX300 eye tracker system defined fixation as the amount of time participants did not deviate their gaze from a defined area of interest (AOI). AOI for the photo and word stimuli was established based on the previous studies [3,21]. To assess the attentional engagement to different stimuli, the total gaze duration for each stimulus (i.e., the averages of total fixation durations within an AOI during the specified time) was calculated. The 3000 ms presentation time was selected to observe maintained attention [3].

2.4. Procedure

After arrival at the laboratory, participants completed the written consent. Prior to the experiment, participants were told to view photos and words on the screen as if they were watching television or reading a magazine. During the experiment, research assistants instructed participants to minimize their head motion and avoid talking for the entire experiment, which lasted 25 min. After the experiment, participants completed the questionnaires. The debriefing of the present study and monetary reward were provided after participants completed the questionnaire. Before each participant left the laboratory, handouts containing information regarding some relaxation techniques (i.e., diaphragmatic breathing, guided imagery) were provided and participants were assisted in learning and practicing relaxation techniques by two research assistants if participants expressed their interest in practicing those techniques.

2.5. Statistical Analysis

Correlational analyses among demographic information, pain-related outcomes, psychological factors, and total fixation durations toward pain, anger, neutral linguistic and pictorial stimuli were conducted. Pain and anger stimuli were compared with neutral stimuli by performing t-tests, and similarities and differences between the pictorial stimuli and linguistic stimuli were examined. Repeated measurement analyses of variance (ANOVAs) with the within-factors 'time' (0–500 ms vs. 500–1000 ms vs. 1000–1500 ms vs. 1500–2000 ms vs. 2000–2500 ms vs. 2500–3000 ms) and 'stimulus type' (pain vs. neutral, anger vs. neutral) were conducted for pictorial stimuli and linguistic stimuli to investigate the time-course of matained attentional patterns toward pain and anger stimuli. Lastly, ANOVAs were performed to test the role of pain catastrophizing on pain attentional bias for the pictorial and linguistic stimuli separately.

3. Results

3.1. Participant Characteristics

Table 1 shows descriptive statistics for the demographic characteristics of the participants (i.e., age, gender, smoking, drinking), pain-related variables (i.e., usage of pain medications, chronic pain durations, current and 3-month pain intensity, pain days per month, pain disability index, chronic pain locations), and pain catastrophizing.

Table 1. Descriptive statistics of demographic information, pain-related variables, and psychological variables.

Variables	Mean (SD)
Age	46.58 (16.26)
Gender	
Male	37.5%
Female	62.5%
Smoking	
Yes	20.0%
No	80.0%
Drinking	
Yes	42.5%
No	57.5%
Pain Medication	
Yes	60.0%
No	40.0%
Chronic pain duration (months)	57.51 (79.92)
Current pain intensity (1–10)	5.40 (2.31)
Average pain intensity in past 3 months (1–10)	6.75 (1.86)
Pain days per month	16.42 (7.40)
Pain disability index	38.38 (14.01)
Pain catastrophizing	25.68 (11.26)
Chronic Pain Location	
Arm	10%
Leg	15%
Shoulder	2.5%
Back	50%
Neck	12.5%
Pelvis	5%
Entire body	5%

We conducted inter-correlation analyses among demographic information (i.e., age, gender), pain-related variables (i.e., pain duration, pain frequency, pain disability index), pain catastrophizing, and gaze duration variables (i.e., total gaze duration toward pain stimulus in pain–neutral facial expression pairs and anger stimulus in anger–neutral facial expression pairs, total gaze duration toward pain words in pain–neutral word pairs and anger words in anger–neutral word pairs). The results revealed no significant correlations between demographic variables (i.e., age, gender) and other variables including pain catastrophizing, pain-related variables, and gaze duration variables; except age was positively correlated with pain duration ($r = 0.347$, $p = 0.028$). Pain catastrophizing was positively correlated with pain duration ($r = 0.383$, $p = 0.015$), total gaze duration for pain-related words in pain–neutral pairs ($r = 0.376$, $p = 0.018$) and total gaze duration for anger-related words in anger–neutral pairs ($r = 0.381$, $p = 0.017$). These results indicated that participants who reported high levels of pain catastrophizing were more likely to report longer pain duration and display higher total gaze duration for pain-related words and anger-related words compared to participants with low levels of pain catastrophizing.

ANOVA and chi-squared tests were performed to determine whether there were significant differences in demographic information and pain-related variables between high catastrophizing group and low catastrophizing group. Table 2 shows that no significant differences were found except for pain catastrophizing scores.

Table 2. Descriptive statistics of demographic information and pain-related variables by two pain catastrophizing scale (PCS) groups.

Variables	Mean (SD)		F/χ^2
	Low PCS ($n = 19$)	High PCS ($n = 21$)	
Age	42.84 (16.02)	49.95 (16.11)	1.953
Gender			0.327/0.567
Male	42.10%	33.30%	
Female	57.90%	66.70%	
Chronic pain duration (month)	34.79 (38.39)	78.07 (100.97)	3.082
Pain frequency	19.63 (9.34)	17.19 (9.83)	0.645
Average pain intensity in past 3 months	6.53 (2.09)	6.95 (1.66)	0.5158
Pain catastrophizing	16.00 (4.40)	34.43 (7.79)	82.459 ***
Pain disability index	34.84 (12.64)	41.57 (14.71)	2.383

Note: low PCS = low catastrophizing group; high PCS = high catastrophizing group. *** $p < 0.001$.

3.2. Total Gaze Patterns toward Different Pairs: Comparison between Pictorial and Linguistic Stimuli

As shown in Table 3, opposite attentional patterns were observed between facial expressions and word stimuli. For facial expressions, attentional preferences toward neutral stimuli in pain–neutral and anger–neutral pairs were observed, while the reverse was seen in word stimuli with preferential attentional patterns toward threat-related stimuli in pain–neutral and anger–neutral pairs.

Table 3. Means/SD and *t*-test results of the gaze durations.

ST	Expression		t	p	Cohen's D
	Pain M (SD)	Neutral M (SD)			
Picture	1.1899 (0.351)	1.3661 (0.417)	−2.017	0.051	0.401
Word	1.2366 (0.447)	1.0718 (0.388)	2.507	0.017 *	0.403
	Anger M (SD)	Neutral M (SD)	t	p	
Picture	1.2117 (0.348)	1.3679 (0.397)	−2.128	0.040 *	0.340
Word	1.1945 (0.386)	1.1030 (0.380)	1.222	0.229	0.204

Note: ST = Stimulus type. * $p < 0.05$

In order to further investigate any potential interactions between stimulus type (word vs. picture) and expression type (pain vs. neutral, anger vs. neutral), ANOVA was conducted. Table 4 revealed that a significant result was found only for the interaction effect ($F(1, 152) = 7.018$, $p < 0.001$, $\eta^2 = 0.044$) for pain and neutral pairs. Regarding anger and neutral pairs, a significant main effect for stimulus type ($F(1, 152) = 5.427$, $p < 0.05$, $\eta^2 = 0.034$) and an interaction effect ($F(1, 152) = 4.184$, $p < 0.05$, $\eta^2 = 0.027$) were found.

Table 4. Summary of ANOVA with 2 stimulus type (word vs. picture) × 2 expressions (pain vs. neutral, anger vs. neutral).

Total Gaze (Pain–neutral)	F	p	η^2
Stimulus type	3.696	0.056	0.024
Expression type	0.008	0.929	0.000
Stimulus × Expression type	7.018	0.000***	0.044
Total Gaze (Anger–neutral)	F	p	η^2
Stimulus type	5.427	0.021*	0.034
Expression type	0.286	0.593	0.002
Stimulus × Expression type	4.184	0.043*	0.027

Note: Stimulus type (word vs. picture). Expression type (pain vs. neutral; anger vs, neutral). * $p < 0.05$, *** $p < 0.001$.

As shown in Figures 1 and 2, the interaction effects were plotted. These plots showed that chronic pain patients gravitated significantly more toward pain- or anger-related words compared to neutral words while the opposite pattern was true for facial expressions (i.e., participants gravitated significantly more toward neutral facial expressions compared to pain- or anger-related facial expressions).

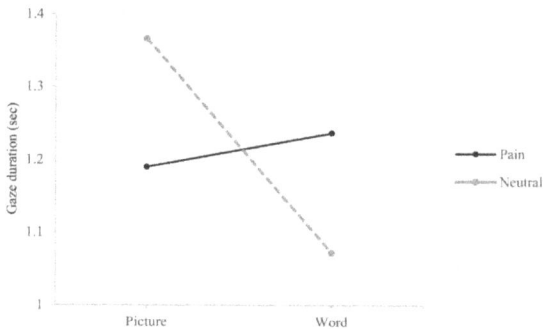

Figure 1. Interaction plot between stimulus type and expression type for pain–neutral pairs.

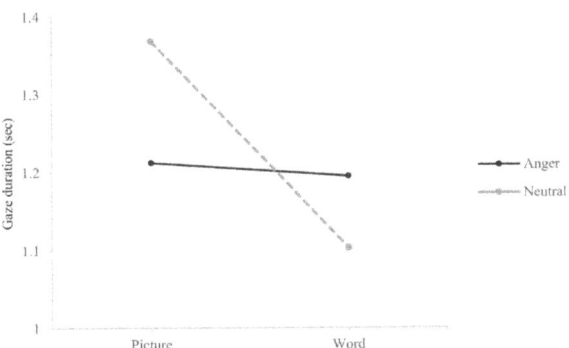

Figure 2. Interaction plot between stimulus type and expression type for anger–neutral pairs.

3.3. Time Course of Gaze Durations

Repeated measure ANOVAs with within-factors 'time' (0–500 ms vs. 500–1000 ms vs. 1000–1500 ms vs. 1500–2000 ms vs. 2000–2500 ms vs. 2500–3000 ms) and 'stimulus type' (pain–neutral vs. anger–neutral) were performed separately for different facial expression and word pairs. As shown in the Table 5, a significant effect was found on time ($F (5, 185) = 37.058$, $p < 0.001$, $\eta^2 = 0.500$) for pain and neutral facial expression pairs. Regarding anger–neutral facial expression pairs, a significant effect was found on time ($F (5, 190) = 38.800$, $p < 0.001$, $\eta^2 = 0.505$) and interaction between time and stimulus type ($F (5, 190) = 2.715$, $p < 0.05$, $\eta^2 = 0.067$). For word stimulus, there were significant effects on time for pain–neutral word pairs ($F (5, 185) = 13.486$, $p < 0.001$, $\eta^2 = 0.267$) and for anger–neutral word pairs ($F (5, 185) = 11.300$, $p < 0.001$, $\eta^2 = 0.234$).

Table 5. Summary of repeated measure ANOVA for pain–neutral pairs and anger–neutral pairs.

Face (Pain–Neutral)	F	p	η^2
Time	37.058	0.000 ***	0.500
Stimulus type	4.079	0.051	0.099
Time × Stimulus type	1.772	0.145	0.046
Face (Anger–Neutral)	**F**	**p**	**η^2**
Time	38.800	0.000 ***	0.505
Stimulus type	3.444	0.071	0.083
Time × Stimulus type	2.715	0.034 *	0.067
Word (Pain–Neutral)	**F**	**p**	**η^2**
Time	13.486	0.000 ***	0.267
Stimulus type	1.381	0.247	0.036
Time × Stimulus type	0.455	0.757	0.012
Word (Anger–Neutral)	**F**	**p**	**η^2**
Time	11.300	0.000 ***	0.234
Stimulus type	0.034	0.854	0.001
Time × Stimulus type	0.481	0.754	0.013

Note: * $p < 0.05$, *** $p < 0.001$.

Figure 3 shows that participants gazed at facial expressions displaying pain- and anger-related information less than neutral stimuli although participants gazed at anger expressions more than neutral expressions during the initial phase of attention (500–1000 ms). Figure 4 revealed that participants gazed at pain-related words more than neutral words whereas in anger–neutral word pairs, this pattern was not as distinct: From the initial to mid phase of attention (i.e., 0–1500 ms), participants gazed at anger-related words more than neutral words, however, they gazed at both word stimulus in a similar degree from the mid to later stage of attention (i.e., 1500–3000 ms). In general, attentional engagement toward all facial expression stimuli tended to gradually increase during the entire attentional process but for word stimuli, attentional engagement increased from the early stage to middle stage of attention and was maintained during the later stage of attention.

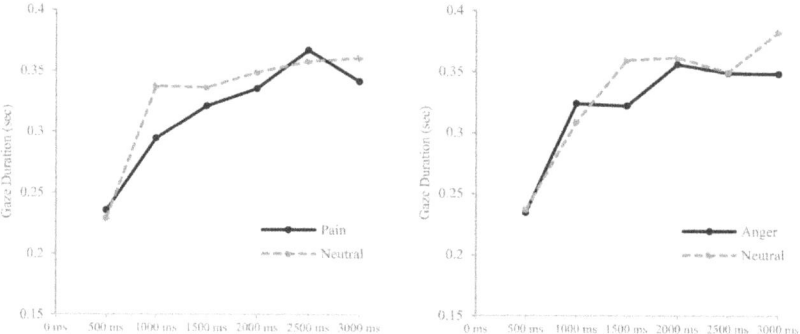

Figure 3. Means of gaze durations for pain and anger faces compared with neutral faces over six times.

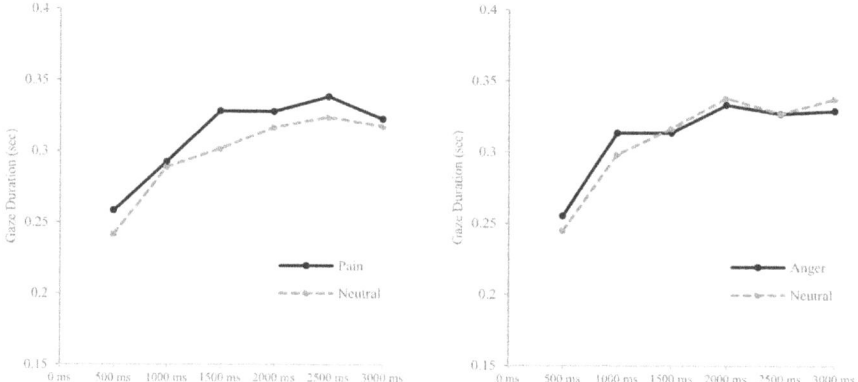

Figure 4. Means of gaze durations for pain and anger-related words compared with neutral words over six times.

ANOVA was performed with dependent variables: bias scores (pain–neutral word bias score, anger–neutral word bias score, pain–neutral facial expression bias score, anger–anger facial expression bias score) and an independent variable (pain catastrophizing group). Bias scores were calculated by subtracting the total fixation durations of neutral stimuli from the total fixation duration of either pain- or anger-related stimuli. To investigate the role of pain catastrophizing on attentional bias toward pain stimuli, participants were divided into a high pain catastrophizing group ($n = 21$) and a low pain catastrophizing group ($n = 19$) using the median split of scores obtained by pain catastrophizing scale (PCS). As shown in Table 6, significant effects were found on pain–neutral word bias score ($F (1,38) = 5.183, p < 0.05$) and anger–neutral word bias score ($F (1,38) = 4.432, p < 0.05$). These results indicated that the high pain catastrophizing group gazed significantly more at pain- or anger-related words rather than neutral words compared to the low pain catastrophizing group.

Table 6. Summary of ANOVA with pain catastrophizing group as an independent variable, and pain–neutral bias scores and anger–neutral bias scores as dependent variables.

	BS M (SD)	BS Std. Error	M (SD)	M (SD)	F	p
	Pain–Neutral W	Pain–Neutral W	Pain W	Neutral W		
High CATA	0.3033 (0.5185)	0.12097	1.3585 (0.5377)	1.0552 (0.4808)	5.183	0.029 *
Low CATA	0.0190 (0.1684)	0.03864	1.1083 (0.2869)	1.0893 (0.2692)		
	Anger–Neutral W	Anger–Neutral W	Anger W	Neutral W	4.432	0.042 *
High CATA	0.2384 (0.5319)	0.12516	1.3199 (0.4373)	1.0815 (0.4355)		
Low CATA	−0.0633 (0.3359)	0.07705	1.0624 (0.2767)	1.1257 (0.3226)		
	Pain–Neutral F	Pain–Neutral F	Pain F	Neutral F		
High CATA	−0.0578 (0.5516)	0.12914	1.2399 (0.4109)	1.2977 (0.4908)	1.983	0.167
Low CATA	−0.3009 (0.5247)	0.12037	1.1372 (0.2749)	1.4381 (0.3188)		
	Anger–Neutral F	Anger–Neutral F	Anger F	Neutral F		
High CATA	−0.1169 (0.4204)	0.09898	1.2138 (0.4255)	1.3308 (0.4777)	0.296	0.590
Low CATA	−0.1976 (0.5035)	0.11552	1.2094 (0.2531)	1.4070 (0.2966)		

Note: CATA = catastrophizing; BS = bias Score, W = word stimuli; F = facial expression stimuli. * $p < 0.05$.

4. Discussion

The current study investigated the attentional engagement to pain-related stimuli for different types of pain-related stimuli among chronic pain patients with musculoskeletal disorders. Results revealed attentional preference toward pain-related words when those stimuli were paired with neutral words, which was consistent with previous studies. Previous studies [26,27] discussed attentional inclination toward threat-related information including pain- and anger-related stimuli for healthy individuals and described this attentional pattern as a natural response to threat. In the present study, results also revealed the attentional preference toward anger-related words when those stimuli were paired with neutral words. However, this result did not reach to the level of significance. The discrepancy in gaze durations between threat-related word stimuli and neutral stimuli was greater for pain–neutral linguistic stimuli pairs compared to anger–neutral linguistic stimuli pairs. This result may indicate that chronic pain patients gravitate toward pain-related words because pain word stimuli were relevant to their pain experience and pain-related word stimuli, like negative thoughts in rumination process among depressed patients, might have activated the attentional process where chronic pain patients had difficulty disengaging from pain-related word stimuli. However, follow-up studies should be conducted to support for the pain-specific attentional bias for the word stimuli among chronic pain patients with musculoskeletal disorders.

The first hypothesis of the present study was only partially supported because the attentional pattern observed for facial expression stimuli (i.e., attentional preference toward neutral stimuli) when pain and anger facial expression stimuli were paired with neutral stimuli, was the opposite pattern observed in previous studies [3,28]. This was a puzzling result particularly because our previous studies [3] utilized similar research methods (i.e., same pictorial stimuli and similar experimental design) as the current study. There were few differences between our previous study [3] and the current study. First, in the previous study [3], subjects were young college students who reported various chronic pain issues whereas the subjects in the present study were an older population who were in treatment for their musculoskeletal disorders in the outpatient clinics of the university hospital. Even though seeing photos that contain pained and angry facial expressions on the computer screen is not as anxiety-provoking and threatening as being in situations where individuals anticipate high levels of pain, visual stimuli that evoke immediate responses may increase fear and anxiety of pain more rapidly for chronic pain patients who are in treatment for their chronic pain. Chronic pain patients in the present study may have diverted their attention away from threat-related facial expression stimuli in order to decrease their distress because they struggled more with pain management and experienced higher level of concerns about their pain than young college students who were not in the treatment for their chronic pain in the previous study [3]. However, current results revealed no significant difference between pain and neutral facial expression stimuli, so the evidence for attentional avoidance from pain-related information is inconclusive based on current results. Second, participants in current study had to view both pictorial stimuli and linguistic stimuli for the viewing trials whereas the previous study [3] only had to view pictorial stimuli. Even though the sequence of presenting two types of stimuli was randomized for each participant and the participants had a break between trials, fatigue may have influenced the attentional process of participants (who were older and more physically challenged due to their chronic pain) in the present study.

A previous study [26] argued that presenting pain-related stimuli longer than 2000 ms could provide an opportunity for researchers to observe an attentional pattern to pain-stimuli more clearly, however, studies that examined maintained attention to pain-related information over 2000 ms by utilizing eye tracking methods are lacking. Thus, the present study investigated the time course of attentional engagement toward pain-related information between pictorial and linguistic stimuli across 3000 ms by utilizing an eye tracking method. Consistent with the previous study [3], the attentional engagement toward threat-related information, particularly pain-related information, was maintained across 3000 ms regardless of stimulus type. This result supported the second hypothesis of the present study and provided evidence for the maintained attention toward pain-related information among individuals with musculoskeletal disorders who are in treatment for their chronic pain in the hospital.

The current study showed that higher pain catastrophizing levels are related to greater levels of attentional engagement to pain- and anger-related words. This result may not be consistent with fear-avoidance attentional patterns shown among individuals with chronic pain in previous studies, however, this result may reflect the tendency of chronic pain patient with high levels of pain catastrophizing to ruminate threat-related thoughts. High levels of ruminations for threat-related thoughts may increase attentional engagement to pain- and anger-related words. The maintaining of attention toward pain-related information shown in previous studies is an attentional bias (e.g., rumination process) similar to the negative thoughts observed in depressed individuals [1]. This implies that repetitive negative thoughts related to pain among chronic pain patients with high levels of pain catastrophizing can intensify and maintain the attention of threat-related information. This is an interesting result as the present study only used sensory pain words and excluded emotional pain words for word stimuli, which indicates that high levels of pain catastrophizing may increase attention toward not only word stimuli that suggest threat or negative emotions but also word stimuli that indicate sensory pain.

The same patterns were not observed for the facial expression stimuli. This result was not consistent with previous research suggesting that pain catastrophizing influences pain perceptions by increasing attention toward pain-related facial expression stimuli [10,29]. Either those who were recently diagnosed as chronic pain [10] or those who were suffering from chronic pain but were not seeking treatment (community or college sample) [3,4] may be differently affected by visual stimuli such as facial expressions of pain than those who were experiencing more severe pain and were receiving treatment in a hospital setting for their musculoskeletal disorders. The greater severity, or perhaps the more prolonged experience of pain may cause altered response to pain stimuli compared to community or college samples.

The current research may inform pain psychology therapy by allowing therapists to provide psychoeducation to chronic patients, informing them that their brain may naturally focus more on pain related words. Once patients are made aware, they may be able to alter this automatic reactive response. We can encourage patients to monitor their observation of pain terms and in the future, potentially implement other empirically validated interventions such as cognitive thought stopping, meditation, distraction, mindfulness to non-pain related stimuli, or some new intervention that has yet to be developed to retrain the brain's response to pain words. Clinicians or health care providers who treat chronic pain patients with musculoskeletal disorders should also be mindful that patients with high levels of pain catastrophizing may experience in difficulty in disengaging from repetitive negative thoughts about pain. Interventions that target to decrease rumination (e.g., behavioral techniques, cognitive restructuring, acceptance and commitment therapy, mindfulness exercises) can be helpful to assist these individuals in decreasing their distress levels and in increasing their capacity to cope with their chronic pain.

Despite the contributions of the present study, there are limitations. First, the study's limited sample size requires a cautious interpretation of results. However, a power analysis was conducted prior to data collection, and the result indicated that 28 participants were sufficient to address the primary study question. Also, the present study differed from previous studies that investigated attentional bias of non-clinic samples with a variety of chronic pain conditions. The present study focused on chronic pain patients with musculoskeletal disorders in the hospital. Second, chronic pain groups were divided according to their scores of pain catastrophizing, and the statistical method utilized was a median split. Researchers raised concerns about using this method because it can increase type I errors and make it harder to detect possible interaction effects [30]. Recent research has found, however, that the median split is a legitimate statistical method when independent variables are uncorrelated [31]. Lastly, the present study did not include a pain-free control group. Previous studies utilizing eye tracking method either found no attentional bias to pain-related information among healthy individuals [5] or found that healthy individuals reduced their attentional engagement to pain-related stimuli significantly during the later stage of attention [26]. However, future studies may confirm this finding further by including a pain-free control group to compare with a chronic pain group to determine whether the maintained attention toward pain-related information is specific to chronic pain groups.

5. Conclusions

The present study expanded previous studies by directly comparing pictorial stimuli (i.e., pained facial expressions) with that of linguistic visual stimuli (i.e., pain-related words) in investigating attentional engagement to pain-related information and the role of pain catastrophizing on attentional engagement to pain-related information. Studies that investigate the time course of maintained attention toward pain-related information on both linguistic and pictorial stimuli were lacking. The current results may underscore the importance of investigating how different modalities of stimuli can differently influence attentional engagement to pain-related information for chronic pain patients. Lastly, consistent with previous studies, the present study supported the role of pain catastrophizing on attentional engagement to pain-related information. The results of the present study can provide useful information for both clinicians and researchers to develop effective psychological interventions for the chronic pain patients with musculoskeletal disorders.

Author Contributions: J.E.L.: First author, conception, acquisition of data, experimental design, data analysis, and data interpretation, manuscript development. J.H.L. (corresponding author): supervision, experimental design, data analysis and interpretation, manuscript development. J.B.: acquisition of data, experimental design. S.Y.C.: acquisition of data, experimental design, and data analysis. S.G.L.: acquisition of data, experimental design, and data analysis. A.W.: consultation for the data analysis and interpretation, and manuscript development.

Funding: This work was supported by the Ministry of Education of the Republic of Korea and the National Research Foundation of Korea (NRF-2017S1A5B5A07063274). AW efforts were supported by the National Institutes of Health (NIDA #K23DA030397).

Conflicts of Interest: The authors declare that there is no conflict of interest regarding the publication of this paper.

References

1. Crombez, G.; van Ryckeghem, D.M.; Eccleston, C.; Van Damme, S. Attentional bias to pain-related information: A meta-analysis. *Pain* **2013**, *154*, 497–510. [CrossRef] [PubMed]
2. Schoth, D.E.; Nunes, V.D.; Liossi, C. Attentional bias towards pain-related information in chronic pain: A meta-analysis of visual-probe investigations. *Clin. Psychol. Rev.* **2012**, *32*, 13–25.3. [CrossRef] [PubMed]

3. Lee, J.E.; Kim, S.H.; Shin, S.K.; Wachholtz, A.; Lee, J.H. Attentional Engagement for Pain-Related Information among Individuals with Chronic Pain: The Role of Pain Catastrophizing. *Pain. Res. Manag.* **2018**, *2018*. [CrossRef] [PubMed]
4. Vervoort, T.; Trost, Z.; Prkachin, K.M.; Mueller, S.C. Attentional processing of other's facial display of pain: An eye tracking study. *Pain* **2013**, *154*, 836–844. [CrossRef] [PubMed]
5. Franklin, Z.; Holmes, P.; Fowler, N. Eye gaze markers indicate visual attention to threatening images in individuals with chronic back pain. *J. Clin. Med.* **2019**, *8*, 31. [CrossRef] [PubMed]
6. Sharpe, L.; Haggman, S.; Nicholas, M.; Dear, B.F.; Refshauge, K. Avoidance of affective pain stimuli predicts chronicity in patients with acute low back pain. *Pain* **2014**, *155*, 45–52. [CrossRef] [PubMed]
7. Lautenbacher, S.; Huber, C.; Schöfer, D.; Kunz, M.; Parthum, A.; Weber, P.G. Attentional and emotional mechanisms related to pain as predictors of chronic postoperative pain: A comparison with other psychological and physiological predictors. *Pain* **2010**, *151*, 722–731. [CrossRef]
8. De Boer, M.J.; Steinhagen, H.E.; Versteegen, G.J. Mindfulness, acceptance and catastrophizing in chronic pain. *PLoS ONE* **2014**, *9*, 1–5. [CrossRef]
9. Drahovzal, D.N.; Stewart, S.H.; Sullivan, M.J. Tendency to catastrophize somatic sensations: Pain catastrophizing and anxiety sensitivity in predicting headache. *Cogn. Behav. Ther.* **2016**, *35*, 226–235. [CrossRef]
10. Sullivan, M.J.; Thorn, B.; Rodgers, W. Path model of psychological antecedents to pain experience: Experimental and clinical findings. *Clinic. J. Pain* **2004**, *20*, 164–173. [CrossRef]
11. Paivio, A. Dual coding theory: Retrospect and current status. *Can. J. Psychol./Rev. Can. De Psychol.* **1991**, *45*, 2559. [CrossRef]
12. Azizian, A.; Watson, T.D.; Parvaz, M.A.; Squires, N.K. Time course of processes underlying picture and word evaluation: An event-related potential approach. *Brain Topogr.* **2006**, *18*, 213–222. [CrossRef] [PubMed]
13. Khateb, A.; Pegna, A.; Michel, C.M.; Landis, T.; Annoni, J. Dynamics of brain activation during an explicit word and image recognition task: An electrophysiological study. *Brain Topogr.* **2002**, *14*, 197–213. [CrossRef]
14. Schlochtermeier, L.H.; Kuchinke, L.; Pehrs, C.; Urton, K.; Kappelhoff, H.; Jacobs, A.M. Emotional picture and word processing: An fMRI study on effects of stimulus complexity. *PLoS ONE* **2013**, *8*, e55619. [CrossRef] [PubMed]
15. Cho, S.K.; Kim, H.Y.; Lee, J.H. Validation of the Korean version of the Pain Catastrophizing Scale in patients with chronic non-cancer pain. *Qual. Life Res.* **2013**, *22*, 1767–1772. [CrossRef] [PubMed]
16. Sullivan, M.J.; Bishop, S.R.; Pivik, J. The pain catastrophizing scale: Development and validation. *Psychol. Assess.* **1995**, *7*, 524. [CrossRef]
17. Pollard, C.A. Preliminary validity study of the pain disability index. *Percept. Mot. Ski.* **1984**, *59*, 974. [CrossRef] [PubMed]
18. Hong, M.S. A study on types of pain belief, and related factors of pain among chronic shoulder pain patients. (Unpublished). Master's Thesis, Korea University, Seoul, Korea, 2010. Unpublished.
19. Lee, T.H.; Lee, K.; Lee, K.Y.; Choi, J.S.; Kim, H.T. *The Korea University Facial Expression Collection: KUFEC. Lab.*; Lab. of Behavioral Neuroscience, Dept. of Psychology: Seoul, Korea, 2006.
20. Bae, S.J.; Cho, S. Attentional bias in breakthrough pain and moderating effect of gender: A preliminary study. (Unpublished). Master's Thesis, Chungnam University, Daejeon, 2017.
21. Lee, E.O.; Yun, S.N.; Song, M.S. A Study for Development of Ratio Scale Measuring Pain Using Korean Pain Terms. *J. Nurses Acad. Soc.* **1984**, *14*, 93–114. [CrossRef]
22. Fashler, S.R.; Katz, J. More than meets the eye: Visual attention biases in individuals reporting chronic pain. *J. Pain Res.* **2014**, *7*, 557. [CrossRef] [PubMed]
23. Kim, S.J.; Lee, J.H. Time course of attentional bias for health-related information in individuals with health anxiety. *J. Health Psychol.* **2016**, *21*, 1527–1535. [CrossRef] [PubMed]
24. Rösler, A.; Ulrich, C.; Billino, J.; Sterzer, P.; Weidauer, S.; Bernhardt, T.; Steinmetz, H.; Frölich, L.; Kleinschmidt, A. Effects of arousing emotional scenes on the distribution of visuospatial attention: Changes with aging and early subcortical vascular dementia. *J. Neurol. Sci.* **2005**, *229*, 109–116. [CrossRef] [PubMed]
25. LaBar, K.S.; Mesulam, M.; Gitelman, D.R.; Weintraub, S. Emotional curiosity: Modulation of visuospatial attention by arousal is preserved in aging and early-stage Alzheimer's disease. *Neuropsychologia* **2000**, *38*, 1734–1740. [CrossRef]

26. Priebe, J.A.; Messingschlager, M.; Lautenbacher, S. Gaze behavior when monitoring pain faces: An eye-tracking study. *Eur. J. Pain* **2014**, *19*, 817–825. [CrossRef]
27. Baum, C.; Schneider, R.; Keogh, E.; Lautenbacher, S. Different stages in attentional processing of facial expressions of pain: A dot-probe task modification. *J. Pain* **2016**, *14*, 223–232. [CrossRef] [PubMed]
28. Khatibi, A.; Dehghani, M.; Sharpe, L.; Asmundson, G.J.; Pouretemad, H. Selective attention towards painful faces among chronic pain patients: Evidence from a modified version of the dot-probe. *Pain* **2009**, *142*, 42–47. [CrossRef] [PubMed]
29. Gracely, R.H.; Geisser, M.E.; Giesecke, T.; Grant, M.A.B.; Petzke, F.; Williams, D.A.; Clauw, D.J. Pain catastrophizing and neural responses to pain among persons with fibromyalgia. *Brain* **2004**, *127*, 835–843. [CrossRef] [PubMed]
30. Aiken, L.S.; West, S.G.; Reno, R.R. *Multiple Regression: Testing and Interpreting Interactions*; Sage: London, UK, 1991.
31. Iacobucci, D.; Posavac, S.S.; Kardes, F.R.; Schneider, M.J.; Popovich, D.L. The median split: Robust, refined, and revived. *J. Consum. Psychol.* **2015**, *25*, 690–704. [CrossRef]

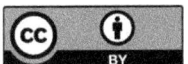

© 2019 by the authors. Licensee MDPI, Basel, Switzerland. This article is an open access article distributed under the terms and conditions of the Creative Commons Attribution (CC BY) license (http://creativecommons.org/licenses/by/4.0/).

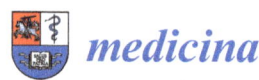

Article

Empathic Accuracy in Chronic Pain: Exploring Patient and Informal Caregiver Differences and Their Personality Correlates

Carlos Suso-Ribera [1,*], Verónica Martínez-Borba [1], Alejandro Viciano [1], Francisco Javier Cano-García [2] and Azucena García-Palacios [1]

1. Department of Personality, Assessment, and Psychological Treatments, Jaume I University, 12071 Castellón de la Plana, Spain
2. Department of Personality, Assessment, and Psychological Treatments, University of Seville, 41018 Seville, Spain
* Correspondence: susor@uji.es; Tel.: +34-964-387-643

Received: 26 June 2019; Accepted: 21 August 2019; Published: 27 August 2019

Abstract: *Background and objectives:* Social factors have demonstrated to affect pain intensity and quality of life of pain patients, such as social support or the attitudes and responses of the main informal caregiver. Similarly, pain has negative consequences on the patient's social environment. However, it is still rare to include social factors in pain research and treatment. This study compares patient and caregivers' accuracy, as well as explores personality and health correlates of empathic accuracy in patients and caregivers. *Materials and Methods:* The study comprised 292 chronic pain patients from the Pain Clinic of the Vall d'Hebron Hospital in Spain (main age = 59.4 years; 66.8% females) and their main informal caregivers (main age = 53.5 years; 51.0% females; 68.5% couples). *Results:* Patients were relatively inaccurate at estimating the interference of pain on their counterparts ($t = 2.16$; $p = 0.032$), while informal caregivers estimated well the patient's status (all differences $p > 0.05$). Empathic accuracy on patient and caregiver status did not differ across types of relationship (i.e., couple or other; all differences $p > 0.05$). Sex differences in estimation only occurred for disagreement in pain severity, with female caregivers showing higher overestimation ($t = 2.18$; $p = 0.030$). Patients' health status and caregivers' personality were significant correlates of empathic accuracy. Overall, estimation was poorer when patients presented higher physical functioning. Similarly, caregiver had more difficulties in estimating the patient's pain interference as patient general and mental health increased ($r = 0.16$, $p = 0.008$, and $r = 0.15$, $p = 0.009$, respectively). Caregiver openness was linked to a more accurate estimation of a patient's status ($r = 0.20$, $p < 0.001$), while caregiver agreeableness was related to a patient's greater accuracy of their caregivers' pain interference ($r = 0.15$, $p = 0.009$). *Conclusions:* Patients poorly estimate the impact of their illness compared to caregivers, regardless of their relationship. Some personality characteristics in the caregiver and health outcomes in the patient are associated with empathic inaccuracy, which should guide clinicians when selecting who requires more active training on empathy in pain settings.

Keywords: empathic accuracy; chronic pain; informal caregiver; spouse; health status; personality

1. Introduction

According to epidemiological studies, chronic pain, which is defined as recurrent pain lasting for long periods of time (i.e., over three months according to the literature) [1], is becoming alarmingly frequent. Specifically, this disease is currently estimated to affect between 20 and 30% of the population globally [2–5] and, with the age distribution changing towards the elderly, the incidence of chronic pain is likely to raise in the coming years due to the increased prevalence of this disease in the elderly [6].

Historically, chronic pain research and theories have embraced different perspectives, from clearly reductionist considerations to complex multidimensional approaches to the pain experience [7]. The more traditional view considered pain as a symptom of illness and assumed that pain severity was proportional to the amount of tissue damage. This reductionist approach has now been substituted by a more comprehensive view of pain as a complex and unpleasant sensory and emotional experience [8] that can only be understood as an interplay between sensory, cognitive, emotional, and social components [9]. As a consequence of this, a biopsychosocial approach to pain is currently considered the gold standard model to understand the pain experience [10–12] and interdisciplinary treatments of chronic pain have become the recommended approach to this disease [10,13,14].

Indeed, important milestones have been reached in the development and incorporation of the psychological perspective in this biopsychosocial approach to pain and the importance of psychological therapies for pain management is well-supported [15–17]. The literature investigating the role of the "social" part has also received attention, but not to the same extent. There is evidence to suggest that environmental elements, such as social support [18–21] and spouse-patient interactions [22–25], are important factors associated with patient outcomes, including functioning despite pain, emotional well-being, and quality of life, among others.

Another interesting line of research into the social determinants of patient adjustment to pain is the study of empathic accuracy, which has some tradition in the chronic pain literature. Empathic accuracy is conceptualized as an individual's interpersonal ability to judge the other person's status and differs from the traditional affective form of empathy [26]. Research into empathic accuracy can be included in a tradition of studies exploring the experience of pain from a caregiver's perspective, which includes not only spouse appraisals about the other's status (i.e., empathic accuracy) but also perceptions about one's status (i.e., caregiving burden) and emotional and behavioral reactions to pain (e.g., validating or critical responses) [27,28]. Two types of empathic accuracy have been traditionally tested, both relying on self-reports. On the one hand, correlational accuracy indicates how well self-reported patient pain is associated with the observer's perception of a patient's pain. This perspective is frequently used when patient and observer ratings are based on different response scales, but its interest is limited because it does not provide information about the size and the direction of inaccuracy. An alternative to this is the paired comparison accuracy, which evaluates the extent to which observers are accurate at estimating the other's status (i.e., overestimation and underestimation) [29]. As noted earlier, this requires the use of the same response scale in patients and observers, but provides more detailed information about empathic accuracy. Thus, the latter will be preferred in the present investigation.

In the chronic pain field, empathic accuracy has been usually defined as the caregiver's or, more frequently, the spouse's accuracy to decode the patient's pain severity; it. is considered to be an important interpersonal process in the patient's adaptation to chronic pain [28]. Accordingly, most research into empathic accuracy in chronic pain settings has focused on the exploration of health and adaptation correlates of empathic accuracy in a couple's context. So far, the literature suggests that spouses are quite accurate in estimating their partner's pain levels [30] irrespective of spousal sex characteristics [31] and supports the aforementioned idea that a spouse's accuracy in estimating a patient's pain levels is associated with positive outcomes in the patient, such as emotional well-being [32–34] and patient satisfaction with spousal support [35]. A recent meta-analysis also indicated that informal caregivers are more accurate than physicians and revealed that pain is more frequently underestimated in male patients [29].

The existing literature that has looked into the relationship between empathic accuracy and patient outcomes is encouraging, but important questions in this field remain unanswered. For instance, spouse and patient predictors of accuracy in the field of pain have rarely been investigated. So far, some examples of spousal characteristics that have been related to (poorer) empathic accuracy are depression in the spouse, being a male spouse rating a female patient, and reporting high levels of spousal catastrophizing [36,37]. An additional gap in pain literature is that the most research has focused on spouses as important sources of interaction, while the role of other relatives and even friends that are known to play a central role in informal caregiving in chronic patients [38] have been ignored. In chronic pain, because the prevalence of the disease raises dramatically with age [6], being a widow or being in a relationship with a partner that is also disabled is frequent [39], which boosts the need for informal caregivers other than spouses and makes the study of empathic accuracy in populations other than spouses important. Finally, empathic accuracy has traditionally been conceptualized from a patient's perspective (i.e., patient as a recipient of empathy). Because pain is also known to impact negatively on the family [40], investigating the patient's ability to estimate the consequence of pain on their significant others might also render important service to pain literature.

The present study aims to contribute to the social aspect of biopsychosocial literature by exploring how chronic pain correlates with empathic accuracy for both patienst and informal caregivers, including spouses and other main caregivers. According to Goubert et al. [28], empathic accuracy is determined by contextual factors (e.g., type of relationship and affinity), top-down mechanisms (e.g., the observer's personality characteristics and past learning experiences), and bottom-up influences (e.g., the observed person's characteristics). In the present study, contextual, top-down and bottom-up mechanisms will be included. Specifically, the explored correlates of empathic accuracy will include the personality characteristics of patients (i.e., bottom-up factor) and informal caregivers (i.e., top-down factor) because there is a large tradition of research showing a relationship between personality and empathy in social psychology research, but not in chronic pain [31,37,41]. While many personality characteristics exist, we chose to evaluate the five core dimensions of the Five Factor Model of personality because this model is cross-culturally robust and has been repeatedly and reliably associated with important study variables (i.e., health status and empathy) across different populations [42,43], including chronic pain [44]. In doing so, we will also explore the association between empathic accuracy and patient (i.e., bottom-up factor)/caregiver (i.e., top-down factor) health status in order to investigate whether existing findings are replicated in our sample. Specifically, we expect to replicate, for empathic accuracy in the patient's pain severity and interference, the correlations between certain personality traits (i.e., agreeableness and openness to experience) and empathy and to find empathic accuracy in the patient to be associated with the patient's health status. We also anticipate that informal caregivers will be quite accurate in estimating a patient's pain and interference levels. Patients' empathic accuracy in relation to the pain's impact on the caregiver, patient and caregiver empathic accuracy differences as a function of the type of relationship (i.e., contextual factor), and the relationship between patient and spouse empathic accuracy and the caregivers' health status will be investigated in an exploratory manner.

Ultimately, with the current investigation, we expect to help guide interdisciplinary interventions in a more effective manner by exploring social factors that could be incorporated in current treatments for pain. Including empathic accuracy training in such interventions would be beneficial for a number of reasons. Empathic accuracy is argued to lead to prosocial and support-related behaviors [45], proximity feelings in a relationship [46], and adaptive solution of conflicts in romantic relationships [47]. In fact, empathic accuracy has been argued to have a survival value for the patient as it would enhance assistance from others in the presence of pain (i.e., affective and behavioral responses) [28,31]. On the contrary, poor estimation by spouses might lead to inadequate support from a caregiver [48], which might ultimately exert a negative impact on a patient's ability to manage pain [32]. By exploring contextual, bottom-up, and bottom-down correlations of empathic accuracy, the present study aims at contributing to the important existing literature on social factors involved in the chronic pain experience.

2. Materials and Methods

2.1. Sample and Procedures

In this study, potential participants were patients with a prospective appointment from the beginning of 2014 to the end of 2015 at the pain clinic of a tertiary hospital in Spain (Vall d'Hebron Hospital in Barcelona) and their informal caregivers. Participants were recruited via postal mailing. A letter was sent to patients' home approximately one month prior to their medical consultation at the pain clinic. The letter included two protocols: one for the patient and one for the main informal caregiver. Each protocol included a study information sheet, an informed consent form, and questionnaires. Patients and informal caregivers were asked to complete the questionnaires separately and were given two additional envelopes. The completed questionnaires had to be returned separately in the corresponding sealed envelope the day of the prospective consultation, together with the signed informed consent forms, either to a physician or to the lead researcher, Carlos Suso-Ribera. Participants were officially enrolled at this stage by collecting the informed consent form and ensuring that eligibility was met.

In total, 335 dyads were willing to participate and returned the signed informed consent form. However, when revising the questionnaires, 81 protocols were found to contain incomplete data. Missing information from 38 of these dyads could be obtained with phone calls, but 53 cases were lost due to difficulties in contacting informal caregivers. As a result of this, the final sample with complete data was composed of 292 patients and their main informal caregivers.

Inclusion criteria for patients included experiencing recurrent pain over the last three months (i.e., chronic pain), being aged 18 or over, completing the questionnaires separately from the caregiver, and providing written informed consent to participate. Eligibility criteria for informal caregivers were being over 18 years of age, acting as the main informal caregiver for the patient, completing the questionnaires separately from the patient, and returning the written informed consent. We verified that caregivers were indeed the main informal caregivers when the patient or both returned the questionnaires during the medical appointment. Because the information letter was very clear at this stage, all patients confirmed that their main caregiver responded to the questionnaires. We also verbally confirmed that the questionnaires were completed separately and ensured that the questionnaires were returned in separate and sealed envelopes.

The Ethics Review Committee of the Vall d'Hebron Hospital in Barcelona approved the present study and all its procedures (PR(ATR)59/2010; approval date 8 May 2010).

2.2. Measures

Pain severity and pain interference in the last 24 h were measured with a numerical rating scale (NRS) ranging from 0 = no pain/interference to 10 = worst possible pain/interference, which was adapted from the Brief Pain Inventory [49]. Regarding pain severity, patients were asked to rate their own pain and informal caregivers were requested to estimate the pain of the patients. Pain interference was rated by both the patient and the caregiver as perceived interference on oneself and estimated interference of the patient's pain on the other.

The personality of patients and informal caregivers was evaluated with the NEO-Five-Factor-Inventory (NEO-FFI) [50,51], which evaluates the five core traits of the Five Factor Model of personality, namely neuroticism, extraversion, openness to experience, agreeableness, and conscientiousness. This comprehensive personality model is the most widely used in different settings [42], including chronic pain [44]. Neuroticism refers to a tendency to experience negative emotional states, such as depression, anxiety, and anger. Extraversion reflects a predisposition to be talkative, lively, enthusiast, and dynamic. Openness to experience characterizes curious, untraditional persons with a variety of interests and high sensitivity to arts. Agreeableness defines altruistic, honest, and helpful individuals. Finally, high conscientiousness scores are obtained by individuals prone to hard work, achievement-directed, and meticulous [50]. The Five Factor Model comprises 60 statements (12 per personality dimension) using a 5-point Likert scale that range from 0 = totally disagree to 4 = completely agree. For each personality dimension, scores range from 0 to 48. The NEO-FFI has obtained good internal consistency indices in previous ($0.66 < \alpha < 0.81$) [51], as well as in the present study for both patients ($0.70 < \alpha < 0.85$) and informal caregivers ($0.67 < \alpha < 0.84$).

The health status of patients and informal caregivers was assessed with the Short Form-36, which contains 36 items referring to eight dimensions of an individual's perceived health [52,53]. These include physical functioning (i.e., the ability to perform in daily activities), physical role (i.e., the capacity to perform in work-related duties), bodily pain (i.e., average pain severity in the last four weeks), general health (i.e., perception of present and future health), vitality (i.e., perceived personal energy), social functioning (i.e., interference of health in interpersonal relationships), role emotional (i.e., interference of emotions on functioning), and mental health (i.e., overall mental well-being) [54]. Two composite scores (i.e., overall physical and mental health) can be computed with the aforementioned subscales [53]. However, the use of subscales was preferred in the present study due to a number of reasons. First, because being retired or unemployed is frequent in chronic pain populations [55], including the present one, the physical role scale is of little relevance. Additionally, the use of the physical composite score would also be problematic because it would contain the measure of bodily pain, which would contaminate the relationship between the dependent variable (i.e., empathic accuracy in pain severity) and the independent variable (i.e., physical health status). To minimize the number of statistical comparisons, which is important to reduce type I errors, we selected three of the eight indicators of patient and spouse health status that represent different dimensions of perceived health, namely physical functioning, general health, and mental health [54]. In the Short Form-36, all scales are standardized and scores range from 0 to 100, with higher rating indicating better health. Previous research had evidence good internal consistency estimates of these scales ($0.78 < \alpha < 0.94$) [52], which was replicated for both patients ($0.78 < \alpha < 0.90$) and informal caregivers ($0.87 < \alpha < 0.95$) in the present investigation.

2.3. Data Analysis

The analytic strategy included a descriptive analysis of the sample, followed by an analysis of differences in patient and caregiver empathic accuracy by means of Student t-tests and a series of Pearson bivariate correlations between patient and caregiver empathic accuracy, personality, and health status both from the patient and the caregiver perspective. Specifically, differences in patient and caregiver empathic accuracy were investigated between patients and caregivers and between partners and non-partners, as well as between men and women because the existing literature shows the importance of sex in the pain experience [56,57].

Several measures of patient and caregiver empathic accuracy were calculated, which is in line with past research [58]. First, we calculated the disagreement in patient pain severity (patient self-perceived pain severity and informal caregiver's perception of patient pain severity), disagreement in patient pain interference (patient self-perceived interference of pain and informal caregiver's perception of pain interference on the patient), and the disagreement in informal caregiver pain interference (informal caregiver self-perceived interference of pain and patient's perception of pain interference on the caregiver). In all cases, a positive score reflected underestimation of the other's status, while a negative value were interpreted as overestimation of the other person's status. These three variables will be the main outcomes in the study. However, we calculated three additional variables for each of these three outcomes (i.e., disagreement in patient pain severity, disagreement in patient pain interference, and disagreement in informal caregiver pain interference). Namely, the three additional variables were the absolute value of each difference (i.e., poor estimation irrespective of the direction of the disagreement) and a dichotomous variable for overestimation and underestimation (where "0 = disagreement lower than 1 SD from the average score" and "1 = estimation with a disagreement of over 1 SD from the average disagreement score above and below the mean, respectively"). These additional outcomes were used in the correlation analyses to facilitate the interpretation of the relationship between patient and caregiver empathic accuracy and personality and health status. Finally, a linear multivariate regression analysis was computed to explore the unique associations between study predictors and the three main outcomes (i.e., empathic accuracy on patient pain severity and interference and empathic accuracy on caregiver pain interference). For each of the three regressions, the multivariate regression included sex and the patient and spouse personality and health characteristics that are found to significantly correlate with study outcomes.

Because of the large number of comparisons made in the Pearson correlation analyses, a more conservative p value of 0.01 was used as a cut-off for the interpretation of the bivariate associations to minimize the risk of type I errors and to reduce overestimation of unimportant correlations. The new alpha level was calculated using a Holm-Bonferroni sequential correction, a less restrictive correction than the original Bonferroni correction [59]. Because multiple comparison corrections often leads to rare occurrences of significant values, effect sizes (Cohen's d) were reported to facilitate the interpretation of mean differences analyses (t-tests) and the strength of the bivariate correlations (r values) and multivariate regressions (standardized β coefficients and explained variance) will be discussed too [60]. All analyses were conducted with SPSS version 25 [61].

3. Results

3.1. Sample Characteristics

Table 1 shows the demographic characteristics of the sample. In total, 584 individuals provided complete dyadic data (292 patients and 292 main informal caregivers). The majority of patients were characterized by experiencing musculoskeletal pain, mostly in the low back and the neck, but patients with any type of non-cancer pain were included in the study (i.e., to obtain a representative sample of the population treated at a specialized pain clinic). An analysis of sex distribution revealed that the majority of patients were females (66.8%), while men and women were similarly represented in the sample of informal caregivers (51.0% of females and 49.0% of males). The most frequent relationship between patients and informal caregivers was being a couple (68.5%). Other frequent relationships included being the patient's child (20.2%), being a sibling (4.1%), and being the patient's parent (2.7%). Overall, patients were slightly older than informal caregivers (59.35 years vs. 53.52 years, $t = 4.63$, $p < 0.001$). Informal caregivers had a higher educational level (25.3% of patients and 34.6% of informal caregivers had more than 12 years of education, $\chi^2 = 16.60$, $p < 0.001$) and were more likely to be working at the time of assessment (32.5% of patients and 52.4% of caregivers were active workers, $\chi^2 = 18.56$, $p < 0.001$). The majority of patients and informal caregivers were Spanish (95.2% and 95.5%, respectively).

Table 1. Sociodemographic characteristics of the sample ($n = 292$).

	Patient n (%)	Caregiver n (%)
Sex		
Women	195 (66.8)	149 (51.0)
Men	97 (33.2)	143 (49.0)
Age Mean (SD)	59.35 (15.76)	53.52 (14.69)
Marital Status		
In a relationship	202 (69.2)	226 (77.4)
Not in a relationship	90 (30.8)	66 (22.6)
Educational level		
<12 years	218 (74.7)	191 (65.4)
>12 years	74 (25.3)	101 (34.6)
Employment		
Working	95 (32.5)	153 (52.4)
Not working	197 (67.5)	139 (47.6)
Nationality		
Spanish	278 (95.2)	279 (95.5)
Non-Spanish	14 (4.8)	13 (4.5)
Relationship		
Partner/Spouse	-	200 (68.5)
Other [1]	-	92 (31.5)

[1] Other = Child (20.2%), sibling (4.1%), parent (2.7%), friend (1.0%), grandchild (0.7%), nephew (0.7%), mother-in-law (0.3%), aunt (0.3%), and child-in-law (0.3%).

3.2. Empathic Accuracy in Patients and Informal Caregivers

Differences between self and other reported pain severity and interference (i.e., empathic accuracy) are reported in Table 2. Informal caregivers were good at estimating a patient's pain severity ($t = 0.57$, $p = 0.573$) and interference ($t = -0.24$, $p = 0.814$). Conversely, patients underestimated the interference of pain in the life of their caregiver ($t = 2.16$, $p = 0.032$).

Table 2. Pain severity and interference characteristics and differences in empathic accuracy between patients and caregivers ($n = 292$).

	Patient Report Mean (SD)	Caregiver Report Mean (SD)	t	p	d
Patient pain severity	7.80 (1.66)	7.87 (1.57)	0.57	0.573	0.04
Patient pain interference	8.15 (1.58)	8.12 (1.59)	−0.24	0.814	0.02
Caregiver pain interference	7.02 (2.39)	7.42 (2.09)	2.16	0.032	0.18

Next, we compared patient and caregiver empathic accuracy according to the type of caregiver-patient relationship (Table 3). There were no significant differences in empathic accuracy of patients and caregivers depending on whether the main caregiver was the partner or not (all $p > 0.050$).

Table 3. Empathic accuracy as a function of partner relationship ($n = 292$).

	Partner/Spouse $n = 200$ Mean (SD)	Not Partner $n = 92$ Mean (SD)	t	p	d
Disagreement in patient pain severity	−0.16 (1.40)	0.10 (1.37)	−1.44	0.150	0.19
Disagreement in patient pain interference	<0.01 (1.52)	0.10 (1.30)	−0.54	0.593	0.06
Disagreement in caregiver pain interference	0.39 (2.19)	0.43 (2.48)	−0.17	0.863	0.02

Note. Disagreement is calculated by subtracting the other's estimation to self-report (i.e., patient's report of patient pain severity-caregiver's report of patient pain severity). Values close to "0" indicate a good estimation.

3.3. Sex Differences in Empathic Accuracy

The results on male-to-female differences in patient and caregiver empathic accuracy are indicated in Table 4. Male and female patients were similarly accurate at estimating the interference of their own pain on the caregiver ($t = 1.76$, $p = 0.080$). This was also the case of male and female caregivers when patient pain interference was the outcome ($t = 0.85$, $p = 0.394$). Conversely, female caregivers were more prone to overestimate their pain severity compared to male caregivers ($t = 2.18$, $p = 0.030$).

Table 4. Empathic accuracy as a function of sex ($N = 292$).

	Male Estimator Mean (SD)	Female Estimator Mean (SD)	t	p	d
Estimator = caregiver	$n = 143$	$n = 149$			
Disagreement in patient pain severity	−0.10 (1.43)	−0.25 (1.34)	2.18	0.030	0.11
Disagreement in patient pain interference	0.10 (1.62)	−0.04 (1.27)	0.85	0.394	0.10
Estimator = patient	$n = 97$	$n = 195$			
Disagreement in caregiver pain interference	0.73 (2.01)	0.24 (2.39)	1.76	0.080	0.22

Note: Disagreement is calculated by subtracting the other's estimation to self-report (i.e., patient's report of patient pain severity-caregiver's report of patient pain severity). Values close to "0" indicate a good estimation.

3.4. Personality Correlates of Empathic Accuracy and Associations with Health Outcomes

Personality and health associations with empathic accuracy outcomes are presented in Table 5. As noted earlier, four dimensions of empathic accuracy were computed: (i) overall disagreement, which can range from −10 (maximum overestimation) to +10 (maximum underestimation) and is calculated as the difference between self-reported pain severity/interference and the other's estimate; (ii) disagreement in absolute value, which can take values between 0 and +10 and reflects poor estimation irrespective of the direction of the misestimation; (iii) overestimation, which reflects the amount of individuals for whom disagreement was over 1 SD below the mean of disagreement; and (iv) underestimation, which reflects the amount of individuals for whom disagreement was over 1 SD above the mean of disagreement.

Overall, the patient's personality was not associated with any form of empathic accuracy (all $p > 0.01$). We found a number of associations between patient health status and patient and caregiver empathic accuracy. Overall, estimation was more difficult as patient status, mostly physical functioning, improved. Specifically, the quality of estimation (i.e., disagreement in absolute value) of patient pain severity ($r = 0.20$; $p < 0.001$), patient pain interference ($r = 0.29$; $p < 0.001$), and caregiver pain interference ($r = 0.19$; $p = 0.001$) worsened as patient physical functioning increased. Similarly, the estimation of patient pain interference (i.e., disagreement in absolute value) was also more challenging as patient overall health status ($r = 0.16$; $p = 0.008$) and mental health ($r = 0.15$; $p = 0.009$) improved. The most frequent judgment error when patient pain status was favorable was overestimation. For instance, good physical functioning was associated with higher overestimation of patient pain severity ($r = 0.15$ $p = 0.009$) and patient pain interference ($r = 0.17$; $p = 0.005$), while general health ($r = 0.16$; $p = 0.008$) and mental health ($r = 0.19$; $p = 0.002$) were positively linked to overestimation of patient pain interference.

Contrary to patient personality, spouse personality characteristics, notably openness to experience, were related to empathic accuracy. Caregiver openness to experience was associated with a better estimation of the patient's pain severity (i.e., less disagreement in absolute value; $r = -0.17$; $p = 0.004$), as well as negatively linked to overestimation ($r = -0.27$; $p < 0.001$). The positive association between disagreement in pain ratings and caregiver openness to experience ($r = 0.20$; $p < 0.001$) should be interpreted as showing that caregivers reporting high openness were more likely to underestimate a patient's pain reports compared to caregivers with a low openness profile, who were more prone to overestimate a patient's pain severity. In addition to caregiver's openness, the analyses also revealed that estimation of the interference of pain on the caregivers varied as a function of caregiver agreeableness. Similar to openness, the positive association between disagreement in caregiver pain interference and caregiver agreeableness ($r = 0.15$; $p = 0.009$) should be interpreted as indicating that underestimation of the caregiver's pain interference was more frequent when caregivers reported high agreeableness, compared to caregivers with a low agreeableness profile, with whom overestimation of pain interference was more frequent. Again, contrary to the patient findings, caregiver health status was not linked to empathic accuracy (all $p > 0.01$).

3.5. Multivariate Associations between Patient and Caregiver Predictors and Outcomes

As revealed in the bivariate analyses, estimation of patient and caregiver status was mostly associated with patient health status (i.e., physical functioning, general health, and mental health) and caregiver personality (i.e., openness and, to a lesser extent, agreeableness). Sex differences in empathic accuracy were also revealed in Table 3. Therefore, patient and caregiver sex, patient health status, and caregiver personality (i.e., openness and agreeableness) were included in the regression predicting (i) empathic accuracy towards the patient's pain severity, (ii) empathic accuracy towards the patient's pain interference, and (iii) empathic accuracy towards the caregiver's pain interference. The findings are reported in Table 6.

Table 5. Means and standard deviations of study variables and Pearson bivariate associations between empathic accuracy measures and patient and caregiver personality characteristics and health status.

	Mean (SD)/n (%)	Patient Personality					Patient Health Status			Caregiver Personality					Caregiver Health Status		
		N	E	O	A	C	PF	GH	MH	N	E	O	A	C	PH	GH	MH
Patient pain severity																	
Disagreement	−0.08 (1.39)	0.06	0.06	−0.01	0.02	0.01	−0.07	−0.11	−0.15	−0.06	0.06	0.20 **	−0.07	0.02	0.08	0.06	0.05
|Disagreement|	0.92 (1.04)	0.06	−0.01	0.04	0.01	−0.06	0.20 **	0.12	0.07	0.12	−0.10	−0.17 *	−0.04	−0.04	−0.03	−0.01	−0.01
Overestimation	31 (10.6%)	−0.03	0.04	−0.07	0.04	−0.05	0.15 *	0.13	0.13	0.10	−0.01	−0.27 **	0.04	0.01	−0.07	−00.04	−0.04
Underestimation	26 (8.9%)	0.12	−0.01	−0.06	0.01	−0.06	0.06	−0.07	−0.06	0.02	−0.01	−0.01	−0.05	0.02	−0.05	.05	0.07
Patient pain interference																	
Disagreement	0.03 (1.45)	0.07	0.01	0.08	−0.01	0.04	0.02	−0.06	−0.11	−0.03	0.07	0.10	−0.04	−0.02	0.01	−0.03	−0.03
|Disagreement|	0.98 (1.07)	−0.03	0.06	0.06	0.03	0.08	0.29 **	0.16 *	0.15 *	0.10	−0.03	0.01	−0.05	−0.04	0.05	0.05	0.04
Overestimation	32 (11%)	−0.12	0.06	−0.06	0.06	0.05	0.17 *	0.16 *	0.19 *	0.10	−0.08	−0.09	−0.04	−0.04	0.06	0.05	0.05
Underestimation	36 (12.3%)	0.06	0.01	0.07	−0.02	0.04	0.16 *	0.07	−0.03	0.11	0.01	0.03	−0.07	−0.08	0.01	−0.02	−0.08
Caregiver pain interference																	
Disagreement	0.40 (2.28)	−0.05	<0.01	−0.04	0.05	<0.01	0.10	−0.02	0.14	0.11	−0.04	−0.08	0.15 *	0.05	−0.11	−0.08	−0.07
|Disagreement|	1.54 (1.73)	0.01	−0.02	0.09	−0.03	0.04	0.19 *	0.10	0.09	0.01	−0.01	0.02	0.05	0.04	0.02	0.02	0.06
Overestimation	40 (13.7%)	0.05	−0.01	0.03	−0.05	0.04	0.03	0.07	−0.09	−0.14	0.05	0.10	−0.11	−0.04	0.13	0.09	0.11
Underestimation	46 (15.8%)	−0.09	0.01	−0.02	0.05	0.06	0.15	0.10	0.14	0.09	−0.01	−0.04	0.06	0.03	−0.04	−0.05	−0.01
Mean (SD)		24.66 (8.88)	26.28 (7.73)	22.50 (6.90)	31.82 (6.27)	30.97 (7.34)	32.77 (23.73)	34.23 (18.68)	50.23 (19.76)	19.92 (8.45)	27.82 (7.67)	24.81 (7.16)	30.98 (5.92)	32.02 (6.94)	77.11 (28.44)	61.40 (23.44)	66.60 (20.57)

Note. For "over/underestimation" variables values in the first column represent "frequencies (percentage)" of individuals who overestimate or underestimate, respectively (0 = "Estimates well, ±1SD from the disagreement mean" and 1 ="Over/Underestimates, over ±1SD from the disagreement mean"). The symbol "||" reflects absolute values. N = Neuroticism; E = Extraversion; O = Openness to experience; A = Agreeableness; C = Conscientiousness; PF = Physical Functioning; GH = General Health; MH = Mental Health. ** $p < 0.001$, * $p < 0.01$.

Table 6. Linear multivariate regression analyses predicting empathic accuracy from patient and caregiver characteristics.

	|Disagreement| in Patient Pain Severity			|Disagreement| in Patient Pain Interference			|Disagreement| in Caregiver Pain Interference		
	B (95% CI)	SE	t	B (95% CI)	SE	t	B (95% CI)	SE	t
Patient sex	0.08 (−0.21, 0.37)	0.15	0.56	−0.03 (−0.33, 0.27)	0.15	−0.20	−0.10 (−0.59, 0.40)	0.25	−0.38
Caregiver sex	0.08 (−0.22, 0.38)	0.15	0.52	0.05 (−0.26, 0.36)	0.16	0.32	0.07 (−0.44, 0.59)	0.26	0.27
Patient physical functioning	0.01 (<0.01, 0.02)	<.01	2.96 *	0.01 (0.01, 0.02)	<0.01	3.94 **	0.01 (<0.01, 0.02)	0.01	2.61 *
Patient general health	<0.01 (−0.01, 0.01)	<0.01	0.87	<0.01 (−0.01, 0.01)	<0.01	0.14	<0.01 (−0.01, 0.01)	0.01	0.09
Patient mental health	>−0.01 (−0.01, 0.01)	<0.01	−0.34	<0.01 (−0.01, 0.01)	<0.01	0.72	<0.01 (−0.01, 0.01)	0.01	0.25
Caregiver openness	−0.03 (−0.05, −0.01)	0.01	−3.41 **	>−0.01 (−0.02, 0.01)	0.01	−0.39	<0.01 (−0.03, 0.03)	0.01	0.09
Caregiver agreeableness	−0.01 (−0.03, 0.01)	0.01	−0.74	−0.01 (−0.03, 0.01)	0.01	−0.66	0.02 (−0.02, 0.05)	0.02	1.00
F	3.57 *			3.95 **			0.10		
R^2	5.8%			6.6%			1.7%		

** $p < 0.001$, * $p < 0.01$. R^2 is adjusted. Betas are unstandardized. Higher |disagreement| should be interpreted as poorer empathic accuracy.

Even though different forms of inaccuracy have been calculated in the study (i.e., overall disagreement, disagreement in absolute value, overestimation, and underestimation), we computed the linear multivariate regressions with disagreement in absolute value only (i.e., any form of poor estimation). This decision was based on the fact that this was the type of estimation with which most simultaneous bivariate associations occurred and because this represents well a general measure of poor empathic accuracy irrespective of the direction of such disagreement.

Overall, the explored models contributed significant variance to the prediction of |disagreement| in patient pain status, namely pain severity ($R^2 = 5.8\%$, $F = 3.57$, $p = 0.001$) and pain interference ($R^2 = 6.6\%$, $F = 3.95$, $p < 0.001$), but not in the prediction of caregiver status ($R^2 = 1.7\%$, $F = 0.10$, $p = 0.102$).

Regarding the contribution of predictors on outcomes, the analyses revealed that patient (increased) physical functioning was associated with all study outcomes, namely poor empathic accuracy towards patient's pain severity ($B = 0.01$, $t = 2.96$, $p = 0.003$, 95% CI = 0.003, 0.015) and interference ($B = 0.01$, $t = 3.94$, $p < 0.001$, 95% CI = 0.006, 0.018) and empathic inaccuracy towards the caregiver's pain interference status ($B = 0.01$, $t = 2.61$, $p = 0.009$, 95% CI = 0.003, 0.023). Additionally, (increased) caregiver openness was uniquely associated with more accurate estimation of the patient's pain severity status ($B = -0.03$, $t = -3.41$, $p < 0.001$, 95% CI = -0.045, -0.012).

4. Discussion

In this study, we wanted to contribute to the body of literature that examines how social factors are involved in the chronic pain experience. In the current investigation, we explored how patient and caregiver personality correlates to empathic accuracy. Further, we investigated differences in empathic accuracy between partners and other main caregivers and across sex groups, including not only patients but also informal caregivers as recipients of empathic accuracy. First, the study revealed that chronic pain patients are likely to be less accurate in estimating the interference of pain on the others than informal caregivers. Additionally, it showed that empathic accuracy is comparable irrespective of the type of partnership (i.e., couple or not a couple) and indicated that sex differences should be considered in empathic accuracy of pain severity. Finally, the results indicated that patient but not spouse health status is associated with empathic accuracy and, on the contrary, it revealed caregiver but not patient personality correlations with the accuracy of estimations.

Past research has associated poor empathic accuracy and non-empathic spouse responses with deleterious outcomes in the pain patient, such as lower perceived social support, emotional distress, and marital satisfaction [30,35,62], which suggests that empathic accuracy is an important variable to be considered in pain research. Consistent with the present study, there is research to suggest that informal caregivers (i.e., spouses in existing previous studies) are good at estimating the patient's pain severity [30–32] or at least better than other observers, including healthcare professionals [29]. However, contrary to the current investigation findings, there are also a number of other studies that have indicated an overall overestimation of patients' pain severity and disability [36] and a poor estimation of the patient's interference of pain [30]. While many factors, including smaller sample sizes compared to the present investigation ($84 \leq n \leq 109$) or differences in sample characteristic (i.e., ethnic or age differences, among others), might influence the discrepancies in empathic accuracy across investigations, an interesting finding in the present study was that caregiver personality, particularly openness to experience, was linked to precision in pain severity estimations. Therefore, it is possible that differences in the distribution of caregiver openness profiles in the studied samples might as well contribute to discrepancies in empathic accuracy of pain severity ratings.

To the best of our knowledge, this is the first investigation to explore personality correlates of empathic accuracy in pain literature. Past research associated empathy with agreeableness, conscientiousness, and openness, but not with neuroticism [63]. The same pattern of associations was found between the FFM of personality and perspective taking, which, similar to empathic accuracy, requires taking another perspective and viewing things from their point of view [64]. While the traditional view of empathy might slightly differ from empathic accuracy in pain research, they both certainly bear important similarities, such as the emphasis on interpersonal perspective-taking [26]. Contrary to the aforementioned literature findings, which revealed that conscientiousness was significantly associated with empathy, our study showed how only openness to experience and agreeableness were related to empathic accuracy. Importantly, the association between openness and empathic accuracy towards the patient's pain severity status remained significant even after controlling for the contribution of sex and patient health status. These findings are consistent with a recent meta-analysis showing a significant association between openness and interpersonal sensitivity, which suggests that openness to experience might be an important factor associated with empathic accuracy [65]. Openness to experience defines individuals with a great variety of interests, who tend to be curious, original, and sensitive to art. On the contrary, people who scored low in openness are more traditional and conservative in their values. Regarding agreeableness, high scores in this personality trait are obtained by altruist, careful, and cooperative individuals. On the opposite pole, we found hostility, egoism, and dominance [66]. Different to openness, the aforementioned meta-analysis [65] failed to obtain a robust association between agreeableness and interpersonal sensitivity, which would explain why agreeableness was only weakly and not uniquely associated with empathic accuracy in our study. While agreeableness has been argued to be a prosocial personality characteristic [67], there seems to be something unique in open individuals that is important for empathic accuracy and not necessarily shared by agreeable persons. Ultimately, what the present study findings suggest is that the personality profile of informal caregivers should not be ignored due to its potential association with empathic ability. Specifically, in the light of the study findings caregivers characterized by a low openness and, to a lesser extent, low agreeableness profile should be considered as target populations for empathic training in pain settings.

Different to the aforementioned conclusion about caregiver personality, the present study did not reveal a set of personality characteristics in the patient that were associated with empathic accuracy, which suggests that good estimates can be reached irrespective of patient personality characteristics and places the focus on caregiver personality traits in empathic accuracy research. Interestingly, though, associations between empathic accuracy and patient characteristics did emerge for patient health status (i.e., poorer estimation of patient pain severity and patient and caregiver pain interference emerged as patient physical functioning improved and the associations were robust to the inclusion of other covariates). So far, the literature has revealed that spousal accuracy in estimating a patient's pain severity decreased as patient status (i.e., pain severity, pain interference, and disability) improved [31]. Thus, it is possible that estimating the patient status becomes more challenging when a patient is less physically impaired by pain. Another possibility, though, is that empathic accuracy is perceived as less important when patient status is favorable. Accurately inferring the feelings or states of the pain patient implies an important physical and emotional exhaustion in the caregiver [68], which could be minimized by being imprecise if the situational demands are low (i.e., patient status is better). Due to the non-experimental and cross-sectional nature of the data, it is not possible to conclude whether these associations occurred because better health impacts perceptions of pain, the other way around, or both. Therefore, the proposed interpretations of these findings remain speculative at this stage and require more investigation as the findings may have important implications for care (i.e., whether empathic accuracy should be encouraged or not).

Contrary to patient health status, caregiver health characteristics were not associated with precision of pain severity and interference estimates. There has been scarce research into the caregiver health contributors of empathic accuracy. So far, distressed spouses have been found to overestimate the patient's pain severity and interference [30,33], but not its physical and psychosocial disability [30]. Our results are in line with the latter study indicating a lack of association between caregiver health status and their empathic accuracy. Further research with larger sample sizes (i.e., sample sizes before the present study completion have been relatively small) and exploring empathic accuracy of important caregivers other than spouses will be needed to clarify whether imprecision is indeed associated with caregiver health status so that this is used to select couples at risk for poor empathic outcomes.

In addition to the study of personality and health correlates of empathic accuracy, important contributions of the present investigation included the study of sex differences in precision and the inclusion of partners and other main caregivers altogether. In relation to sex differences, it has been argued that women are more precise in estimating the physical and emotional states of their counterparts, arguably due to differences in motivation and socialization but not in ability [26,69]. Consistent with this idea, male spouses of chronic pain patients have been found to underestimate the patient's physical disability, while female spouses have been shown to accurately estimate such disability [36]. Contrary to this idea, another investigation indicated that male and female spouses were comparably good at inferring the care recipient's pain severity [31] and a recent experimental study revealed that male-to-female differences in accuracy are more likely to be due to stereotypes than to real differences [70]. In our investigation, men and women were very similar at estimating the interference of pain on the other (both when the recipient of empathic accuracy was the patient and the caregiver), which would be in line with research indicating no sex differences in empathic accuracy [31]. If, indeed, motivational reasons are key predictors explaining sex differences in empathy, one possible explanation for male-to-female similarities in judgment is that, in situations where empathy is perceived as important (i.e., in the presence of illness), men and women might become similarly motivated to estimate the status of their counterparts, thus leading to comparable empathic accuracy estimates. Surprisingly, though, our study revealed that female caregivers were more likely to overestimate the severity of a patient's pain compared to male caregivers. Research has shown that spouse catastrophizing, which is a tendency to worry and focus on the worst possible pain-related scenarios [71], is associated with increased perceptions of patient pain severity [72]. This tendency to ruminate and magnify the threat value of pain is more marked in women [73], which might provide with a tentative explanation for the higher tendency to present increased pain severity estimates of female caregivers in the sample. Again, because of the novelty of these findings and the differences in sample composition, sample size, and together with other methodological differences between the current and past similar research (i.e., measures and constructs evaluated), replication studies will be crucial to obtaining a reliable body of research into the social components into pain research.

As noted in the previous paragraph, the inclusion of caregivers other than spouses is novel in empathic accuracy literature. Past research has already highlighted the important supportive role of informal caregivers other than spouses in pain settings [74]. However, the study of informal caregiver associations with patient outcomes is dominated by research on spouses [27]. Similar to the literature into other chronic conditions [75], the present study indicated that, while spouses of chronic pain patients are likely to play a key role in daily care of pain patients, other actors, particularly children, are also likely to gain prominence in pain research studies. Interestingly, our results evidenced similar empathic accuracy estimates across partners and non-partners, even though both groups are likely to differ in a number of important characteristics (i.e., age, sex distribution, working status, and number of hours spent together, among others). As noted before, it is possible that high motivation to help a person in need might explain that all agents were similarly effective in estimating the patient's pain status. However, the information available in the present study does not allow us to draw further conclusions and they only provide initial interesting findings in relation to empathic accuracy similarities between partners and other relatives/friends acting as main caregivers of pain patients.

While acknowledging the aforementioned strengths of the present investigation, there are also shortcomings in the study. First, because this is a cross-sectional and observational study, causal and temporary inferences cannot be derived from the results and should be interpreted with caution. The same conclusion applies to the novelty of some of the questions investigated in the study, which will need further replication. Additionally, the patient sample was characterized by experiencing chronic musculoskeletal pain. While this is a frequent practice in pain research into empathic accuracy due to the representativeness of such samples of the populations attending specialized pain clinics [31,33,39], this clearly prevents us from generalizing the findings to specific pain populations. Another limitation of this study is that the list of variables that might be associated with empathic accuracy is far from complete. For instance, time spent together could be an interesting variable to be explored in empathic accuracy research, but our question ("What is the average number of hours you spend with the patient daily?") was left blank by many caregivers and was misinterpreted by others (i.e., some people reported "24 h" to reflect that they spent all day together, while others did not count sleeping hours or were more conservative and reported less hours despite spending all day together). Another variable that has been linked with empathy in the literature but has not been investigated in the present study is depression [36]. An additional shortcoming has been that we could not visually confirm that patients and caregivers indeed completed to the questionnaires separately. While we did visually confirm that the questionnaires were returned in separate, sealed envelopes and we observed differences in patient-to-caregiver estimates (i.e., patients slightly underestimated the caregivers' status), which would suggest that the measures were indeed completed separately, we cannot firmly conclude this. As a final remark, the reader should note that all effect sizes were small (i.e., significant correlations and Cohen's d were all <0.03) and the explored multivariate models contributed little variance to the prediction of empathic accuracy (i.e., less than 7%), so the strength of the presented associations and mean differences should not be overestimated.

While acknowledging the aforementioned shortcomings, it should be noted that the present investigation explored important contextual, bottom-up and top-down correlates of empathic accuracy described in the empathic accuracy model of pain by Dr. Goubert and her team [28]. Specifically, we found support for top-down mechanisms (i.e., the observer's openness to experience and, to a lesser extent, agreeableness) and bottom-up factors (i.e., patient health status, mostly physical functioning) associations with empathic accuracy. Conversely, empathic accuracy differences were not revealed as a function of the type of relationship (i.e., contextual factor). As noted earlier, replicating these findings and exploring different sets of mechanisms will be fundamental to provide more robust evidence for the model proposed by Goubert et al. [28]. However, the present study findings make a significant contribution into the literature on empathic accuracy and provide further support for the need of pain models that account for both personal and interpersonal mechanisms that are activated to respond to pain.

5. Conclusions

This study contributes to the existing literature on the social context of chronic pain in a number of ways. First, because it revealed that empathic accuracy, which has been argued to be a protective factor for patient well-being, should not only consider patients as recipients of empathy but also caregivers. Next, because it highlighted that sex differences in empathic accuracy might take unexpected directions when considering larger sample sizes and indicated that informal caregivers other than spouses should be incorporated in research into social contributors of the pain experience. Last but not least, an important finding in the present investigation was that caregiver characteristics (i.e., low openness and low agreeableness) and patient health status (notably increased physical functioning) might be significant factors associated with difficulties in empathic accuracy in pain settings. Ultimately, the importance of these findings lies in their applicability in clinical settings. For instance, in light of our results, target populations for empathic training would be non-agreeable and non-open caregivers, together with dyads in which the patient status is favorable, irrespective of the type of relationship between patients and caregivers (i.e., couples or non-couples). Thus, the present study findings might help guide biopsychosocial interventions in a more effective manner by providing a set of recommendations to be included in the social part of multidimensional treatments for pain management.

Author Contributions: All listed authors significantly contributed to the present investigation. C.S.-R., A.G.-P., and V.M.-B. were in charge of study conceptualization and the design of the methodology. C.S.-R., A.V., and V.M.-B. took care of data curation and formal analyses. C.S.-R. and A.G.-P. were responsible for funding acquisition.

C.S.-R. was responsible for investigation and validation. All authors contributed to the methodology selection. C.S.-R. and A.G.-P. were in charge of project administration and resources. C.S.-R. and V.M.-B. were responsible for visualization. A.Z.-G. and F.J.C.-G. supervised the study. The original draft was prepared by C.S.-R., in collaboration with V.M.-B. F.J.C.-G., A.V., and A.G.-P. reviewed and edited the text, which was then discussed by all authors. A final version was prepared and approved by all listed authors.

Funding: This research was partially funded by the Spanish Government (grant FPU-AP2010-5585) and the Jaume I University (grant POSDOC/2016/15).

Acknowledgments: The authors want to thank the team of the pain clinic of the Vall d'Hebron Hospital, particularly Maria Victoria Ribera Canudas, for their support in data collection.

Conflicts of Interest: The authors declare no conflict of interest to disclose.

References

1. Treede, R.D.; Rief, W.; Barke, A.; Aziz, Q.; Bennett, M.I.; Benoliel, R.; Cohen, M.; Evers, S.; Finnerup, N.B.; First, M.B.; et al. A classification of chronic pain for ICD-11. *Pain* **2015**, *156*, 1003–1007. [CrossRef] [PubMed]
2. Larsson, C.; Hansson, E.E.; Sundquist, K.; Jakobsson, U. Chronic pain in older adults: Prevalence, incidence, and risk factors. *Scand. J. Rheumatol.* **2017**, *46*, 317–325. [CrossRef] [PubMed]
3. Nahin, R.L. Estimates of Pain Prevalence and Severity in Adults: United States, 2012. *J. Pain* **2015**, *16*, 769–780. [CrossRef] [PubMed]
4. Langley, P. The prevalence, correlates and treatment of pain in the European Union. *Curr. Med. Res. Opin.* **2011**, *27*, 463–480. [CrossRef] [PubMed]
5. Azevedo, L.F.; Costa-Pereira, A.; Mendonça, L.; Dias, C.C.; Castro-Lopes, J.M. Epidemiology of Chronic Pain: A Population-Based Nationwide Study on Its Prevalence, Characteristics and Associated Disability in Portugal. *J. Pain* **2012**, *13*, 773–783. [CrossRef] [PubMed]
6. Miró, J.; Paredes, S.; Rull, M.; Queral, R.; Miralles, R.; Nieto, R.; Huguet, A.; Baos, J. Pain in older adults: A prevalence study in the Mediterranean region of Catalonia. *Eur. J. Pain* **2007**, *11*, 83. [CrossRef] [PubMed]
7. Gatchel, R.J.; Peng, Y.B.; Peters, M.L.; Fuchs, P.N.; Turk, D.C. The biopsychosocial approach to chronic pain: Scientific advances and future directions. *Psychol. Bull.* **2007**, *133*, 581–624. [CrossRef] [PubMed]
8. Merskey, H. Classification of chronic pain: Descriptions of chronic pain syndromes and definitions of pain terms. *Pain* **1986**, *3*, 226.
9. Williams, A.C.; Craig, K.D. Updating the definition of pain. *Pain* **2016**, *157*, 2420–2423. [CrossRef]
10. Gatchel, R.J.; McGeary, D.D.; McGeary, C.A.; Lippe, B. Interdisciplinary chronic pain management: Past, present, and future. *Am. Psychol.* **2014**, *69*, 119–130. [CrossRef]
11. Cheatle, M.D. Biopsychosocial Approach to Assessing and Managing Patients with Chronic Pain. *Med. Clin. N. Am.* **2016**, *100*, 43–53. [CrossRef] [PubMed]
12. Johnson, M.I. The Landscape of Chronic Pain: Broader Perspectives. *Medicina (B Aires)* **2019**, *55*, 182. [CrossRef] [PubMed]
13. Turk, D.C.; Wilson, H.D.; Cahana, A. Treatment of chronic non-cancer pain. *Lancet* **2011**, *377*, 2226–2235. [CrossRef]
14. Kamper, S.J.; Apeldoorn, A.T.; Chiarotto, A.; Smeets, R.J.E.M.; Ostelo, R.W.J.G.; Guzman, J.; Van Tulder, M.W. Multidisciplinary biopsychosocial rehabilitation for chronic low back pain: Cochrane systematic review and meta-analysis. *BMJ* **2015**, *350*, h444. [CrossRef]
15. Williams, A.; Eccleston, C.; Morley, S. Psychological therapies for the management of chronic pain (excluding headache) in adults. *Cochrane Database Syst. Rev.* **2013**. [CrossRef] [PubMed]
16. Eccleston, C.; Morley, S.J.; Williams, A.C.D.C. Psychological approaches to chronic pain management: Evidence and challenges. *Br. J. Anaesth.* **2013**, *111*, 59–63. [CrossRef]
17. McCracken, L. Psychological approaches to chronic pain management: Where are we coming from and where might we go? *Rev. Soc. Española Dolor* **2017**, *24*, 57–63. [CrossRef]
18. López-Martínez, A.E.; Esteve-Zarazaga, R.; Ramírez-Maestre, C. Perceived Social Support and Coping Responses Are Independent Variables Explaining Pain Adjustment Among Chronic Pain Patients. *J. Pain* **2008**, *9*, 373–379. [CrossRef]
19. Osborne, T.L.; Jensen, M.P.; Ehde, D.M.; Hanley, M.A.; Kraft, G. Psychosocial factors associated with pain intensity, pain-related interference, and psychological functioning in persons with multiple sclerosis and pain. *Pain* **2007**, *127*, 52–62. [CrossRef]

20. Lee, J.E.; Kahana, B.; Kahana, E. Social support and cognitive functioning as resources for elderly persons with chronic arthritis pain. *Aging Ment. Health* **2016**, *20*, 370–379. [CrossRef]
21. Matos, M.; Bernardes, S.F.; Goubert, L.; Beyers, W. Buffer or amplifier? Longitudinal effects of social support for functional autonomy/dependence on older adults' chronic pain experiences. *Health Psychol.* **2017**, *36*, 1195–1206. [CrossRef] [PubMed]
22. Newton-John, T.R.; Williams, A.C.D.C. Chronic pain couples: Perceived marital interactions and pain behaviours. *Pain* **2006**, *123*, 53–63. [CrossRef] [PubMed]
23. Cunningham, J.L.; Hayes, S.E.; Townsend, C.O.; Laures, H.J.; Hooten, W.M. Associations Between Spousal or Significant Other Solicitous Responses and Opioid Dose in Patients with Chronic Pain. *Pain Med.* **2012**, *13*, 1034–1039. [CrossRef] [PubMed]
24. Raichle, K.A.; Romano, J.M.; Jensen, M.P. Partner responses to patient pain and well behaviors and their relationship to patient pain behavior, functioning, and depression. *Pain* **2011**, *152*, 82–88. [CrossRef] [PubMed]
25. Leonard, M.T.; Chatkoff, D.K.; Maier, K.J. Couples' Relationship Satisfaction and Its Association with Depression and Spouse Responses Within the Context of Chronic Pain Adjustment. *Pain Manag. Nurs.* **2018**, *19*, 400–407. [CrossRef] [PubMed]
26. Ickes, W. Empathic Accuracy: Its Links to Clinical, Cognitive, Developmental, Social, and Physiological Psychology. In *Social Neuroscience Empathy*; Decety, J., Ickes, W., Eds.; MIT Press: Cambridge, MA, USA, 2009; pp. 57–70.
27. Leonard, M.T.; Cano, A.; Johansen, A.B. Chronic Pain in a Couples Context: A Review and Integration of Theoretical Models and Empirical Evidence. *J. Pain* **2006**, *7*, 377–390. [CrossRef] [PubMed]
28. Goubert, L.; Craig, K.D.; Vervoort, T.; Morley, S.; Sullivan, M.J.; Williams, D.C.; Cano, A.; Crombez, G. Facing others in pain: The effects of empathy. *Pain* **2005**, *118*, 285–288. [CrossRef]
29. Ruben, A.M.; Blanch-Hartigan, D.; Shipherd, J.C. To Know Another's Pain: A Meta-analysis of Caregivers' and Healthcare Providers' Pain Assessment Accuracy. *Ann. Behav. Med.* **2018**, *52*, 662–685. [CrossRef]
30. Cano, A.; Johansen, A.B.; Franz, A. Multilevel analysis of couple congruence on pain, interference, and disability. *Pain* **2005**, *118*, 369–379. [CrossRef]
31. Gauthier, N.; Thibault, P.; Sullivan, M.J.L. Individual and Relational Correlates of Pain-related Empathic Accuracy in Spouses of Chronic Pain Patients. *Clin. J. Pain* **2008**, *24*, 669–677. [CrossRef]
32. Cremeans-Smith, J.K.; Stephens, M.A.P.; Franks, M.M.; Martire, L.M.; Druley, A.J.; Wojno, W.C. Spouses' and physicians' perceptions of pain severity in older women with osteoarthritis: Dyadic agreement and patients' well-being. *Pain* **2003**, *106*, 27–34. [CrossRef]
33. Geisser, M.E.; Cano, A.; Leonard, M.T. Factors Associated with Marital Satisfaction and Mood among Spouses of Persons with Chronic Back Pain. *J. Pain* **2005**, *6*, 518–525. [CrossRef] [PubMed]
34. Riemsma, R.P.; Taal, E.; Rasker, J.J. Perceptions about perceived functional disabilities and pain of people with rheumatoid arthritis: Differences between patients and their spouses and correlates with well-being. *Arthritis Rheum.* **2000**, *13*, 255–261. [CrossRef]
35. Martire, L.M.; Keefe, F.J.; Schulz, R.; Ready, R.; Beach, S.R.; Rudy, T.E.; Starz, T.W. Older spouses' perceptions of partners' chronic arthritis pain: Implications for spousal responses, support provision, and caregiving experiences. *Psychol. Aging* **2006**, *21*, 222–230. [CrossRef] [PubMed]
36. Cano, A.; Johansen, A.B.; Geisser, M. Spousal congruence on disability, pain, and spouse responses to pain. *Pain* **2004**, *109*, 258–265. [CrossRef] [PubMed]
37. Leonard, M.T.; Issner, J.H.; Cano, A.; Williams, A.M. Correlates of Spousal Empathic Accuracy for Pain-related Thoughts and Feelings. *Clin. J. Pain* **2013**, *29*, 324–333. [CrossRef]
38. Goldberg, A.; Rickler, K.S. The role of family caregivers for people with chronic illness. *Med. Health Rhode Isl.* **2011**, *94*, 41–42.
39. Leonard, M.T.; Cano, A. Pain affects spouses too: Personal experience with pain and catastrophizing as correlates of spouse distress. *Pain* **2006**, *126*, 139–146. [CrossRef]
40. Strunin, L.; Boden, I.L. Family consequences of chronic back pain. *Soc. Sci. Med.* **2004**, *58*, 1385–1393. [CrossRef]
41. Sims, C.M. Do the Big-Five Personality Traits Predict Empathic Listening and Assertive Communication? *Int. J. List* **2017**, *31*, 163–188. [CrossRef]

42. John, O.P.; Naumann, L.P.; Soto, C.J. Paradigm Shift to the Integrative Big-Five Trait Taxonomy: History, Measurement, and Conceptual Issues. In *Handbook of Personality: Theory and Research*, 3rd ed.; John, O.P., Robins, R.W., Pervin, L.A., Eds.; Guilford Press: New York, NY, USA, 2008; pp. 114–158.
43. Melchers, M.C.; Li, M.; Haas, B.W.; Reuter, M.; Bischoff, L.; Montag, C. Similar Personality Patterns Are Associated with Empathy in Four Different Countries. *Front. Psychol.* **2016**, *7*, 13. [CrossRef] [PubMed]
44. Suso-Ribera, C.; Gallardo-Pujol, D. Personality and health in chronic pain: Have we failed to appreciate a relationship? *Pers. Individ. Differ.* **2016**, *96*, 7–11. [CrossRef]
45. Verhofstadt, L.L.; Buysse, A.; Ickes, W.; Davis, M.; Devoldre, I. Support provision in marriage: The role of emotional similarity and empathic accuracy. *Emotion* **2008**, *8*, 792–802. [CrossRef] [PubMed]
46. Simpson, J.A.; Oriña, M.M.; Ickes, W. When Accuracy Hurts, and When It Helps: A Test of the Empathic Accuracy Model in Marital Interactions. *J. Pers. Soc. Psychol.* **2003**, *85*, 881–893. [CrossRef] [PubMed]
47. Kilpatrick, S.D.; Bissonnette, V.L.; Rusbult, C.E. Empathic accuracy and accommodative behavior among newly married couples. *Pers. Relatsh.* **2002**, *9*, 369–393. [CrossRef]
48. Craig, K.D. Toward the Social Communication Model of Pain. *Soc. Interpers. Dyn. Pain* **2018**, *50*, 23–41.
49. Cleeland, C.S.; Ryan, K.M. Pain assessment: Global use of the Brief Pain Inventory. *Ann. Acad. Med. Singap.* **1994**, *23*, 129–138.
50. Costa, P.T.; McCrae, R.R. *Revised NEO Personality Inventory (NEO-PI-R) and the NEO Five-Factor Inventory (NEO-FFI) Professional Manual*; Odessa, F.L., Ed.; Psychological Assessment Resources: Odessa, Florida, 1992.
51. Solé i Fontova, M.D. *Validació i Estandarització Espanyola del Neo-Pi-R, Neo-Ffi, Neo-Ffi-R I Escales de Schinka, en Mostres Universitèries i Població General*; Universitat de Lleida: Lleida, Spain, 2006.
52. Alonso, J.; Regidor, E.; Barrio, G.; Prieto, L.; Rodrigues, C.; de la Fuente, L. Valores poblacionales de referencia de la versión española del Cuestionario de Salud SF-36 [Population-based reference values for the Spanish version of the health Survey SF-36]. *Med. Clin.* **1998**, *111*, 410–416.
53. McHorney, C.; Ware, J.; Raczek, A. The MOS 36-Item Short-Form Health Survey (SF-36): II. Psychometric and clinical tests of validity in measuring physical and mental health constructs. *Med. Care* **1993**, *31*, 247–263. [CrossRef]
54. Bergman, S.; Jacobsson, L.T.H.; Herrström, P.; Petersson, I.F. Health status as measured by SF-36 reflects changes and predicts outcome in chronic musculoskeletal pain: A 3-year follow up study in the general population. *Pain* **2004**, *108*, 115–123. [CrossRef]
55. De Sola, H.; Salazar, A.; Dueñas, M.; Ojeda, B.; Failde, I. Nationwide cross-sectional study of the impact of chronic pain on an individual's employment: Relationship with the family and the social support. *BMJ Open* **2016**, *6*. [CrossRef]
56. Alabas, O.; Tashani, O.; Johnson, M.; Tashani, O. Gender role expectations of pain mediate sex differences in cold pain responses in healthy Libyans. *Eur. J. Pain* **2012**, *16*, 300–311. [CrossRef] [PubMed]
57. Zagni, E.; Simoni, L.; Colombo, D. Sex and Gender Differences in Central Nervous System-Related Disorders. *Neurosci. J.* **2016**, *2016*, 1–13. [CrossRef] [PubMed]
58. Johansen, A.B.; Cano, A. A Preliminary Investigation of Affective Interaction in Chronic Pain Couples. *Pain* **2007**, *132*, S86–S95. [CrossRef] [PubMed]
59. Holm, S. A simple sequential rejective method procedure. *Scand. J. Stat.* **1979**, *6*, 65–70.
60. Nakagawa, S. A farewell to Bonferroni: The problems of low statistical power and publication bias. *Behav. Ecol.* **2004**, *15*, 1044–1045. [CrossRef]
61. IBM. *IBM SPSS Statistics for Windows*, version 25.0; IBM: Armonk, NY, USA, 2017.
62. Cano, A.; Barterian, J.A.; Heller, J.B. Empathic and Nonempathic Interaction in Chronic Pain Couples. *Clin. J. Pain* **2008**, *24*, 678–684. [CrossRef]
63. Barrio, V.; del Aluja, A.; García, L.F. Relationship between Empathy and The Big Five Personality Traits in A Sample of Spanish Adolescents. *Soc. Behav. Pers. Int. J.* **2004**, *32*, 677–681. [CrossRef]
64. Song, Y.; Shi, M. Associations between empathy and big five personality traits among Chinese undergraduate medical students. *PLoS ONE* **2017**, *12*, e0171665. [CrossRef]
65. Hall, J.A.; Andrzejewski, S.A.; Yopchick, J.E. Psychosocial Correlates of Interpersonal Sensitivity: A Meta-Analysis. *J. Nonverbal Behav.* **2009**, *33*, 149–180. [CrossRef]
66. McCrae, R.R.; John, O.P. An Introduction to the Five-Factor Model and Its Applications. *J. Pers.* **1992**, *60*, 175–215. [CrossRef] [PubMed]

67. Graziano, W.G.; Habashi, M.M.; Sheese, B.E.; Tobin, R.M. Agreeableness, Empathy, and Helping: A Person × Situation Perspective. *J. Pers. Soc. Psychol.* **2007**, *93*, 583–599. [CrossRef] [PubMed]
68. Cano, A. Pain catastrophizing and social support in married individuals with chronic pain: The moderating role of pain duration. *Pain* **2004**, *110*, 656–664. [CrossRef] [PubMed]
69. Ickes, W.; Gesn, P.R.; Graham, T. Gender differences in empathic accuracy: Differential ability or differential motivation? *Pers. Relatsh.* **2000**, *7*, 95–109. [CrossRef]
70. Baéz, S.; Flichtentrei, D.; Prats, M.; Mastandueno, R.; García, A.M.; Cetkovich, M.; Ibáñez, A. Men, women . . . who cares? A population-based study on sex differences and gender roles in empathy and moral cognition. *PLoS ONE* **2017**, *12*, e0179336. [CrossRef]
71. Suso-Ribera, C.; García-Palacios, A.; Botella, C.; Ribera-Canudas, M.V. Pain Catastrophizing and Its Relationship with Health Outcomes: Does Pain Intensity Matter? *Pain Res. Manag.* **2017**, *2017*, 1–8. [CrossRef] [PubMed]
72. Gauthier, N.; Thibault, P.; Sullivan, M.J.L. Catastrophizers with chronic pain display more pain behaviour when in a relationship with a low catastrophizing spouse. *Pain Res. Manag.* **2011**, *16*, 293–299. [CrossRef]
73. Sullivan, M.J.L.; Tripp, D.A.; Santor, D. Gender Differences in Pain and Pain Behavior: The Role of Catastrophizing. *Cogn. Ther. Res.* **2000**, *24*, 121–134. [CrossRef]
74. Bambara, J.K.; Turner, A.P.; Williams, R.M.; Haselkorn, J.K. Social support and depressive symptoms among caregivers of veterans with multiple sclerosis. *Rehabil. Psychol.* **2014**, *59*, 230–235. [CrossRef]
75. Blyth, F.M.; Cumming, R.G.; Brnabic, A.J.M.; Cousins, M.J. Caregiving in the presence of chronic pain. *J. Gerontol. Ser. A Biol. Sci. Med. Sci.* **2008**, *63*, 399–407. [CrossRef]

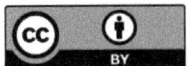

© 2019 by the authors. Licensee MDPI, Basel, Switzerland. This article is an open access article distributed under the terms and conditions of the Creative Commons Attribution (CC BY) license (http://creativecommons.org/licenses/by/4.0/).

MDPI
St. Alban-Anlage 66
4052 Basel
Switzerland
www.mdpi.com

Medicina Editorial Office
E-mail: medicina@mdpi.com
www.mdpi.com/journal/medicina

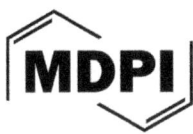

Disclaimer/Publisher's Note: The statements, opinions and data contained in all publications are solely those of the individual author(s) and contributor(s) and not of MDPI and/or the editor(s). MDPI and/or the editor(s) disclaim responsibility for any injury to people or property resulting from any ideas, methods, instructions or products referred to in the content.

www.ingramcontent.com/pod-product-compliance
Lightning Source LLC
LaVergne TN
LVHW070146100526
838202LV00015B/1904